Essentials of
Anaesthetic Equipment

To our wives and families

For Elsevier:
Commissioning Editor: *Michael Parkinson*
Project Manager: *Elouise Ball*
Development Editor: *Alison McMurdo*
Senior Designer: *Erik Bigland*
Illustration Manager: *Gillian Richards*
Illustrator: *Martin Woodward*

Essentials of Anaesthetic Equipment

Third edition

Baha Al-Shaikh FCARCSI, FRCA

Consultant Anaesthetist, Ashford, Kent UK
Honorary Senior Lecturer, GKT Medical School, University of London, UK

Simon Stacey FRCA

Consultant Anaesthetist, Bart's and The London NHS Trust, London, UK

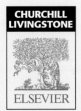

CHURCHILL
LIVINGSTONE

ELSEVIER

Edinburgh London New York Oxford Philadelphia St Louis Sydney Toronto 2007

CHURCHILL
LIVINGSTONE
ELSEVIER

First published 1995
Reprinted 1996, 1999
Second edition 2002
Reprinted 2002, 2003, 2004, 2005
Third edition 2007
Reprinted 2007, 2008

ISBN 13: 9780443100871

British Library Cataloguing in Publication Data
A catalogue record for this book is available from the British Library

Library of Congress Cataloging in Publication Data
A catalog record for this book is available from the Library of Congress

Working together to grow
libraries in developing countries
www.elsevier.com | www.bookaid.org | www.sabre.org

ELSEVIER   BOOK AID International   Sabre Foundation

your source for books,
journals and multimedia
in the health sciences
www.elsevierhealth.com

The publisher's policy is to use paper manufactured from sustainable forests

Printed in China

Contents

Preface

After the publication of the first edition in 1995 and the second edition in 2001, the demands and the standards of the anaesthetist have not stood still. This totally updated third edition has had all its artwork redrawn in colour, in addition to many new colour photographic illustrations. Much of the text has been rewritten and more MCQs have also been added. New references, at the end of each chapter, offer additional reading pointers. The popular standardized format for each piece of equipment has been retained, as have the summary boxes.

We have tried to concentrate on the equipment seen in everyday practice, rather than the esoteric. We hope that the scope of this concise book will be adequate for the trainee sitting the FRCA, or similar examinations. We do hope that this book will continue to be a very useful reference tool, not only for the trainee anaesthetist, but also for our nursing and operating department practitioner colleagues.

BAS, Ashford, Kent.
SGS, London.
2006

Acknowledgements

We are extremely grateful to the many manufacturing companies who have supplied the necessary data and illustrations for this book. Space will not allow an extensive list of companies deserving our gratitude for each illustration. However a list of manufacturers that have helped us, is to be found in Appendix F at the back of the book. Without their help, this third edition could not have gone ahead in its current format.

The extra cost for colour illustrations has been met again by Smiths Medical. Ken Crowe of Smiths Medical deserves a special mention for his unflagging help with all things photographic. Thanks also to Dr John Nelson and Dr M Rothwell for additional photographic help. We are also grateful to the Association of Anaesthetists of Great Britain and Ireland for granting permission to reproduce their machine checklist and monitoring recommendations.

Finally, we would like to thank especially the brilliant Alison McMurdo who resurrected this edition and the staff at the Edinburgh office of Elsevier for their hard work.

Chapter 1

Medical gas supply

Gas supply

Medical gas supply takes the form of either cylinders or a piped gas system, depending on the requirements of the hospital.

Cylinders

Components

1. Cylinders are made of thin-walled seamless molybdenum steel in which gases and vapours are stored under pressure. They are designed to withstand considerable internal pressure.
2. The top end of the cylinder is called the neck, and this ends in a tapered screw thread into which the valve is fitted. The thread is sealed with a material that melts if the cylinder is exposed to intense heat. This allows the gas to escape so reducing the risk of an explosion.
3. There is a plastic disc around the neck of the cylinder. The year when the cylinder was last examined can be identified from the shape and colour of the disc.
4. Cylinders are manufactured in different sizes (A to J). Sizes A and H are not used for medical gases. Cylinders attached to the anaesthetic machine are usually size E (Figs 1.1–1.4), while size J cylinders are commonly used for cylinder manifolds. Size E oxygen cylinder contains 680 litres, whereas size E nitrous oxide can release 1800 litres. The smallest sized cylinder, size C, can hold 1.2 litres of water while the largest, L, can hold 50 litres.
5. Lightweight cylinders can be made from aluminium alloy with a fibreglass covering in epoxy resin matrix. These can be used to provide oxygen at home or during transport. They have a flat base to help in storage and handling.

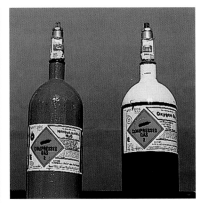

Fig. 1.1 Medical gas cylinders with plastic wrapping intact. A nitrous oxide cylinder (left) and oxygen cylinder (right).

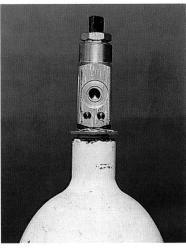

Fig. 1.2 Oxygen cylinder valve and pin index.

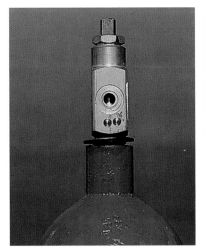

Fig. 1.3 Nitrous oxide cylinder valve and pin index.

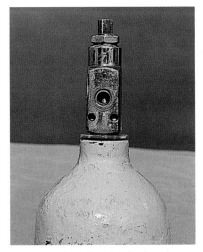

Fig. 1.4 Carbon dioxide cylinder valve and pin index.

- **Gas** exits in the gaseous state at room temperature. Its liquefaction at room temperature is impossible, since the room temperature is above its critical temperature.
- **Vapour** is the gaseous state of a substance below its critical temperature. At room temperature and atmospheric pressure, the substance is liquid.
- **Critical temperature** is the temperature above which a substance can not be liquefied no matter how much pressure is applied. The critical temperatures for nitrous oxide and oxygen are 36.5 and −118°C respectively.

Oxygen is stored as a gas at a pressure of 13 700 kPa whereas nitrous oxide is stored in a liquid phase with its vapour on top at a pressure of 4400 kPa. As the liquid is less compressible than the gas, this means that the cylinder should be only partially filled. The amount of filling is called the **filling ratio**. Partially filling the cylinders with liquid minimizes the risk of dangerous increases in pressure with any increase in the ambient temperature that can lead to an explosion. In the UK, the filling ratio for nitrous oxide and carbon dioxide is 0.75. In hotter climates, the filling ratio is reduced to 0.67.

The filling ratio is the weight of the fluid in the cylinder divided by the weight of water required to fill the cylinder.

A full oxygen cylinder at atmospheric pressure can deliver 130 times its capacity of oxygen.

At constant temperature, a gas-containing cylinder shows a linear and proportional reduction in cylinder pressure as it empties. For a cylinder that contains liquid and vapour, initially the pressure remains constant as more vapour is produced to replace that used. Once all the liquid has been evaporated, the pressure in the cylinder decreases. The temperature in such a cylinder can decrease because of the loss of the latent heat of vaporization leading to the formation of ice on the outside of the cylinder.

Cylinders in use are checked and tested by manufacturers at regular intervals, usually 5 years:

1. *Internal endoscopic examination.*
2. *Flattening, bend and impact tests* are carried out on at least one cylinder in every hundred.
3. *Pressure test*: the cylinder is subjected to high pressures of about 22 000 kPa, which is more than 50% above their normal working pressure.
4. *Tensile test* where strips of the cylinder are cut and stretched. This test is carried out on at least one cylinder in every hundred.

The marks engraved on the cylinders are:

1. Test pressure.
2. Dates of test performed.
3. Chemical formula of the cylinder's content.
4. Tare weight (weight of nitrous oxide cylinder when empty).

Labelling. The cylinder label includes the following details:

- name, chemical symbol, pharmaceutical form, specification of the product, its licence number and the proportion of the constituent gases in a gas mixture
- substance identification number and batch number
- hazard warnings and safety instructions
- cylinder size code
- nominal cylinder contents (litres)
- maximum cylinder pressure (bars)
- filling date, shelf life and expiry date
- directions for use
- storage and handling precautions.

Problems in practice and safety features

1. The gases and vapours should be free of water vapour when stored in cylinders. Water vapour freezes and blocks the exit port when the temperature of the cylinder decreases on opening.
2. The outlet valve uses the pin-index system to make it almost impossible to connect a cylinder to the wrong yoke (Fig. 1.5).
3. Cylinders are colour-coded to reduce accidental use of the wrong gas or vapour. In the UK, the colour-coding is a two-part colour (Table 1.1).
4. Cylinders should be checked regularly whilst in use to ensure that they have sufficient content and that leaks do not occur.

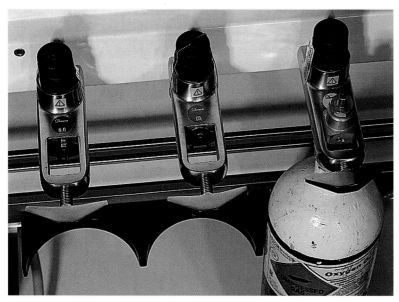

Fig. 1.5 Anaesthetic machine cylinder yokes. For the sake of comparison, the Bodok seal is absent from the nitrous oxide yoke (left).

Cylinders

- Cylinders are made of thin-walled molybdenum steel to withstand high pressures, e.g. 13 700 kPa and 4400 kPa for oxygen and nitrous oxide respectively.
- They are made in different sizes; size E cylinders are used on the anaesthetic machine; size J cylinders are used in cylinder banks.
- Oxygen cylinders contain gas whereas nitrous oxide cylinders contain a mixture of liquid and vapour. In the UK nitrous oxide cylinders are 75% filled with liquid nitrous oxide (filling ratio); this is 67% in hotter climates.
- At a constant temperature, the pressure in a gas cylinder decreases linerally and proportionally as it empties. This is not true in cylinder containing liquid/vapour.
- They are colour-coded.

5. Cylinders should be stored in a purpose built dry, well-ventilated and fireproof room, preferably inside and not subjected to extremes of heat. They should not be stored near flammable materials such as oil or grease or near any source of heat. They should not be exposed to continuous dampness, corrosive chemicals or fumes. This can lead to corrosion of cylinders and their valves.

6. To avoid accidents, full cylinders should be stored separately from empty ones. F, G and J size cylinders are stored upright to avoid damage to the valves. C, D and E size cylinders can be stored horizontally on shelves made of a material that does not damage the surface of the cylinders.

7. Overpressurized cylinders are hazardous and should be reported to the manufacturer.

Cylinder valves

These valves seal the cylinder contents. The chemical formula of the particular gas is engraved on the valve (Fig. 1.6). Other types of

Table 1.1 Colour coding of medical gas cylinders, their pressure when full and their physical state in the cylinder

	Body colour	Shoulder colour	Pressure, kPa (at room temperature)	Physical state in cylinder
Oxygen	Black (Green in USA)	White	13 700	Gas
Nitrous oxide	Blue	Blue	4 400	Liquid/vapour
Carbon dioxide	Grey	Grey	5 000	Liquid/vapour
Air	Grey (Yellow in USA)	White/black quarters	13 700	Gas
Entonox	Blue	White/blue quarters	13 700	Gas
Oxygen/helium (Heliox)	Black	White/brown quarters	13 700	Gas

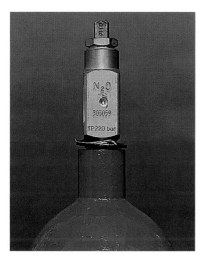

Fig. 1.6 Chemical formula (N₂O) engraved on a nitrous oxide cylinder valve.

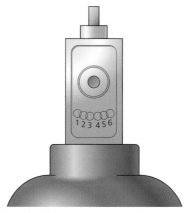

Fig. 1.7 Diagram showing the index positions of a cylinder valve. Oxygen 2 & 5; nitrous oxide 3 & 5; air 1 & 5; carbon dioxide 1 & 6.

valves, the bull nose, the hand wheel and the star, are used under special circumstances.

Components

1. The valve is mounted on the top of the cylinder, screwed into the neck via a threaded connection. It is made of brass and sometimes chromium plated.
2. An on/off spindle is used to open and close the valve by opposing a plastic facing against the valve seating.
3. The exit port for supplying gas to the apparatus (e.g. anaesthetic machine).
4. A safety relief device allows the discharge of cylinder contents to the atmosphere if the cylinder is overpressurized.
5. The non-interchangeable safety system (**Pix-index system**) is used on cylinders of size E or smaller as well as on F and G-size Entonox cylinders. A specific pin configuration exists for each medical gas on the yoke of the anaesthetic machine. The

matching configuration of holes on the valve block allows only the correct gas cylinder to be fitted in the yoke (Figs 1.7 and 1.8). The gas exit port will not seal against the washer of the yoke unless the pins and holes are aligned.
6. A more recent modification where the external part of the valve is designed to allow manual turning

on and off of the cylinder without the need for a key (Fig. 1.9).

Mechanism of action

1. The cylinder valve acts as a mechanism for opening and closing the gas pathway.
2. A compressible yoke sealing washer (**Bodok seal**) must be placed between valve outlet and the apparatus to make a gas-tight joint (Fig. 1.10).

Problems in practice and safety features

1. The plastic wrapping of the valve should be removed just before use. The valve should be slightly opened and closed (cracked) before connecting the cylinder to the anaesthetic machine. This clears particles of dust, oil and grease from the exit port, which would otherwise enter the anaesthetic machine.
2. The valve should be opened slowly when attached to the anaesthetic machine or regulator. This prevents the rapid rise in pressure and the associated rise

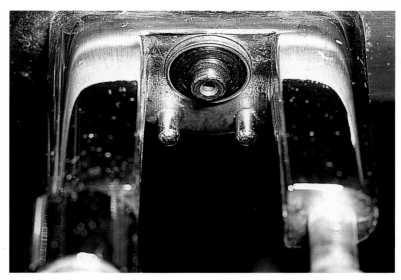

Fig. 1.8 A cylinder yoke and pin index system. Note that a Bodok seal is in position.

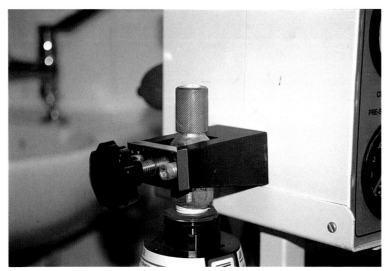

Fig. 1.9 New cylinder valve which allows manual opening and closing.

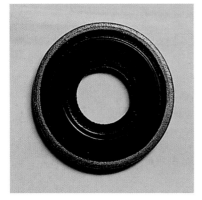

Fig. 1.10 A Bodok seal.

Cylinder valves

- They are mounted on the neck of the cylinder.
- Act as an on/off device for the discharge of cylinder contents.
- Pin index system prevents cylinder identification errors.
- Bodock sealing washer must be placed between the valve and the yoke of the anaesthetic machine.
- A newly designed valve allows keyless manual turning on and off.

---

in temperature of the gas in the machine's pipelines. The cylinder valve should be fully open when in use (the valve must be turned two full revolutions).

3. During closure, overtightening the valve should be avoided. This might lead to damage to the seal between the valve and the cylinder neck.
4. The Bodock seal should be inspected for damage prior to use. Having a spare seal readily available is advisable.

Piped gas supply (piped medical gas and vacuum – PMGV)

PMGV is a system where gases are delivered from central supply points to different sites in the hospital at a pressure of about 400 kPa. Special outlet valves supply the various needs throughout the hospital.

Oxygen, nitrous oxide, Entonox, compressed air and medical vacuum are commonly supplied through the pipeline system.

Components

1. Central supply points such as cylinder banks or liquid oxygen storage tank.
2. Pipework made of special high quality copper alloy, which both prevents degradation of the gases it contains and has bacteriostatic properties. The fittings used are made from brass and are brazed rather than soldered.
3. The size of the pipes differs according to the demand that they carry. Pipes with a 42 mm diameter are usually used for leaving the manifold. Smaller diameter tubes, such as 15 mm, are used after repeated branching.
4. Outlets which are identified by gas colour-coding, gas name and by shape (Fig. 1.11). They accept matching quick connect/disconnect probes, Schrader sockets, (Fig. 1.12) with an indexing collar specific for each gas (or gas mixture).
5. Outlets can be installed as flush-fitting units, surface-fitting units, on booms or pendants, suspended on a hose and gang mounted (Fig. 1.13).
6. Flexible colour-coded hoses connect the outlets to the anaesthetic machine (Fig. 1.14). The anaesthetic machine end should be permanently fixed using a nut and liner union where the thread is gas specific and non-interchangeable (non-interchangeable screw-thread, **NIST** is the British Standard).
7. Isolating valves behind break glass covers are positioned at strategic points throughout the pipeline network. They are also known as AVSUs (Area Valve Service Units) (Fig. 1.15).

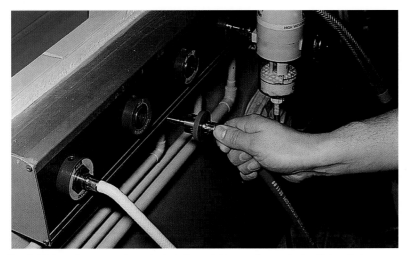

Fig. 1.11 Inserting a remote probe into its matching wall-mounted outlet socket.

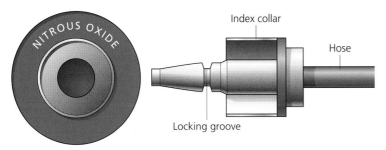

Fig. 1.12 A remote probe and matching outlet socket (not drawn to scale).

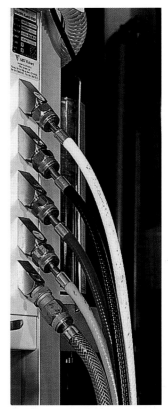

Fig. 1.14 Colour-coded hoses with NIST fittings attached to an anaesthetic machine.

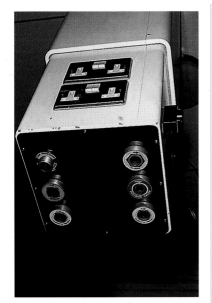

Fig. 1.13 Outlet sockets mounted in a retractable ceiling unit.

Problems in practice and safety features

1. A reserve bank of cylinders is available should the primary supply fail. Low pressure alarms detect gas supply failure (Fig. 1.16).
2. Single hose test is performed to detect cross-connection.
3. Tug test is performed to detect misconnection.
4. Regulations for PMGV installation, repair and modification are enforced.
5. Anaesthetists are responsible for the gases supplied from the terminal outlet through to the anaesthetic machine. Pharmacy, Supplies and Engineering departments share the responsibility for the gas pipelines 'behind the wall'.
6. There is the risk of fire from worn or damaged hoses that are designed to carry gases under pressure from a primary source such as a cylinder or wall mounted terminal to medical devices such as ventilators and anaesthetic machines. Because of heavy wear and tear, the risk of rupture is greatest in oxygen hoses used with transport devices. Regular inspection and replacement, every 2–5 years, of all medical gas hoses is recommended.

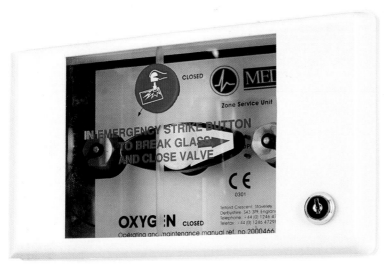

Fig. 1.15 An Area Valve Service Unit (AVSU).

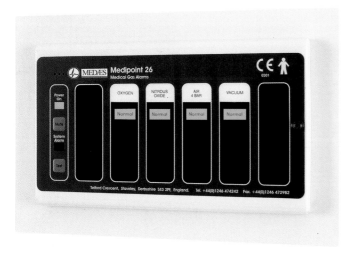

Fig. 1.16 Medical gas alarm panel.

Piped gas supply

- There is a network of copper alloy pipelines throughout the hospital from central supply points.
- The outlets are colour- and shape-coded to accept matching 'Schrader' probes.
- Flexible and colour-coded pipelines run from the anaesthetic machine to the outlets.
- Single hose and tug tests are performed to test for cross-connection and misconnection respectively.
- There is risk of fire from worn and damaged hoses.

Sources of gas supply

The source of supply can be cylinder manifold(s) and, in the case of oxygen, a liquid oxygen storage tank or oxygen concentrator.

CYLINDER MANIFOLD

Manifolds are used to supply nitrous oxide, Entonox and oxygen.

Components

1. Large cylinders (e.g. size J each with 6800 litres capacity) are usually divided into two groups, primary and secondary. The two groups alternate in supplying the pipelines (Fig. 1.17). The number of cylinders depends on the expected demand.
2. All cylinders in each group are connected through non-return valves to a common pipe. This in turn is connected to the pipeline through pressure regulators.

Mechanism of action

1. In either group, all the cylinders' valves are opened. This allows them to empty simultaneously.
2. The supply is automatically changed to the secondary group when the primary group is nearly empty. The changeover is achieved through a pressure-sensitive device that detects when the cylinders are nearly empty.
3. The changeover activates an electrical signalling system to alert staff to the need to change the cylinders.

Problems in practice and safety features

1. The manifold should be housed in a well-ventilated room built of fireproof material away from the main buildings of the hospital.

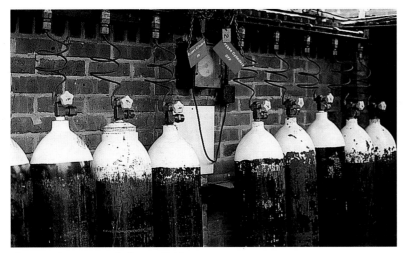

Fig. 1.17 An oxygen cylinder manifold.

2. The manifold room should not be used as a general cylinder store.
3. All empty cylinders should be removed immediately from the manifold room.

LIQUID OXYGEN

A vacuum-insulated evaporator (VIE) (Fig. 1.18) is the most economical way to store and supply oxygen.

Components

1. A thermally insulated double-walled steel tank with a layer of perlite in a vacuum is used as the insulation (Fig. 1.19).
2. A pressure regulator allows gas to enter the pipelines and maintains the pressure through the pipelines at about 400 kPa.
3. A safety valve opens at 1700 kPa allowing the gas to escape when there is a build-up of pressure

within the vessel. This can be caused by underdemand for oxygen.

4. A control valve opens when there is an excessive demand on the system. This allows liquid oxygen to evaporate by passing through superheaters made of uninsulated coils of copper tubing.

Mechanism of action

1. Liquid oxygen is stored (up to 1500 litres) at a temperature of −150° to −170°C (lower than the critical temperature) and at a pressure of 5–10 atmospheres.
2. The temperature of the vessel is maintained by the high-vacuum shell. Evaporation of the liquid oxygen requires heat (latent heat of vaporization). This heat is taken from the liquid oxygen, helping to maintain its low temperature.
3. The storage vessel rests on a weighing balance to measure the mass of the liquid. More recently, a differential pressure gauge which measures the pressure difference between the bottom and top of the liquid oxygen can be used instead. As liquid oxygen evaporates, its mass decreases, reducing

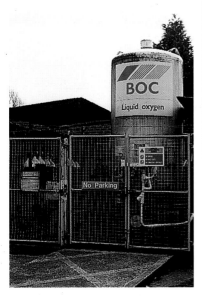

Fig. 1.18 A vacuum-insulated evaporator (VIE).

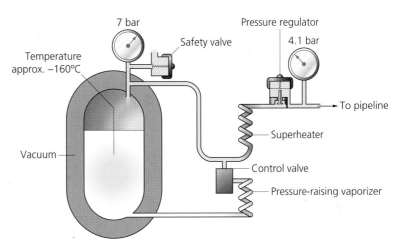

Fig. 1.19 Schematic diagram of a liquid oxygen supply system (reproduced with permission from Parbrook GD et al., Basic Physics and Measurement in Anaesthesia, 3rd edn. Butterworth-Heinemann).

the pressure at the bottom. By measuring the difference in pressure, the contents of the VIE can be calculated. When required, fresh supplies of liquid oxygen are pumped from a tanker into the vessel.

4. The cold oxygen gas is warmed once outside the vessel in a coil of copper tubing. The increase in temperature causes an increase in pressure.

5. At a temperature of 15°C and atmospheric pressure, liquid oxygen can give 842 times its volume as gas.

Problems in practice and safety features

1. Reserve banks of cylinders are kept in case of supply failure.
2. A liquid oxygen storage vessel should be housed away from main buildings due to the fire hazard. The risk of fire is increased in cases of liquid spillage.
3. Spillage of cryogenic liquid can cause cold burns, frostbite and hypothermia.

OXYGEN CONCENTRATORS

Oxygen concentrators extract oxygen from air by differential absorption. These devices may be small, designed to supply oxygen to a single patient (Figs 1.20 and 1.21), or they can be large enough to supply oxygen for a medical gas pipeline system (Fig. 1.22).

Components

A zeolite molecular sieve is used. Zeolites are hydrated aluminium silicates of the alkaline earth metals in a powder or granular form. Many zeolite columns are used.

Mechanism of action

1. Ambient air is filtered and pressurized to about 137 kPa by a compressor.

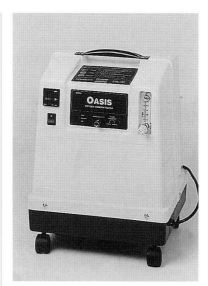

Fig. 1.20 The Oasis home oxygen concentrator (reproduced with permission from Rimmer Alco Ltd).

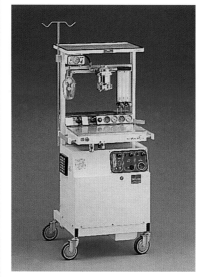

Fig. 1.21 The oxyPac 550 anaesthetic machine which has a built-in oxygen concentrator (reproduced with permission from pneuPac Ltd).

2. Air is exposed to a zeolite molecular sieve column, forming a very large surface area, at a certain pressure.
3. The sieve selectively retains nitrogen and other unwanted components of air. These are released into the atmosphere after heating the column and applying a vacuum.
4. The changeover between columns is made by a time switch.
5. The maximum oxygen concentration achieved is 95% by volume. Argon is the main remaining constituent.

Problems in practice and safety features

Although the oxygen concentration achieved is sufficient for the vast majority of clinical applications, its use with the circle system leads to argon accumulation. To avoid this, higher fresh gas flows are required.

Source of supply

- Cylinder manifold: banks of large cylinders, usually size J, are used.
- Liquid oxygen: a thermally insulated vessel at a temperature of −150° to −170°C and at a pressure of 5–10 atmospheres is used.
- Oxygen concentrator: a zeolite molecular sieve is used.

Entonox (BOC Medical)

This is a compressed gas mixture containing 50% oxygen and 50% nitrous oxide by volume. It is commonly used in the casualty and labour ward settings to provide analgesia. A two-stage pressure demand regulator is attached to the Entonox cylinder when in use (Figs 1.23 and 1.24). As the patient inspires through the mask or mouth piece, gas flow is allowed to occur. Gas flow ceases at the end of an inspiratory effort. Entonox is compressed into cylinders to a pressure of 13 700 kPa.

If the temperature of the Entonox cylinder is decreased to

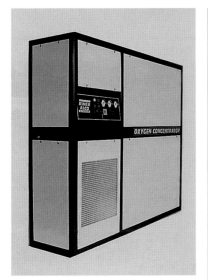

Fig. 1.22 The OC 11 oxygen concentrator (reproduced with permission from Rimmer Alco Ltd).

below −5.5°C, liquefaction and separation of the two components occur (**Poynting effect**). This results in:

1. a liquid mixture containing mostly nitrous oxide with about 20% oxygen dissolved in it

2. above the liquid, a gas mixture of high oxygen concentration.

This means that when used at a constant flow rate, a gas with a high concentration of oxygen is supplied first. This is followed by a gas of decreasing oxygen concentration as the liquid evaporates. This may lead to the supply of hypoxic mixtures, with less than 20% oxygen, as the cylinder is nearly empty.

Rewarming and mixing of both the cylinder and its contents reverses the separation and liquefaction.

Problems in practice and safety features

1. Liquefaction and separation of the components can be prevented by:
   a) cylinders being stored horizontally for about 24 hours at temperatures of or above 5°C before use. The horizontal position increases the area for diffusion. If the contents are well mixed by repeated inversion, cylinders can be used earlier than 24 hours
   b) large cylinders are equipped with a dip tube with its tip ending in the liquid phase. This results in the liquid being used first, preventing the delivery of an oxygen concentration of less than 20%.

2. Prolonged use of Entonox should be avoided because of the effect of nitrous oxide on the bone marrow especially in the critically ill patient. Adequate facilities for scavenging should be provided to protect hospital staff.

Compressed air

Medical air is supplied in a hospital for clinical uses or to drive power tools. The former is supplied at a pressure of 400 kPa and the latter at 700 kPa. The anaesthetic machines and most intensive care ventilator blenders accept a 400 kPa supply. The terminal outlets for the two

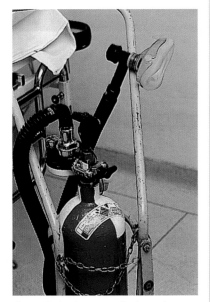

Fig. 1.23 An Entonox cylinder and delivery system.

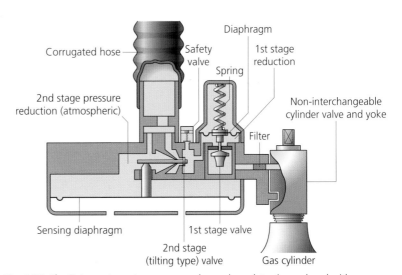

Fig. 1.24 The Entonox two-stage pressure demand regulator (reproduced with permission from Aitkenhead R, Smith G. Textbook of Anaesthesia, 3rd edn. Churchill Livingstone, 1996).

pressures are different to prevent misconnection.

Air may be supplied from cylinder manifolds, or more economically from a compressor. Oil-free medical air is cleaned by filters and separators and then dried before use.

Centralized vacuum system

This system consists of a pump, receiver and a filter. The pump

is capable of creating a negative pressure of –53 kPa (–400 mmHg) and can accommodate an air flow of 40 L/min. It is recommended that there are at least two vacuum outlets per operating theatre, one per anaesthetic room and one per recovery bed.

FURTHER READING

Health Technical Memorandum 2022. Medical gas pipeline systems. London: The Stationery Office, 1997.

Lovell T. Medical gases, their storage and delivery. Anaesthesia and Intensive Care Medicine 2004;5(1):10–14.

MCQs

In the following lists, which of the statements (a) to (e) are true?

1. Concerning cylinders
   a) Oxygen is stored in cylinders as a gas.
   b) The pressure in a half-filled oxygen cylinder is 13 700 kPa.
   c) The pressure in a half-full nitrous oxide cylinder is 4400 kPa.
   d) Nitrous oxide is stored in the cylinder in the gas phase.
   e) Pressure in a full Entonox cylinder is 13 700 kPa.

2. Entonox
   a) Entonox is 50:50 mixture by weight of O_2 and N_2O.
   b) Entonox has a critical temperature of 5.5°C.
   c) Entonox cylinders should be stored upright.
   d) At room temperature, Entonox cylinders contain only gas.
   e) Entonox cylinders have blue bodies and white and blue quarters on the shoulders.

3. Oxygen
   a) For medical use, oxygen is usually formed from fractional distillation of air.
   b) Long-term use can cause bone marrow depression.
   c) In hyperbaric concentrations, oxygen may cause convulsions.
   d) At constant volume, the absolute pressure of oxygen is directly proportional to its absolute temperature.
   e) The critical temperature of oxygen is –118°C.

4. Oxygen concentrators
   a) Oxygen concentrators concentrate O_2 that has been delivered from an oxygen cylinder manifold.
   b) Argon accumulation can occur when oxygen concentrators are used with the circle system.
   c) They are made of columns of a zeolite molecular sieve.
   d) They can achieve O_2 concentrations of up to 100%.
   e) They can only be used in home oxygen therapy.

5. Oxygen
   a) Oxygen is stored in cylinders at approximately 140 bars.
   b) It has a critical temperature of 36.5°C.
   c) It is a liquid in its cylinder.
   d) It may form an inflammable mixture with oil.
   e) It obeys Boyle's law.

6. Concerning cylinders
   a) The filling ratio = weight of liquid in cylinder divided by the weight of water required to fill the cylinder.
   b) The tare weight is the weight of the cylinder plus its contents.
   c) Nitrous oxide cylinders have a blue body and blue and white top.
   d) A full oxygen cylinder has a pressure of approximately 137 bars.
   e) At 40°C, a nitrous oxide cylinder contains both liquid and vapour.

7. Concerning piped gas supply in the operating theatre
   a) Compressed air is supplied only under one pressure.
   b) The NIST system is the British Standard.
   c) Only oxygen and air are supplied.
   d) E-size cylinders are normally used in cylinder manifolds.
   e) Liquid oxygen is stored at temperatures above –100°C.

8. The following statements are true
   a) There is no need for cylinders to undergo regular checks
   b) The only agent identification on the cylinder is its colour
   c) When attached to the anaesthetic machine, the cylinder valve should be opened slowly.
   d) When warmed, liquid oxygen can give 842 times its volume as gas.
   e) Cylinders are made of thick-walled steel to withstand the high internal pressure.

Answers

1. Concerning cylinders
   a) *True.* Oxygen is stored in the cylinder as a gas.
   b) *False.* Oxygen is stored as a gas in the cylinder where gas laws apply. The pressure gauge accurately reflects the contents of the cylinder. A full oxygen cylinder has a pressure of 13 700 kPa. Pressure in a half-full oxygen cylinder is therefore 6850 kPa.
   c) *True.* Nitrous oxide is stored in the cylinder in the liquid form. The pressure of a full nitrous oxide cylinder is about 4400 kPa. As the cylinder is used, the vapour above the liquid is used first. This vapour is replaced by new vapour from the liquid. Therefore the pressure is maintained. So the cylinder is nearly empty before the pressure starts to decrease. For this reason the pressure gauge does not accurately reflect the contents of the cylinder.
   d) *False.* Nitrous oxide is stored in the cylinder as a liquid. The vapour above the liquid is delivered to the patient.
   e) *True.* Entonox is a compressed gas mixture containing 50% oxygen and 50% nitrous oxide by volume.

2. Entonox
   a) *False.* Entonox is a 50:50 mixture of O_2 and N_2O by volume and not by weight.
   b) *False.* The critical temperature of Entonox is $-5.5°C$. At or below this temperature, liquefaction and separation of the two components occurs. This results in a liquid mixture of mainly nitrous oxide and about 20% oxygen. Above the liquid is a gaseous mixture with a high concentration of oxygen.
   c) *False.* This increases the risk of liquefaction and separation of the components. To prevent this, Entonox cylinders should be stored horizontally for about 24 hours at temperatures of or above 5°C. This position increases the area for diffusion. With repeated inversion, Entonox cylinders can be used earlier than 24 hours.
   d) *True.* Liquefaction and separation of nitrous oxide and oxygen occurs at or below $-5.5°C$.
   e) *True.*

3. Oxygen
   a) *True.* Except for oxygen concentrators which use zeolites.
   b) *False.* Long term use of oxygen has no effect on the bone marrow. Long term use of N_2O can cause bone marrow depression especially with high concentrations in critically ill patients.
   c) *True.*
   d) *True.* This is Gay-Lussac's law where pressure = constant × temperature. Oxygen also obeys the other gas laws (Dalton's law of partial pressures, Boyle's and Charles's laws).
   e) *True.* At or below $-118°C$, oxygen changes to the liquid phase. This is used in the design of the vacuum insulated evaporator where oxygen is stored in the liquid phase at temperatures of -150 to $-170°C$.

4. Oxygen concentrators
   a) *False. Oxygen concentrators extract oxygen from air using a zeolite molecular sieve. Many columns of zeolite are used. Zeolites are hydrated aluminium silicates of the alkaline earth metals.*
   b) *True. The maximum oxygen concentration achieved by oxygen concentrators is 95%. The rest is mainly argon. Using low flows with the circle breathing system can lead to the accumulation of argon. Higher fresh gas flows are required to avoid this.*
   c) *True. The zeolite molecular sieve selectively retains nitrogen and other unwanted gases in air. These are released into the atmosphere. The changeover between columns is made by a time switch.*
   d) *False. Oxygen concentrators can deliver a maximum oxygen concentration of 95%.*
   e) *False. Oxygen concentrators can be small delivering oxygen to a single patient or they can be large enough to supply oxygen to hospitals.*

5. Oxygen
   a) *True. Molybdenum steel or aluminium alloy cylinders are used to store oxygen at pressures of approximately 14 000 kPa (140 bars).*
   b) *False. The critical temperature of O_2 is –118°C. Above that temperature, oxygen can not be liquefied however much pressure is applied.*
   c) *False. Oxygen is a gas in the cylinder as its critical temperature is –118°C.*
   d) *True. Oil is flammable while oxygen aids combustion. Oxygen cylinders should be stored away from oil.*
   e) *True. At a constant temperature, the volume of a given mass of oxygen varies inversely with the absolute pressure (volume = constant × 1/pressure). Oxygen obeys other gas laws.*

6. Concerning cylinders
   a) *True. The filling ratio is used when filling cylinders with liquid, e.g. nitrous oxide. As the liquid is less compressible than the gas, the cylinder should be only partially filled. Depending on the ambient temperature, the filling ratio can be from 0.67 to 0.75.*
   b) *False. The tare weight is the weight of the empty cylinder. This is used to estimate the amount of the contents of the cylinder. It is one of the marks engraved on the cylinders.*
   c) *False. Nitrous oxide cylinder have a blue body and top. Entonox cylinders have a blue body and blue and white top.*
   d) *True.*
   e) *False. At 40°C, nitrous oxide exists as a gas only. This is above its critical temperature, 36.5°C, so it can not be liquefied above that.*

7. Concerning piped gas supply in the operating theatre

a) *False. Air is supplied at two different pressures; at 400 kPa when it is delivered to the patient and at 700 kPa when used to operate power tools in the operating theatre.*

b) *True. This stands for non-interchangeable screw thread. This is one of the safety features present in the piped gas supply system. Flexible colour-coded hoses connect the outlets to the anaesthetic machine. The connections to the anaesthetic machine should be permanently fixed using a nut and liner union where the thread is gas-specific and non-interchangeable.*

c) *False. Oxygen, nitrous oxide, air and vacuum can be supplied by the piped gas system.*

d) *False. Larger cylinders, e.g. J size, are normally used in a cylinder manifold. E size cylinders are usually mounted on the anaesthetic machine.*

e) *False. Liquid oxygen has to be stored at temperatures below its critical temperature, –118°C. So oxygen stored at temperatures above –100°C (above its critical temperature) exists as a gas.*

8. The following statements are true

a) *False. Cylinders should be checked regularly by the manufacturers. Internal endoscopic examination, pressure testing, flattening, bending and impact testing and tensile testing are done on a regular basis.*

b) *False. To identify the agent, the name, chemical symbol, pharmaceutical form and specification of the agent, in addition to the colour of the cylinder are used.*

c) *True. When attached to an anaesthetic machine, the cylinder valve should be opened slowly to prevent the rapid rise in pressure within the machine's pipelines.*

d) *True. It is more economical to store oxygen as liquid before supplying it. At a temperature of 15°C and atmospheric pressure, liquid oxygen can give 842 times its volume as gas.*

e) *False. For ease of transport, cylinders are made of thin-walled seamless molybdenum steel. They are designed to withstand considerable internal pressures and tested up to pressures of about 22 000 kPa.*

Chapter 2

The anaesthetic machine

The anaesthetic machine accurately and continuously delivers gas and vapour mixtures of the desired compositions (Figs 2.1 and 2.2). It consists of:

1. gas supplies (see Chapter 1)
2. pressure gauges
3. pressure regulators (reducing valves)
4. flowmeters
5. vaporizers
6. common gas outlet
7. a variety of other features, e.g. high flow oxygen flush, pressure relief valve and oxygen supply failure alarm and suction apparatus
8. most modern anaesthetic machines incorporate a circle breathing system (see Chapter 4) and a bag-in-bottle type ventilator (see Chapter 8).

Safety features of a modern anaesthetic machine to ensure the delivery of a safe gas mixture should include the following:

1. Colour-coded pressure gauges.
2. Colour-coded flowmeters.
3. An oxygen flowmeter controlled by a single touch-coded knob.
4. Oxygen is the last gas to be added to the mixture.
5. Oxygen concentration monitor or analyser.
6. Nitrous oxide is cut off when the oxygen pressure is low.
7. Oxygen: nitrous oxide ratio monitor and controller.
8. Pin index safety system for cylinders and non-interchangeable screw thread (NIST) for pipelines.
9. Alarm for failure of oxygen supply.
10. Ventilator disconnection alarm.
11. At least one reserve oxygen cylinder should be available on machines that use pipeline supply.

Pressure gauge

This measures the pressure in the cylinder or pipeline. The pressure gauges for oxygen, nitrous oxide and medical air are mounted in a front-facing panel on the anaesthetic machine (Fig. 2.3).

Components

1. A robust, flexible and coiled tube which is oval in cross-section (Fig. 2.4). It should be able to withstand the sudden high pressure when the cylinder is switched on.
2. The tube is sealed at its inner end and connected to a needle pointer which moves over a dial.

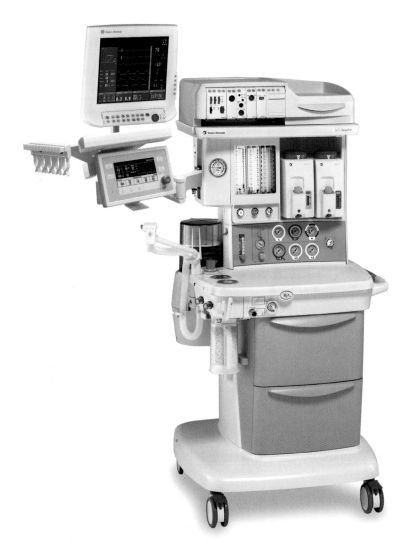

Fig. 2.1 The Datex-Ohmeda Aestiva S/5 anaesthetic machine.

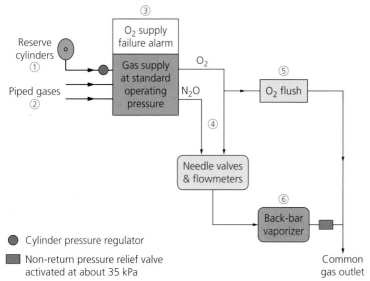

Fig. 2.2 Diagrammatic representation of a continuous flow anaesthetic machine. Pressures throughout the system 1. O_2: 13 700 kPa, N_2O: 4400 kPa; 2. pipeline: about 400 kPa; 3. O_2 supply failure alarm activated at <250 kPa; 4. regulated gas supply at about 400 kPa; 5. O_2: flush 45 L/min at a pressure of about 400 kPa; 6. back-bar pressure: 1–10 kPa (depending on flow rate and type of vaporizer).

● Cylinder pressure regulator

■ Non-return pressure relief valve activated at about 35 kPa

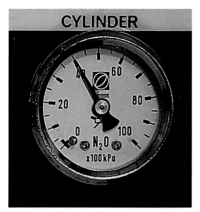

Fig. 2.3 One of the front-facing cylinder pressure gauges. Gauges for both cylinder and pipeline operating pressures are featured.

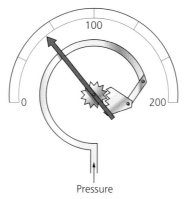

Fig. 2.4 The Bourdon pressure gauge (reproduced with permission from Aitkenhead R, Smith G. Textbook of Anaesthesia, 3rd edn. Churchill Livingstone, 1996).

pressure measured indicates the contents available in an oxygen cylinder. Oxygen is stored as a gas and obeys Boyle's gas law (pressure × volume = constant). This is not the case in a nitrous oxide cylinder since it is stored as a liquid and vapour.

2. A pressure gauge designed for pipelines should not be used to measure cylinder pressure and vice versa. This leads to inaccuracies and/or damage to the pressure gauge.

3. Should the coiled tube rupture, the gas vents from the back of the pressure gauge casing. The face of the pressure gauge is made of heavy glass as an additional safety feature.

Pressure gauge
● Measures pressure in cylinder or pipeline.
● Pressure acts to straighten a coiled tube.
● Colour-coded and calibrated for a particular gas or vapour.

Pressure regulator (reducing valve)

Pressure regulators are used because

● Gas and vapour are stored under high pressure in cylinders. A regulator reduces the variable cylinder pressure to a constant safer operating pressure of about 400 kPa (just below the pipeline pressure) (Fig. 2.5).
● The temperature and pressure of the cylinder contents decrease with use. In order to maintain flow, constant adjustment is required in the absence of regulators.
● Regulators protect the components of the anaesthetic machine against pressure surges.

3. The other end of the tube is exposed to the gas supply.

Mechanism of action

1. The high pressure gas causes the tube to uncoil (Bourdon gauge).
2. The movement of the tube causes the needle pointer to move on

the calibrated dial indicating the pressure.

Problems in practice and safety features

1. Each pressure gauge is colour-coded and calibrated for a particular gas or vapour. The

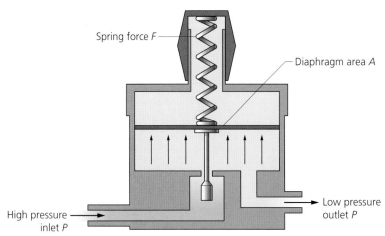

Fig. 2.5 The principles of a pressure regulator (reducing valve) (reproduced with permission from Aitkenhead R, Smith G. Textbook of Anaesthesia, 3rd edn. Churchill Livingstone, 1996).

They are positioned between the cylinders and the rest of the anaesthetic machine (Figs 2.6 and 2.7).

Components

1. An inlet, with a filter, leading to a high pressure chamber with a valve.
2. This valve leads to a low pressure chamber and outlet.
3. A diaphragm attached to a spring is situated in the low pressure chamber.

Mechanism of action

1. Gas enters the high pressure chamber and passes into the low pressure chamber via the valve.
2. The force exerted by the high pressure gas tries to close the valve. The opposing force of the diaphragm and spring tries to open the valve. A balance is reached between the two opposing forces. This maintains a gas flow under a constant pressure of about 400 kPa.

Problems in practice and safety features

1. Formation of ice inside the regulator can occur. If the cylinder contains water vapour, this may condense and freeze as a result of the heat lost when gas expands on entry into the low pressure chamber.
2. The diaphragm can rupture.
3. Relief valves (usually set at 700 kPa) are fitted downstream of the regulators and allow the escape of gas should the regulators fail.
4. A one-way valve is positioned within the cylinder supply line. This prevents backflow and loss of gas from the pipeline supplies should a cylinder not be connected. This one-way valve may be incorporated into the design of the pressure regulator.

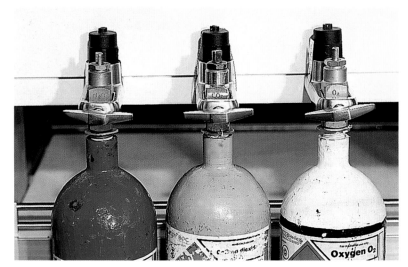

Fig. 2.6 Cylinder pressure regulators (black domes) positioned above the cylinder yokes in the Datex-Ohmeda Flexima anaesthetic machine.

> **Pressure regulator**
> - Reduces pressure of gases from cylinders to about 400 kPa (similar to pipeline pressure).
> - Allows fine control of gas flow and protects the anaesthetic machine from high pressures.
> - A balance between two opposing forces maintains a constant operating pressure.

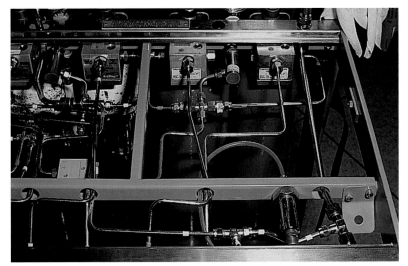

Fig. 2.7 Cylinder pressure regulators (metal boxes at the top of the figure) in the M&IE Cavendish anaesthetic machine. (The machine's tray has been removed.)

Second stage regulators and flow restrictors

The control of pipeline pressure surges can be achieved either by using a second-stage pressure regulator or a flow restrictor (Fig. 2.8) – a constriction, between the pipeline supply and the rest of the anaesthetic machine. A lower pressure (100–200 kPa) is achieved. If there are only flow restrictors and no regulators in the pipeline supply, adjustment of the flowmeter controls is usually necessary whenever there is change in pipeline pressure.

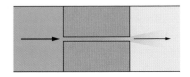

Fig. 2.8 A flow restrictor. The constriction causes a significant pressure drop when there is a high gas flow rate.

Flow restrictors may also be used downstream of vaporizers to prevent back pressure effect (see later).

One-way valve or backflow check valves

These valves are usually placed next to the inlet yoke. Their function is to prevent loss or leakage of gas from an empty yoke. They also prevent accidental transfilling between paired cylinders.

Flow control (needle) valves

These valves control the flow through the flowmeters by manual adjustment. They are positioned at the base of the associated flowmeter tube (Fig. 2.9). Increasing the flow of a gas is achieved by turning the valve in an anticlockwise direction.

Components

1. The body, made of brass, screws into the base of the flowmeter.
2. The stem screws into the body and ends in a needle. It has screw threads allowing fine adjustment.
3. The flow control knobs are labelled and colour-coded.
4. A flow control knobs guard is fitted in some designs to protect against accidental adjustment in the flowmeters.

Flowmeters

Flowmeters measure the flow rate of a gas passing through them. They are individually calibrated for each gas. Calibration occurs at room temperature and atmospheric pressure (sea level). They have an accuracy of about ± 2.5%. For flows above 1 L/min, the units are L/min, and for flows below that, the units are 100 mL/min (Fig. 2.10).

Components

1. A flow control (needle) valve.
2. A tapered (wider at the top), transparent plastic or glass tube.
3. A light weight rotating bobbin or ball. Bobbin-stops at either end of the tube ensure that it is always visible to the operator at extremes of flow.

Mechanism of action

1. When the needle valve is opened, gas is free to enter the tapered tube.
2. The bobbin is held floating within the tube by the gas flow passing around it. The higher the flow rate, the higher the bobbin rises within the tube.
3. The effect of gravity on the bobbin is counteracted by the gas flow. A constant pressure

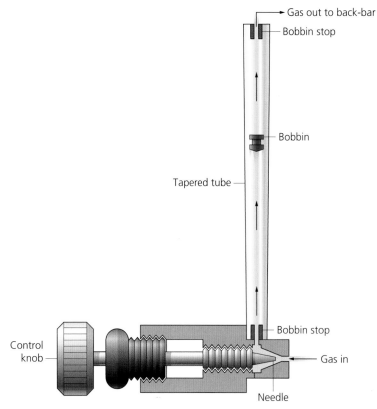

Fig. 2.9 A flow control (needle) valve and flowmeter.

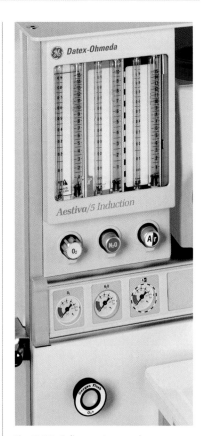

Fig. 2.10 A flowmeter panel.

difference across the bobbin exists as it floats.

4. The clearance between the bobbin and the tube wall widens as the gas flow increases (Fig. 2.11).

5. At low flow rates, the clearance is longer and narrower, thus acting as a tube. Under these circumstances, the flow is laminar and a function of gas viscosity (Poiseuille's Law).

6. At high flow rates the clearance is shorter and wider, thus acting as an orifice. Here, the flow is turbulent and a function of gas density.

7. The top of the bobbin has slits (flutes) cut into its side. As gas flows past it, the slits cause the bobbin to rotate. A dot on the bobbin indicates to the operator

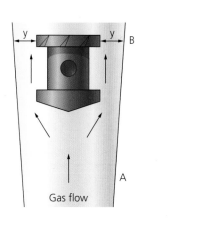

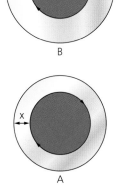

Fig. 2.11 Mechanism of action of the flowmeter. As the bobbin rises from A to B, the clearance increases (from x to y).

that the bobbin is rotating and not stuck.

8. The reading of the flowmeter is taken from the top of the bobbin (Fig. 2.12). When a ball is used the reading is generally taken from the midpoint of the ball.

9. When very low flows are required, e.g. in the circle breathing system, an arrangement of two flowmeters in series is used. One flowmeter reads a maximum of 1 L/min allowing fine adjustment of the flow. One flow control per gas is needed for both flowmeters (Fig. 2.13).

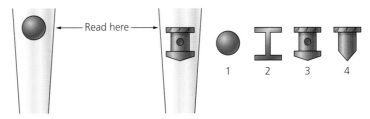

Fig. 2.12 Reading a flowmeter (top). Different types of bobbin: 1. ball; 2. non-rotating H float; 3. skirted; 4. non-skirted.

Problems in practice and safety features

1. The flow control knobs are colour-coded for their respective gases. The oxygen control knob is situated to the left (in the UK) and, in some designs, is larger with larger ridges and has a longer stem than the other control knobs, making it easily recognizable. In the USA and Canada, the oxygen control knob is situated to the right.

2. Some designs make it impossible for nitrous oxide to be delivered without the addition of a fixed percentage of oxygen. This is achieved by using interactive oxygen and nitrous oxide controls. This helps to prevent the possibility of delivering a hypoxic mixture to the patient.

3. A crack in a flowmeter may result in a hypoxic mixture (Fig. 2.14). To avoid this, oxygen is the last gas to be added to the mixture delivered to the back bar.

4. Flow measurements can become inaccurate if the bobbin sticks to the inside wall of the flowmeter. The commonest causes are:
   a) Dirt: this is a problem at low flow rates when the clearance is narrow. The source of the

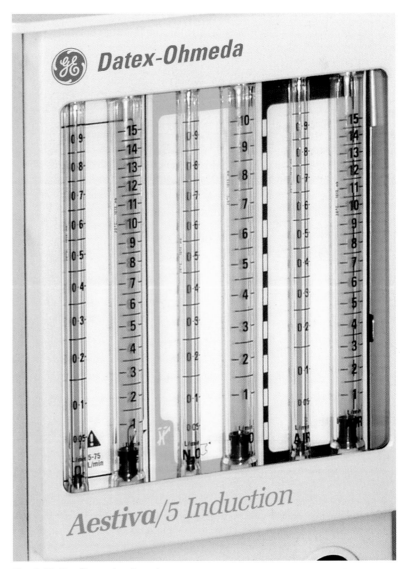

Fig. 2.13 Two flowmeters in series.

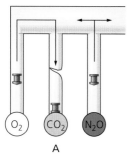
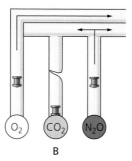

Fig. 2.14 (A) A broken CO_2 flowmeter allows oxygen to escape and a hypoxic mixture to be delivered from the back bar. (B) A possible design measure to prevent this.

dirt is usually a contaminated gas supply. Filters, acting before gas enters the flowmeters, will remove the dirt;

b) Static electricity: the charge usually builds up over a period of time, leading to inaccuracies of up to 35%. Using antistatic materials in flowmeter construction helps to eliminate any build-up of charge. Application of antistatic spray removes any charge present.

5. Flowmeters are designed to be read in a vertical position, so any change in the position of the machine can affect the accuracy.

6. Pressure rises at the common gas outlet are transmitted back to the gas above the bobbin. This results in a drop in the level of the bobbin with an inaccurate reading. This can happen with minute volume divider ventilators as back pressure is exerted as they cycle with inaccuracies of up to 10%. A flow restrictor is fitted downstream of the flowmeters to prevent this occurring.

7. Accidents have resulted from failure to see the bobbin clearly at the extreme ends of the tube. This can be prevented by illuminating the flowmeter bank **and** installing a wire stop at the top to prevent the bobbin reaching the top of the tube.

8. If facilities for the use of carbon dioxide are fitted to the machine, the flowmeter is designed to allow a maximum of 500 mL/min to be added to the fresh gas flow. This ensures that dangerous levels of hypercarbia are avoided.

9. Highly accurate computer controlled gas mixers are available.

> Flowmeter
> • Both laminar and turbulent flows are encountered, making both the viscosity and density of the gas relevant.
> • The bobbin should not stick to the tapered tube.
> • Oxygen is the last gas to be added to the mixture.
> • It is very accurate with an error margin of ± 2.5%.

Vaporizers

A vaporizer is designed to add a controlled amount of an inhalational agent, after changing it from liquid to vapour, to the fresh gas flow. This is normally expressed as a percentage of saturated vapour added to the gas flow.

Characteristics of the ideal vaporizer

1. Its performance is not affected by changes in fresh gas flow, volume of the liquid agent, ambient temperature and pressure, decrease in temperature due to vaporization and pressure fluctuation due to the mode of respiration.
2. Low resistance to flow.
3. Light weight with small liquid requirement.
4. Economy and safety in use with minimal servicing requirements.
5. Corrosion- and solvent-resistant construction.

Vaporizers can be classified according to location:
1. Inside the breathing system. Gases pass through a very low resistance, draw-over vaporizer due to the patient's respiratory efforts (e.g. Goldman, Oxford Miniature Vaporizer OMV).
2. Outside the breathing system. Gases are driven through a plenum (high resistance, unidirectional) vaporizer due to gas supply pressure.

PLENUM VAPORIZER (FIG. 2.15)

Components

1. The case with the filling level indicator and a port for the filling device.
2. Percentage control dial on top of the case.
3. The bypass channel and the vaporization chamber. The latter has wicks or baffles to increase the surface area available for vaporization (Fig. 2.16).
4. The splitting ratio is controlled by a temperature-sensitive valve utilizing a bimetallic strip (Fig. 2.17). The latter is made of two strips of metal with different

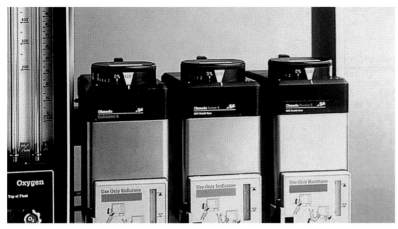

Fig. 2.15 Tec Mk 5 vaporizers mounted on the back bar of an anaesthetic machine.

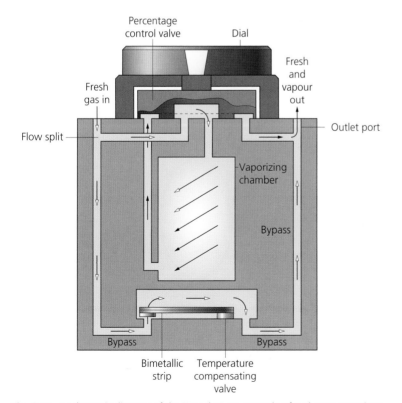

Fig. 2.16 A schematic diagram of the Tec Mk 5, an example of a plenum vaporizer.

coefficients of thermal expansion bonded together. It is positioned inside the vaporization chamber in the Tec Mk 2 whereas in Tec Mk 3, 4 and 5, it is outside the vaporization chamber. An ether-filled bellows is the temperature compensating device in the M&IE Vapamasta Vaporizer 5 and 6. The bellows contracts as the temperature of the vaporizer decreases.

5. The vaporizers are mounted on the back bar (Fig. 2.18) using the interlocking Selectatec system (Fig. 2.19). The percentage control dial cannot be moved unless the locking lever of the system is engaged (in Mk 4 and 5). The interlocking extension rods prevent more than one vaporizer being used at any one time, preventing contamination of the one downstream (in Mk 4 and 5). The fresh gas flow only enters the vaporizer when it is switched on (Fig. 2.20).

Mechanism of action

1. The calibration of each vaporizer is agent-specific.
2. Fresh gas flow is split into two streams on entering the vaporizer. One stream flows through the bypass channel and the other, smaller stream, flows through the vaporizing chamber. The two gas streams reunite as the gas leaves the vaporizer.
3. The vaporization chamber is designed so that the gas leaving it is always fully saturated with vapour before it rejoins the bypass gas stream. This should be achieved despite changes in the fresh gas flow.
4. Full saturation with vapour is achieved by increasing the surface area of contact between the carrier gas and the anaesthetic agent. This is achieved by having wicks saturated by the inhalational agent, a series of baffles or by bubbling the gas through the liquid.

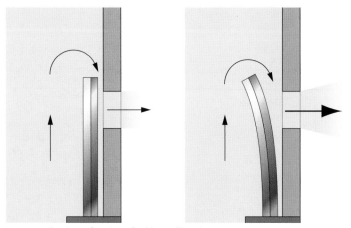

Fig. 2.17 Mechanism of action of a bimetallic strip.

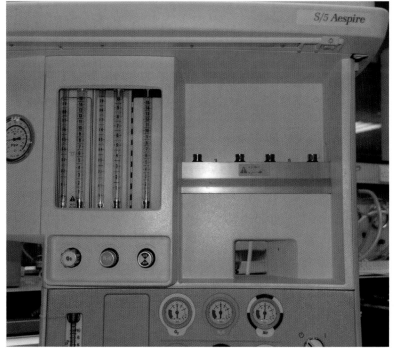

Fig. 2.18 An empty Selectatec back bar of an anaesthetic machine.

and high specific heat capacity with a very high thermal conductivity, e.g. copper. Copper acts as a heat sink, readily giving heat to the anaesthetic agent and maintaining its temperature

b) a temperature sensitive valve (e.g. bimetallic strip or bellows) within the body of the vaporizer automatically adjusts the splitting ratio according to the temperature. It allows more flow into the vaporizing chamber as the temperature decreases.

8. The amount of vapour carried by the FGF is a function of both the saturated vapour pressure of the agent and the atmospheric pressure. At high altitudes, the atmospheric pressure is reduced whereas the saturated vapour pressure remains the same. This leads to an increased amount of vapour whereas the saturation of the agent remains the same. The opposite occurs in hyperbaric chambers. This is of no clinical relevance as it is the partial pressure of the agent in the alveoli that determines the clinical effect of the agent.

Problems in practice and safety features

1. In modern vaporizers (Tec Mk 5), the liquid anaesthetic agent does not enter the bypass channel even if the vaporizer is tipped upside down due to an antispill mechanism. In earlier designs, dangerously high concentrations of anaesthetic agent could be delivered to the patient in cases of agent spillage into the bypass channel. Despite that, it is recommended that the vaporizer is purged with a fresh gas flow of 5 L/min for 30 min with the percentage control dial set at 5%.

2. The Selectatec system increases the potential for leaks. This is due

5. The desired concentration is obtained by adjusting the percentage control dial. This alters the amount of gas flowing through the bypass channel to that flowing through the vaporization chamber.

6. In the modern designs the vapour concentration supplied by the vaporizer is virtually independent of the fresh gas flows between 0.5 and 15 L/min.

7. During vaporization, cooling occurs due to the loss of latent heat of vaporization. Lowering the temperature of the agent makes it less volatile. In order to compensate for temperature changes:

a) the vaporizer is made of a material with high density

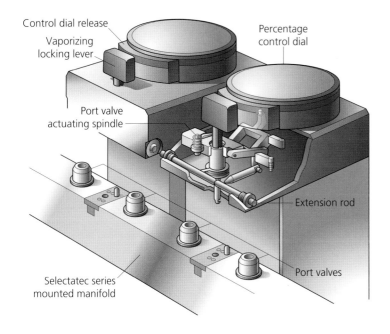

Fig. 2.19 The Selectatec vaporizer interlock mechanism. See text for details (reproduced with permission from Datex-Ohmeda).

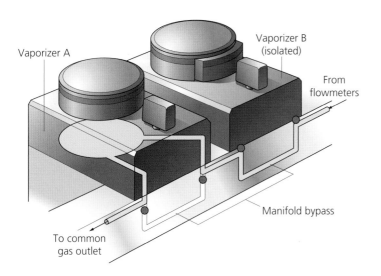

Fig. 2.20 The Selectatec series mounted manifold bypass circuit. Only when a vaporizer is locked in position and turned on can fresh gas enter. Vaporizer B is turned off and is isolated from the fresh gas which only enters vaporizer A which is turned on. If no vaporizer is fitted the port valves are closed (reproduced with permission from Datex-Ohmeda).

to the risk of accidental removal of the O-rings with changes of vaporizers.

3. Minute volume divider ventilators exert back pressure as they cycle. This pressure forces some of the gas exiting the outlet port back into the vaporizing chamber, where more vapour is added. Retrograde flow may also contaminate the bypass channel. These effects cause an increase in the inspired concentration of the agent which may be toxic. These pressure fluctuations can be compensated for by:
   a) long inlet port into the vaporizing chamber as in Tec Mk 3. This ensures that the bypass channel is not contaminated by retrograde flow from the vaporizing chamber;
   b) downstream flow restrictors are used to maintain the vaporizer at a pressure greater than any pressure required to operate commonly used ventilators;
   c) both the bypass channel and the vaporizing chamber are of equal volumes so gas expansion and compression are equal.

4. Preservatives, such as thymol in halothane, accumulate on the wicks of vaporizer with time. Large quantities may interfere with the function of the vaporizer. Thymol can also cause the bimetallic strip in the Tec Mk 2 to stick. Enflurane and isoflurane do not contain preservative.

5. A pressure relief valve downstream of the vaporizer opens at about 35 kPa. This prevents damage to flowmeters or vaporizers if the common gas outlet is blocked.

6. The bimetallic strip has been situated in the bypass channel since the Tec Mk 3. It is possible for the chemically active strip to corrode in a mixture of oxygen and the inhalational agent within the vaporizing chamber (Tec Mk 2).

Vaporizers

- The case is made of copper which is a good heat sink.
- Consists of a bypass channel and vaporization chamber. The latter has wicks to increase the surface area available for vaporization.
- A temperature-sensitive valve controls the splitting ratio. It is positioned outside the vaporizing chamber in Tec Mk 3, 4 and 5.
- The gas leaving the vaporizing chamber is fully saturated.
- The effect of back pressure is compensated for.

Vaporizer filling devices

These are agent specific being geometrically coded (keyed) to fit the safety filling port of the correct vaporizer and anaesthetic agent supply bottle (Fig. 2.21). They prevent the risk of adding the wrong agent to the wrong vaporizer and decrease the extent of spillage. The safety filling system, in addition, ensures that the vaporizer can not overflow. Fillers used for desflurane and sevoflurane have valves that are only opened when fully inserted into their ports. This prevents spillage.

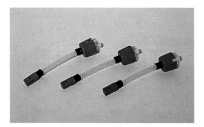

Fig. 2.21 Agent-specific, colour-coded, keyed filling devices.

The fillers are colour-coded:

Red	Halothane
Orange	Enflurane
Purple	Isoflurane
Yellow	Sevoflurane
Blue	Desflurane

A recent design feature is the antipollution cap allowing the filler to be left fitted to the bottle between uses to prevent the agent from vaporizing. It also eliminates air locks, speeding up vaporizer filling, and ensures that the bottle is completely emptied, reducing wastage.

Non-return pressure relief safety valve

This is situated downstream of the vaporizers either on the back bar itself or near the common gas outlet (Fig. 2.22).
1. Its non-return design helps to prevent back pressure effects commonly encountered using minute volume divider ventilators.

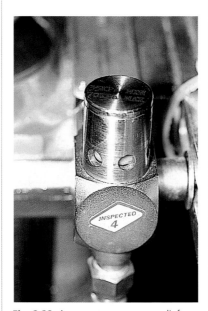

Fig. 2.22 A non-return pressure relief valve situated at the end of the back bar.

2. It opens when the pressure in the back bar exceeds about 35 kPa. Flowmeter and vaporizer components can be damaged at higher pressures.

Emergency oxygen flush

Usually activated by a non-locking button (Fig. 2.23). When pressed, pure oxygen is supplied from the outlet of the anaesthetic machine. The flow bypasses the flowmeters and the vaporizers. A flow of about 35–75 L/min at a pressure of about 400 kPa is expected.

Problems in practice and safety features

1. The high operating pressure and flow of the oxygen flush puts the patient at a higher risk of barotrauma.
2. When the emergency oxygen flush is used inappropriately, it leads to dilution of the

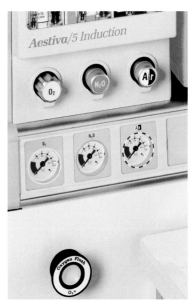

Fig. 2.23 The emergency oxygen flush button situated below the flowmeters.

anaesthetic gases and possible awareness.
3. It should not be activated while ventilating a patient using a minute volume divider ventilator.

Compressed oxygen outlet(s)

One or more compressed oxygen outlets used to provide oxygen at about 400 kPa (Fig. 2.24). It can be used to drive ventilators or a manually controlled jet injector.

Oxygen supply failure alarm

There are many designs available (Fig. 2.25) but the characteristics of the ideal warning device are:
1. Activation depends on the pressure of oxygen itself.
2. It requires no batteries or mains power.

3. It gives an audible signal of a special character and of sufficient duration and volume to attract attention.
4. It should give a warning of impending failure and a further alarm that failure has occurred.
5. It should have pressure-linked controls which interrupt the flow of all other gases when it comes into operation. Atmospheric air is allowed to be delivered to the patient, without carbon dioxide accumulation. It should be impossible to resume anaesthesia until the oxygen supply has been restored.
6. The alarm should be positioned on the reduced pressure side of the oxygen supply line.
7. It should be tamper proof.
8. It is not affected by back-pressure from the anaesthetic ventilator.

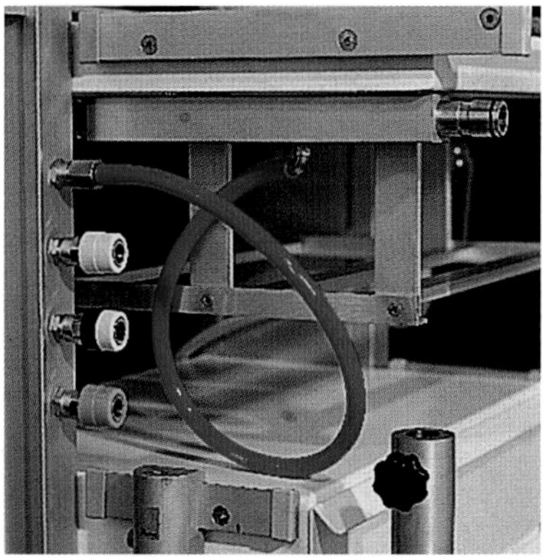

Anti-hypoxic safety features
These features are designed to prevent the delivery of gaseous mixtures with oxygen concentrations of less than 25%. This can be achieved by:

- *Mechanical means*: a chain links the oxygen and nitrous oxide flow control valves. Increasing the flow rate of nitrous oxide leads to a proportional increase in oxygen flow rate.
- *Pneumatic means*: a pressure sensitive diaphragm measuring the changes in oxygen and nitrous oxide concentrations.
- *A paramagnetic oxygen analyser* continuously measuring the oxygen concentration. Nitrous oxide flow is switched off automatically when oxygen concentration falls under 25%.

Other modifications and designs

1. Desflurane Tec Mk 6 vaporizer (Figs 2.26 and 2.27). Desflurane is an inhalational agent with a saturated vapour pressure of 664 mmHg at 20°C and a boiling point of 23.5°C at atmospheric pressure. In order to overcome these physical properties, Tec Mk 6 design is completely different from the previous Tec series despite the similar appearance. It is mounted on the Selectatec system.
   a) An electrically heated desflurane vaporization chamber (sump) with a capacity of 450 mL. The desflurane is heated to a temperature of 39°C with a pressure of 1550 mmHg (about two atmospheric pressures).
   b) A fixed restriction is positioned in the fresh gas flow path.

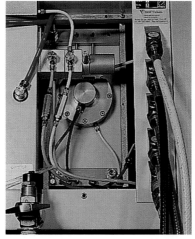

Fig. 2.24 The common gas outlet (red), compressed oxygen (white), compressed air (black and white) and medical vacuum (yellow) outlets on an anaesthetic machine.

Fig. 2.25 The oxygen supply failure alarm in the Datex-Ohmeda Flexima anaesthetic machine.

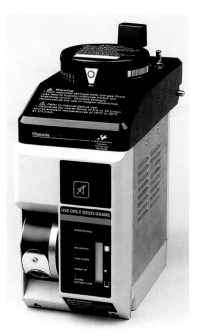

Fig. 2.26 The Tec Mk 6 vaporizer (reproduced with permission from Datex-Ohmeda).

c) A percentage control dial with a rotary valve controls the flow of desflurane vapour into the fresh gas flow. The dial calibration is from 0 to 18%

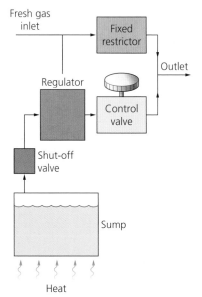

Fig. 2.27 A schematic diagram of the Tec Mk 6 vaporizer (reproduced with permission from Datex-Ohmeda).

with 1% graduation from 0 to 10%; and 2% graduation from 10 to 18%.

d) A differential pressure transducer adjusts a pressure regulating valve at the outlet of the vaporization chamber. The transducer senses pressure at the fixed restriction on one side and the pressure of desflurane vapour upstream to the pressure-regulating valve on the other side. This transducer ensures that the pressure of desflurane vapour upstream of the control valve equals the pressure of fresh gas flow at the fixed restriction.

e) The fresh gas flow does not enter the vaporization chamber. The vaporizer does not operate until the temperature of vaporization chamber has reached 39°C. A period of 5 to 10 minutes warm-up time is required to reach operating temperature.

f) The vaporizer incorporates malfunction alarms (auditory and visual). There is a back-up 9 volt battery should there be a mains failure.

g) A rotating filling port in the front of the vaporizer.

2. Since most of the anaesthetic machine is made from metal, it should not be used close to an MRI scanner. Distorted readings and physical damage to the scanner are possible, because of the attraction of the strong magnetic fields. Newly designed anaesthetic machines made of totally non-ferrous material solve this problem (Fig. 2.28).

3. Newly designed anaesthetic machines are more sophisticated than that described above. Many important components have become electrically or electronically controlled as an integrated system. Thermistors can be used to measure the flow of gases. Gas flow causes changes in temperature which are measured by the thermistors. Changes in temperature are calibrated to measure flows of gases.

4. Quantiflex Anaesthetic Machine (Fig. 2.29). This machine has the following features:
   a) Two flowmeters, one for oxygen and one for nitrous oxide, with one control knob for both flowmeters.

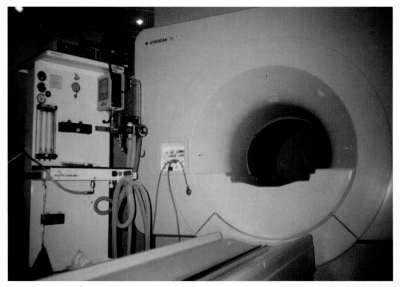

Fig. 2.28 A non-ferrous MRI compatible anaesthetic machine.

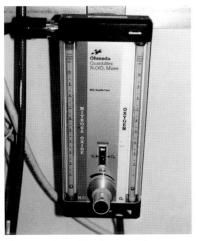

Fig. 2.29 Quantiflex Anaesthetic Machine.

b) The oxygen flowmeter is situated to the right, whereas the nitrous oxide flowmeter is situated to the left.

c) The relative concentrations of oxygen and nitrous oxide are adjusted by a mixture control wheel. The oxygen concentration can be adjusted in 10% steps from 30% to 100%.

d) This design prevents the delivery of hypoxic mixtures.

e) It is mainly used in dental anaesthesia.

Some newly designed anaesthetic machines have an extra outlet with its own flowmeter to deliver oxygen to conscious or lightly sedated patients via a face mask. This can be used in patients undergoing surgery under regional anaesthesia with sedation.

Anaesthesia in remote areas

The apparatus used must be compact, portable and robust. The Triservice apparatus is suitable for use in remote areas where supply of compressed gases and vapours is difficult (Figs 2.30 and 2.31).

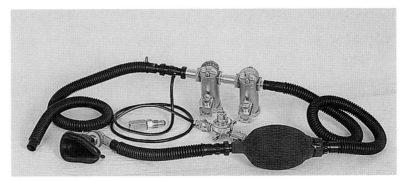

Fig. 2.30 The Triservice apparatus.

Components

1. A face mask with a non-rebreathing valve fitted.
2. A short length of tubing leading to a self-inflating bag.
3. A second length of tubing leading from the self-inflating bag to two Oxford Miniature Vaporizers (OMV).
4. An oxygen cylinder can be connected upstream of the vaporizers. A third length of tubing acts as an oxygen reservoir during expiration.

Mechanism of action

1. The Triservice apparatus can be used for both spontaneous and controlled ventilation.
   a) The patient can draw air through the vaporizers. The exhaled gases are vented out via the non-rebreathing valve.
   b) The self-inflating bag can be used for controlled or assisted ventilation.
2. The Oxford Miniature Vaporizer is a draw-over vaporizer with a capacity for 50 mL of anaesthetic

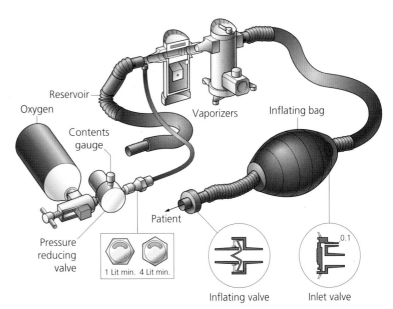

Fig. 2.31 Mechanism of action of the Triservice apparatus.

agent. The wick is made of metal with no temperature compensation features. There is an ethylene glycol jacket acting as a heat sink to help to stabilize the vaporizer temperature. The calibration scale on the vaporizer can be detached allowing the use of different inhalational agents. A different inhalational agent can be used after blowing air for 10 minutes and rinsing the wicks with the new agent. The vaporizer casing has extendable feet fitted.

3. The downstream vaporizer is traditionally filled with trichloroethylene to compensate for the absence of the analgesic effect of nitrous oxide.

Problems in practice and safety features

1. The vaporizers' heat sink (ethylene glycol jacket) is not suitable for prolonged use at high gas flows. The vapour concentration decreases as the temperature decreases.
2. During use, accidental tipping of the vaporizer can spill liquid agent into the breathing system. The vaporizer is spillproof when turned off.

Triservice apparatus

- Consists of two OMVs, self-inflating bag and non-rebreathing valve.
- The apparatus is suitable for both spontaneous and controlled breathing.
- OMV is a draw-over vaporizer with no temperature compensation. It has a heat sink. It can be used with different inhalational agents.

FURTHER READING

Ehrenwerth J, Eisenkraft JB. Anesthesia Equipment, Principles and Applications, 1st edn. St Louis: Mosby-Year Book, 1993.

MCQs

In the following lists, which of the following statements (a) to (e) are true?

1. Flowmeters in an anaesthetic machine
   a) N_2O may be used in an O_2 flowmeter without a change in calibration.
   b) Flowmeters use a tube and bobbin.
   c) They are example of a variable orifice device.
   d) They have a linear scale.
   e) Both laminar and turbulent flows are encountered.

2. Vaporizers
   a) Manual ventilation using a VIC (vaporizer in circle) causes a reduction in the inspired concentration of the inhalational agent.
   b) A Tec Mark 3 vaporizer can be used as a VIC.
   c) Gas flow emerging from the vaporizing chamber should be fully saturated with the inhalational agent.
   d) The bimetallic strip valve in Tec Mark 5 is in the vaporizing chamber.
   e) The inhalational agent concentration delivered to the patient gradually decreases the longer the vaporizer is used due to cooling of the agent.

3. Pressure gauges on an anaesthetic machine
   a) Use the Bourdon pressure gauge principle.
   b) The pressure reflects accurately the cylinders' contents for both oxygen and nitrous oxide.
   c) Can be interchangeable between oxygen and nitrous oxide.
   d) The same pressure gauge can be used for both cylinder and pipeline gas supply.
   e) They are colour-coded for a particular gas or vapour.

4. Laminar flow
   a) It is directly proportional to the square root of pressure.
   b) Halving the radius results in a flow equivalent to a 16th of the original laminar flow.
   c) It is related to the density of the fluid.
   d) The flow is greatest in the centre.
   e) Laminar flow changes to turbulent when Reynold's number exceeds 2000.

5. Flowmeters on an anaesthetic machine
   a) They have an accuracy of ± 2.5%.
   b) They have a tapered tube with a narrow top.
   c) Oxygen is the first gas to be added to the mixture at the back bar.
   d) At high flows, the density of the gas is important in measuring the flow.
   e) The reading of the flow is from the top of the bobbin.

6. Concerning the Triservice apparatus
   a) Two plenum vaporizers are used.
   b) It can be used for both spontaneous and controlled ventilation.
   c) An inflating bag and a one-way valve are used.
   d) The Oxford Miniature Vaporizer has a metal wick and a heat sink.
   e) Supplementary oxygen can be added to the system.

7. Pressure regulators
   a) They are only used to reduce pressure of gases.
   b) They maintain a gas flow at a constant pressure of about 400 kPa.
   c) Their main purpose is to protect the patient.
   d) Relief valves open at 700 kPa in case of failure.
   e) Flow restrictors can additionally be used in pipeline supply.

8. The safety features found in an anaesthetic machine include
   a) Oxygen supply failure alarm.
   b) Colour-coded flowmeters.
   c) Vaporizer level alarm.
   d) Ventilator disconnection alarm.
   e) Two vaporizers can be safely used at the same time.

9. The non-return valve on the
   back bar of an anaesthetic
   machine between the vaporizer
   and common gas outlet
   a) Decreases the pumping effect.
   b) Often is incorporated with
      a pressure relief valve on
      modern machines.
   c) Is designed to protect the
      patient.
   d) Is designed to protect the
      machine.
   e) Opens at a pressure of
      70 kPa.

10. The oxygen emergency flush on
    an anaesthetic machine
    a) Operates at 20 L/min.
    b) Is always safe to use during
       anaesthesia.
    c) Operates at 40 L/min.
    d) Increases risk of awareness
       during anaesthesia.
    e) Can be safely used with
       a minute volume divider
       ventilator.

Answers

1. Flowmeters in an anaesthetic machine
   a) *False*. *The flowmeters in an anaesthetic machine are calibrated for the particular gas(es) used taking into consideration the viscosity and density of the gas(es). N_2O and O_2 have different viscosities and densities so unless the flowmeters are re-calibrated, false readings will result.*
   b) *True*. *They are constant pressure, variable orifice flowmeters. A tapered transparent tube with a lightweight rotating bobbin. The bobbin is held floating in the tube by the gas flow. The clearance between the bobbin and the tube wall widens as the flow increases. The pressure across the bobbin remains constant as the effect of gravity on the bobbin is countered by the gas flow.*
   c) *True*. *See above.*
   d) *False*. *The flowmeters do not have a linear scale. There are different scales for low and high flow rates.*
   e) *True*. *At low flows, the flowmeter acts as a tube, as the clearance between the bobbin and the wall of the tube is longer and narrower. This leads to laminar flow which is dependent on the viscosity (Poiseuille's law). At high flows, the flowmeter acts as an orifice. The clearance is shorter and wider. This leads to turbulent flow which is dependent on density.*

2. Vaporizers
   a) *False*. *During manual (or controlled) ventilation using a VIC vaporizer, the inspired concentration of the inhalational agent is increased. It can increase to dangerous concentrations. Unless the concentration of the inhalational agent(s) is measured continuously, this technique is not recommended.*
   b) *False*. *As the patient is breathing through a VIC vaporizer, it should have very low internal resistance. The Tec Mark 3 has a high internal resistance because of the wicks in the vaporizing chamber.*
   c) *True*. *This can be achieved by increasing the surface area of contact between the carrier gas and the anaesthetic agent. Full saturation should be achieved despite changes in fresh gas flow. The final concentration is delivered to the patient after mixing with the fresh gas flow from the bypass channel.*
   d) *False*. *The bimetallic strip valve in the Tec Mk 5 is in the bypass chamber. The bimetallic strip has been positioned in the bypass chamber since the Tec Mk 3. This was done to avoid corrosion of the strip in a mixture of oxygen and inhalational agent when positioned in the vaporizing chamber.*

   e) *False*. *The concentration delivered to the patient stays constant because of temperature compensating mechanisms. This can be achieved by:*
      • *using a material with high density and high specific thermal conductivity (e.g. copper) which acts as a heat sink readily giving heat to the agent and maintaining its temperature*
      • *a temperature-sensitive valve within the vaporizer which automatically adjusts the splitting ratio according to the temperature, so if the temperature decreases due to loss of latent heat of vaporization, it allows more flow into the vaporizing chamber.*

3. Pressure gauges on an anaesthetic machine
   a) *True. A pressure gauge consists of a coiled tube that is subjected to pressure from the inside. The high pressure gas causes the tube to uncoil. The movement of the tube causes a needle pointer to move on a calibrated dial indicating the pressure.*
   b) *False. Oxygen is stored as a gas in the cylinder hence it obeys the gas laws. The pressure changes in an oxygen cylinder accurately reflect the contents. Nitrous oxide is stored as a liquid and vapour so it does not obey Boyle's gas law. This means that the pressure changes in a nitrous oxide cylinder do not reflect accurately the contents of the cylinder.*
   c) *False. The pressure gauges are calibrated for a particular gas or vapour. Oxygen and nitrous oxide pressure gauges are not interchangeable.*
   d) *False. Cylinders are kept under much higher pressures (13 700 kPa for oxygen and 5400 kPa for nitrous oxide) than the pipeline gas supply (about 400 kPa). Using the same pressure gauges for both cylinders and pipeline gas supply can lead to inaccuracies and/or damage to pressure gauges.*
   e) *True. Colour-coding is one of the safety features used in the use and delivery of gases in medical practice. In the UK, white is for oxygen, blue for nitrous oxide and black for medical air.*

4. Laminar flow
   a) *False. Laminar flow is directly proportional to pressure. Hagen–Poiseuille equation: Flow ∝ pressure × radius⁴/viscosity × length*
   b) *True. From the above equation, the flow ∝ radius⁴.*
   c) *False. Laminar flow is related to viscosity. Turbulent flow is related to density.*
   d) *True. Laminar flow is greatest in the centre at about twice the mean flow rate. The flow is slower nearer to the wall of the tube. At the wall the flow is almost zero.*
   e) *True. Reynold's number is the index used to predict the type of flow, laminar or turbulent. Reynold's number = velocity of fluid × density × radius of tube/viscosity. In laminar flow, Reynold's number is <2000. In turbulent flow, Reynold's number is >2000.*

5. Flowmeters on an anaesthetic machine
   a) *True. The flowmeters on the anaesthetic machine are very accurate with an accuracy of ± 2.5%.*
   b) *False. The flowmeters on an anaesthetic machine are tapered tubes. The top is wider than the bottom.*
   c) *False. Oxygen is the last gas to be added to the mixture at the back bar. This is a safety feature in the design of the anaesthetic machine. If there is a crack in a flowmeter, a hypoxic mixture may result if oxygen is added first to the mixture.*
   d) *True. At high flows, the flow is turbulent which is dependent on density. At low flows, the flow is laminar which is dependent on viscosity.*

   e) *True. When a ball is used, the reading is taken from the midpoint.*

6. Concerning the Triservice apparatus
   a) *False. In the Triservice apparatus, two Oxford Miniature, draw-over, Vaporizers (OMV) are used. Plenum vaporizers are not used due to their high internal resistance. The OMV is light weight and by changing its calibration scale, different inhalational agents can be used easily.*
   b) *True. The system allows both spontaneous and controlled ventilation. The resistance to breathing is low allowing spontaneous ventilation. The self-inflating bag provides the means to control ventilation.*
   c) *True. As above.*
   d) *True. The OMV has a metal wick to increase area of vaporization within the vaporization chamber. The heat sink consists of an ethylene glycol jacket to stabilize the vaporizer temperature.*
   e) *True. Supplementary oxygen can be added to the system from an oxygen cylinder. The oxygen is added to the reservoir proximal to the vaporizer(s).*

7. Pressure regulators
   a) *False. Pressure regulators are used to reduce pressure of gases and also to maintain a constant flow. In the absence of pressure regulators, the flowmeters need to be adjusted regularly to maintain constant flows as the contents of the cylinders are used up. The temperature and pressure of the cylinder contents decrease with use.*
   b) *True. Pressure regulators are designed to maintain a gas flow at a constant pressure of about 400 kPa irrespective of the pressure and temperature of the contents of the cylinder.*
   c) *False. Pressure regulators offer no protection to the patient. Their main function is to protect the anaesthetic machine from the high pressure of the cylinder and to maintain a constant flow of gas.*
   d) *True. In situations where the pressure regulator fails, a relief valve that opens at 700 kPa prevents the build up of excessive pressure.*
   e) *True. Flow restrictors can be used in a pipeline supply. They are designed to protect the anaesthetic machine from pressure surges in the system. They consist of a constriction between the pipeline supply and the anaesthetic machine.*

8. The safety features found in an anaesthetic machine include
   a) *True. This is an essential safety feature in the anaesthetic machine. The ideal design should operate under the pressure of oxygen itself, give a characteristic audible signal, be capable of warning of impending failure and give a further alarm when failure has occurred, be capable of interrupting the flow of other gases and not require batteries or mains power to operate.*
   b) *True. The flowmeters are colour-coded and also the shape and size of the oxygen flowmeter knob is different from the nitrous oxide knob. This allows the identification of the oxygen knob even in a dark environment.*
   c) *False. The vaporizer level can be monitored by the anaesthetist. This is part of the anaesthetic machine checklist. There is no alarm system.*
   d) *True. A ventilator disconnection alarm is essential when a ventilator is used. They are also used to monitor leaks, obstruction and malfunction. They can be pressure and/or volume monitoring alarms. In addition, clinical observation, end-tidal carbon dioxide concentration and airway pressure are also 'disconnection alarms'.*
   e) *False. Only one vaporizer can be used at any one time. This is due to the interlocking Selectatec system where interlocking extension rods prevent more than one vaporizer being used at any one time. These rods prevent the percentage control dial from moving,* *preventing contamination of the downstream vaporizer.*

9. The non-return valve on the back bar of an anaesthetic machine between the vaporizer and common gas outlet
   a) *True. Minute volume divider ventilators exert back pressure as they cycle. This causes reversal of the fresh gas flow through the vaporizer. This leads to an uncontrolled increase in the concentration of the inhalational agent. Also the back pressure causes the fluctuation of the bobbins in the flowmeters as the ventilator cycles. The non-return valve on the back bar prevents these events from happening.*
   b) *True. The non-return valve on the back bar opens when the pressure in the back bar exceeds 35 kPa. Flowmeters and vaporizer components can be damaged at higher pressures.*
   c) *True. By preventing the effects of back pressure on the flowmeters and vaporizer as the minute volume divider ventilator cycles, the non-return valve on the back bar provides some protection to the patient. The flows on the flowmeters and the desired concentration of the inhalational agent can be accurately delivered to the patient.*
   d) *True. See 'b'.*
   e) *False. The non-return valve on the back bar of the anaesthetic machine opens at pressure of 35 kPa.*

10. The oxygen emergency flush on an anaesthetic machine

a) *False. 35–75 L/min can be delivered by activating the oxygen emergency flush on the anaesthetic machine.*

b) *False. The inappropriate use of the oxygen flush during anaesthesia increases risk of awareness (a 100% oxygen can be delivered) and barotrauma to the patient (because of the high flows delivered).*

c) *True. See 'a'.*

d) *True. This can happen by diluting the anaesthetic mixture; see 'b'.*

e) *False. Because of the high FGF (35–70 L/min), the minute volume divider ventilator does not function appropriately.*

Chapter 3

Pollution in theatre and scavenging

Since the late 1960s there has been speculation that trace anaesthetic gases/vapours may have a harmful effect on operating theatre personnel. It has been concluded from currently available studies that there is no association between occupational exposure to trace levels of waste anaesthetic vapours in scavenged operating theatres and adverse health effects. However, it is desirable to vent out the exhaled anaesthetic vapours and maintain a vapour-free theatre environment. A prudent plan for minimizing exposure includes maintenance of equipment, training of personnel and routine exposure monitoring.

Although not universally agreed upon, the recommended maximum accepted concentrations in the UK (issued in 1996), over an (see Table 3.1 for main causes) 8-hour, time-weighted average, are as follows:

- 100 particles per million (ppm) for nitrous oxide
- 50 ppm for enflurane
- 50 ppm for isoflurane
- 10 ppm for halothane.

These levels were chosen because they are well below the levels at which any significant adverse effects occurred in animals and represent levels at which there is no evidence to suggest human health would be affected.

In the United States, the maximum accepted concentrations of any halogenated agent should be less than 2 ppm. When such agents are used in combination with nitrous oxide, levels of less than 0.5 ppm should be achieved. Nitrous oxide, when used as the sole anaesthetic agent, at 8-hour time-weighted average concentrations should be less than 25 ppm during the administration of an anaesthetic.

Holland has a limit of 25 ppm for nitrous oxide, whereas Italy, Sweden, Norway and Denmark set 100 ppm as their limit for exposure to nitrous oxide. The differences illustrate

Table 3.1 Causes of operating theatre pollution

	Causes of operating theatre pollution
Anaesthetic techniques	Incomplete scavenging of the gases from ventilator and/or APL valve Poorly fitting face mask Paediatric breathing systems, e.g. T-piece Failure to turn off fresh gas and/or vaporizer at the end of an anaesthetic Uncuffed tracheal tubes Filling of the vaporizers Exhalation of the gases/vapours during recovery
Anaesthetic machine	Leaks from the various connections used, e.g. 'O' rings, soda lime canister
Others	Cryosurgery units and cardio-pulmonary bypass circuit if a vapour is used

the difficulty in setting standards without adequate data.

Methods used to decrease theatre pollution are listed below.

1. Adequate theatre ventilation and air conditioning, with frequent and rapid changing of the circulating air (15–20 times per hour). This is one of the most important factors in reducing pollution. Theatres that are unventilated are four times as contaminated with anaesthetic gases and vapours compared to those with proper ventilation. A non-recirculating ventilation system is usually used. A recirculating ventilation system is not recommended. In labour wards, where anaesthetic agents including Entonox are used, rooms should be well ventilated with a minimum of 5 air changes per hour.
2. Use of the circle breathing system.
3. Total intravenous anaesthesia.
4. Regional anaesthesia.
5. Avoiding spillage and using fume cupboards during vaporizer filling.
6. Scavenging.

Sampling procedures for evaluating waste anaesthetic vapour concentrations in air should be

conducted for nitrous oxide and halogenated agents on a yearly basis in the UK and on a quarterly basis in the USA in each location where anaesthesia is administered. Monitoring should include:

a) Leak testing of equipment.
b) Sampling air in the theatre personnel breathing zone.

Anaesthetic equipment, gas scavenging, gas supply, flowmeters and ventilation systems must be subject to a *planned preventative maintenance (PPM) programme*. At least once annually, the general ventilation system and the scavenging equipment should be examined and tested by a responsible person.

Pollution in the operating theatre

- In scavenged areas, there is no association between occupational exposure to anaesthetic agents trace levels and adverse health effects.
- There are no agreed international standards of the maximum accepted concentrations of agents in the theatre environment.
- Routine monitoring and testing (PPM) are mandatory.

Scavenging

In any location which inhalation anaesthetics are administered, there should be an adequate and reliable system for scavenging waste anaesthetic gases. A scavenging system is capable of collecting the waste anaesthetic gases from the breathing system and discarding them safely. Un-scavenged operating theatres can show N_2O levels of 400–3000 ppm.

> The ideal scavenging system
> * Should not affect the ventilation and oxygenation of the patient.
> * Should not affect the dynamics of the breathing system.

A well-designed scavenging system should consist of a collecting device for gases from the breathing system/ventilator at the site of overflow, a ventilation system to carry waste anaesthetic gases from the operating theatre, and a method for limiting both positive and negative pressure variations in the breathing system.

The performance of the scavenging system should be part of the anaesthetic machine check.

Scavenging systems can be divided into passive and active systems.

PASSIVE SYSTEM

The passive system is simple to construct with zero running cost.

Components

1. The collecting and transfer system which consists of a shroud connected to the APL valve (or expiratory valve of the ventilator). A 30 mm connector attached to transfer tubing leads to a receiving system (Fig. 3.1).

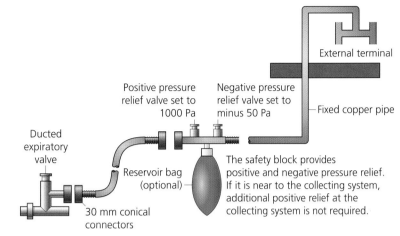

Fig. 3.1 Diagram of a passive scavenging system (reproduced with permission from Aitkenhead R, Smith G. Textbook of Anaesthesia, 3rd edn. Churchill Livingstone, 1996).

2. A receiving system (reservoir bag) can be used. Two spring-loaded valves guard against excessive positive (1000 Pa) or negative (–50 Pa) pressures in the scavenging system.
3. The disposal system is a wide bore copper pipe leading to the atmosphere directly or via the theatre ventilation system.

Mechanism of action

1. The exhaled gases are driven by either the patient's respiratory efforts or the ventilator.
2. The receiving system should be mounted on the anaesthetic machine to minimize the length of transfer tubing.

Problems in practice and safety features

1. Connecting the scavenging system to the exit grille of the theatre ventilation is possible. Recirculation or reversing of the flow is a problem in this situation.
2. Excess positive or negative pressures caused by the wind at the outlet might affect the performance and even reverse the flow.
3. The outlet should be fitted with a wire mesh to protect against insects.
4. Compressing or occluding the passive hose may lead to the escape of gases/vapours into the operating theatre so polluting it. The disposal hose should be made of non-compressible materials and not placed on the floor.

ACTIVE SYSTEM

Components

1. The collecting and transfer system which is similar to that of the passive system (Fig. 3.2).
2. The receiving system (Fig 3.3). A bacterial filter situated downstream and a visual flow indicator positioned between the receiving and disposal systems can be used. A reservoir bag with two spring-loaded safety valves can also be used as a receiving system.
3. The active disposal system consists of a fan or a pump used to generate a vacuum (Fig. 3.4).

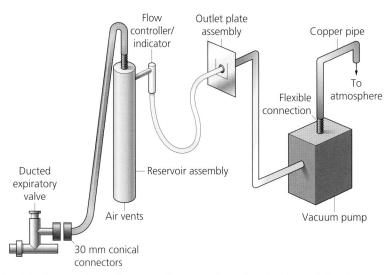

Fig. 3.2 Diagram of an active scavenging system (reproduced with permission from Aitkenhead R, Smith G. Textbook of Anaesthesia, 3rd edn. Churchill Livingstone, 1996).

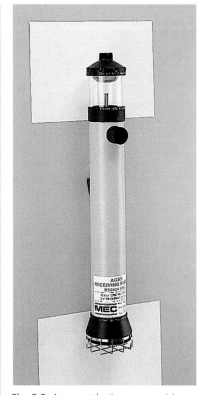

Fig. 3.3 An anaesthetic gases receiving system.

Mechanism of action

1. The vacuum drives the gases through the system. Active scavenging systems are able to deal with a wide range of expiratory flow rates (30–130 L/min).
2. A motorized fan, a pump or a Venturi system is used to generate the vacuum or negative pressure that is transmitted through pipes.
3. The receiving system is capable of coping with changes in gas flow rates. As a result, a uniform gas flow is passed to the disposal system.

Problems in practice and safety features

1. The reservoir is designed to prevent excessive negative or positive pressures being applied to the patient. Excessive negative pressure leads to the collapse of the reservoir bag of the breathing system and the risk of rebreathing. Excessive positive pressure increases the risk of barotrauma should there be an obstruction beyond the receiving system.
2. An independent vacuum pump should be used for scavenging purposes.

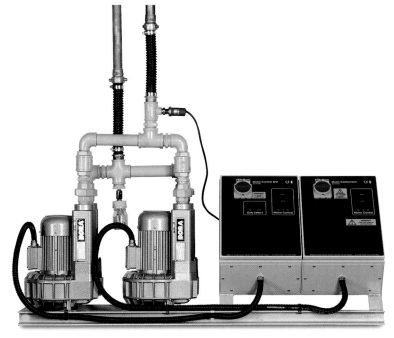

Fig. 3.4 Anaesthetic gases scavenging system (AGSS) vacuum pumps used in an active scavenging system.

Scavenging

- Active or passive systems.
- Consists of a collecting and transfer system, a receiving system and a disposal system.
- Both excessive positive and negative pressure variations in the system are limited.
- Other methods used to reduce theatre pollution: theatre ventilation, circle system, total intravenous and regional anaesthesia.

Cardiff Aldasorber

The Aldasorber is a compact passive scavenging system (Fig. 3.5).

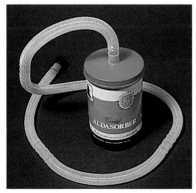

Fig. 3.5 The Cardiff Aldasorber.

Components

1. A canister.
2. Charcoal particles.
3. Transfer tubing connecting the canister to the APL valve of the breathing system or the expiratory valve of the ventilator.

Mechanism of action

1. The charcoal particles absorb the halogenated inhalational agents (halothane, enflurane and isoflurane).
2. The increasing weight of the canister is the only indication that it is exhausted.

Problems in practice and safety features

1. It cannot absorb nitrous oxide.
2. Heating the canister causes the release of the inhalational agents.

Cardiff Aldasorber

- A canister with charcoal granules used to absorb halogenated agents.
- Does not absorb nitrous oxide.
- Its weight indicates the degree of exhaustion.
- When heated, the agents escape back into the atmosphere.

FURTHER READING

Advice on the implementation of the Health and Safety Commission's occupational exposure standards for anaesthetic agents. London: Department of Health, 1996.

Al-Shaikh B. Pollution in theatre and scavenging. CPD Anaesthesia 2003;5(3):137–140.

Anaesthetic Agents: Controlling Exposure Under the Control of Substances Hazardous to Health Regulations (COSHH). London: Health Service Advisory Committee, 1996.

Guidelines for Construction and Equipment of Hospitals and Medical Facilities. Washington, DC: American Institute Architects, 1992.

MCQs

In the following lists, which of the statements (a) to (e) are true?

1. Pollution in theatre
   a) The Cardiff Aldasorber can absorb N_2O and the inhalational agents.
   b) The circulating air in theatre should be changed 15–20 times per hour.
   c) In the scavenging system, excessive positive and negative pressures should be prevented from being applied to the patient.
   d) In the active scavenging system, an ordinary vacuum pump can be utilized.
   e) The maximum accepted concentration of nitrous oxide is 100 ppm.

2. Important factors in reducing pollution in the operating theatre
   a) Scavenging.
   b) Low flow anaesthesia using the circle system.
   c) Adequate theatre ventilation.
   d) The use of fume cupboards when filling vaporizers.
   e) Cardiff Aldasorber.

3. Passive scavenging system
   a) Is easy to build and maintain.
   b) Is efficient.
   c) There is no need to have positive or negative relief valves in the collecting system.
   d) The exhaled gases are driven by the patient's respiratory effort or the ventilator.
   e) Commonly uses 15 mm connectors in the United Kingdom.

4. Concerning anaesthetic agents pollution
   a) There is an international standard for the concentrations of trace inhalational agents in the operating theatre environment.
   b) In the UK, monitoring of inhalational agents concentration in the operating theatre is done annually.
   c) PPM stands for *particles per million*.
   d) An un-scavenged operating theatre would have less than 100 particles per million of nitrous oxide.
   e) A T-piece paediatric breathing system can cause theatre pollution.

Answers

1. Pollution in theatre
   a) *False. Cardiff Aldasorber can only absorb the inhalational agents but not nitrous oxide. This limits its use in reducing pollution in the operating theatre.*
   b) *True. Changing the circulating air in the operating theatre 15–20 times per hour is one of the most effective methods of reducing pollution. An unventilated theatre is about four times more polluted compared to a properly ventilated one.*
   c) *True. The patient should be protected against excessive positive and negative pressures being applied by the scavenging system. Excessive positive pressure puts the patient under the risk of barotrauma. Excessive negative pressure causes the reservoir in the breathing system to collapse thus leading to incorrect performance of the breathing system.*

   d) *False. Because of the nature of the flow of the exhaled gases, the scavenging system should be capable of tolerating high and variable gas flows. The flow of exhaled gases is very variable during both spontaneous and controlled ventilation. An ordinary vacuum pump might not be capable of coping with such variable flows, from 30 to 120 L/min. The active scavenging system is a high flow, low pressure system. A pressure of −0.5 cmH$_2$O to the patient breathing system is needed. This can not be achieved with an ordinary vacuum pump (low flow, high pressure system).*
   e) *True. In the UK, the maximum accepted concentration of nitrous oxide is 100 ppm over an 8-hour time-weighted average.*

2. Important factors in reducing pollution in the operating theatre
   a) *True. In any location in which inhalation anaesthetics are administered, there should be an adequate and reliable system for scavenging waste anaesthetic gases. Un-scavenged operating theatres can show 400–3000 ppm of N$_2$O, which is much higher than the maximum acceptable concentration.*
   b) *True.*
   c) *True. One of the most important factors in reducing pollution is adequate theatre ventilation. The circulating air is changed 15–20 times per hour. Unventilated theatres are four times more contaminated than properly ventilated theatres.*
   d) *False. Modern vaporizers use agent-specific filling keys which limit spillage.*
   e) *False. Cardiff Aldasorber absorbs the inhalational agents but not nitrous oxide.*

3. Passive scavenging system
   a) *True*. A passive scavenging system is easy and cheap to build and costs nothing to maintain. There is no need for a purpose-built vacuum pump system with the necessary maintenance required.
   b) *False*. The passive system is not an efficient system. Its efficiency depends on the direction of the wind blowing at the outlet. Negative or positive pressure might affect the performance and even reverse the flow.
   c) *False*. The positive pressure relief valve protects the patient against excessive pressure build up in the breathing system and barotrauma. The negative pressure relief valve prevents the breathing system reservoir from being exhausted, ensuring correct performance of the breathing system.
   d) *True*. The driving forces for gases in the passive system are the patient's respiratory effort or the ventilator. For this reason the transfer tubing should be made as short as possible to reduce resistance to flow.
   e) *False*. 30 mm connectors are used in the UK as a safety feature to prevent misconnection.

4. Concerning anaesthetic agents pollution
   a) *False*. There is not an international standard for the concentrations of trace inhalational agents in the operating theatre environment. This is mainly because of unavailability of adequate data. Different countries set their own standards but there is an agreement on the importance of maintaining a vapour-free environment in the operating theatre.
   b) *True*. Monitoring of inhalational agents concentration in the operating theatre is done annually in the UK and on a quarterly basis in the USA in each location where anaesthesia is administered.
   c) *False*. PPM (capitals) stands for planned preventative maintenance, whereas ppm (small letters) stands for particles per million.
   d) *False*. An un-scavenged operating theatre would have 400–3000 particles per million of nitrous oxide. In the UK, the recommended maximum accepted concentration over an 8-hour time-weighted average is 100 ppm of nitrous oxide.
   e) *True*. A T-piece paediatric breathing system can cause theatre pollution because of the open-ended reservoir. A modified version has an APL valve allowing scavenging of the anaesthetic vapours (see Chapter 4).

Chapter 4

Breathing systems

There are several breathing systems used in anaesthesia. Mapleson classified them into A, B, C, D and E. After further revision of the classification, a Mapleson F breathing system was added (Fig. 4.1). Currently only systems A, D, E and F and their modifications are commonly used during anaesthesia. Mapleson B and C systems are used more frequently during the recovery period and in emergency situations.

The fresh gas flow rate required to prevent rebreathing of alveolar gas is a measure of the efficiency of a breathing system.

Properties of the ideal breathing system

1. Simple and safe to use.
2. Delivers the intended inspired gas mixture.
3. Permits spontaneous, manual and controlled ventilation in all age groups.
4. Efficient, requiring low fresh gas flow rates.
5. Protects the patient from barotrauma.
6. Sturdy, compact and lightweight in design.
7. Permits the easy removal of waste exhaled gases.
8. Easy to maintain with minimal running costs.

Components of the breathing systems

ADJUSTABLE PRESSURE LIMITING (APL) VALVE

A valve which allows the exhaled gases and excess fresh gas flow to leave the breathing system (Fig. 4.2).

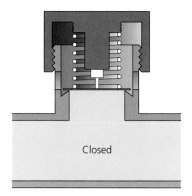

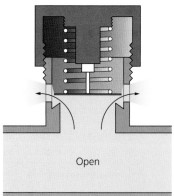

Fig. 4.2 Diagram of an adjustable pressure-limiting (APL) valve (reproduced with permission from Aitkenhead R, Smith G. Textbook of Anaesthesia, 3rd edn. Churchill Livingstone, 1996).

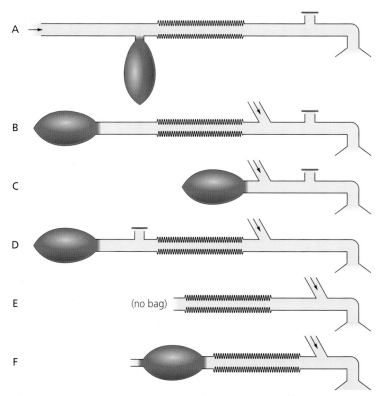

Fig. 4.1 Mapleson classification of anaesthetic breathing systems. The arrow indicates entry of fresh gas to the system (reproduced with permission from Aitkenhead R, Smith G. Textbook of Anaesthesia, 3rd edn. Churchill Livingstone, 1996).

It does not allow room air to enter the breathing system. Synonymous terms for the APL valve are expiratory valve, spill valve and relief valve.

Components

1. Three ports: the inlet, the patient and the exhaust ports. The latter can be open to the atmosphere or connected to the scavenging system using a shroud.
2. A lightweight disc rests on a knife-edge seating. The disc is held onto its seating by a spring. The tension in the spring, and therefore the valve's opening pressure, are controlled by the valve dial.

Mechanism of action

1. This is a one-way, adjustable, spring-loaded valve. The spring is used to adjust the pressure required to open the valve. The disc rests on a knife-edge seating in order to minimize its area of contact.
2. The valve allows gases to escape when the pressure in the breathing system exceeds the valve's opening pressure.
3. During spontaneous ventilation, the patient generates a positive pressure in the system during expiration, causing the valve to open. A pressure of less than $1 cmH_2O$ (0.1 kPa) is needed to actuate the valve when it is in the open position.
4. During positive pressure ventilation, a controlled leak is produced by adjusting the valve dial during inspiration. This allows control of the patient's airway pressure.

Problems in practice and safety features

1. Malfunction of the scavenging system may cause excessive negative pressure. This can lead to the APL valve remaining open throughout respiration. This leads to an unwanted enormous increase in the breathing system's dead space.
2. The patient may be exposed to excessive positive pressure if the valve is closed during assisted ventilation. A pressure relief safety mechanism actuated at a pressure of about $60 cmH_2O$ is present in some designs (Fig. 4.3).
3. Water vapour in exhaled gas may condense on the valve. The surface tension of the condensed water may cause the valve to stick. The disc is usually made of a hydrophobic (water repelling) material, which prevents water condensing on the disc.

Adjustable pressure limiting valve (APL)

- One-way spring-loaded valve with three ports.
- The spring adjusts the pressure required to open the valve.

RESERVOIR BAG

The reservoir bag is an important component of most breathing systems.

Components

1. It is made of antistatic rubber or plastic. Latex-free versions also exist. Designs tend to be ellipsoidal in shape.
2. The standard adult size is 2 litres. The smallest size for paediatric use is 0.5 litre. Volumes from 0.5 to 6 litres exist. Bigger size reservoir bags are useful during inhalational induction, e.g. adult induction with sevoflurane.

Mechanism of action

1. Accommodates the fresh gas flow during expiration acting as a reservoir available for the following inspiration.
2. It acts as a monitor of the patient's ventilatory pattern during spontaneous breathing.

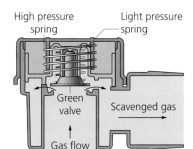
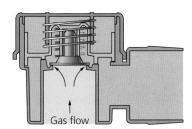
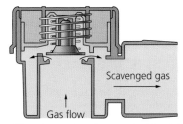

Fig. 4.3 Intersurgical APL valve. In the open position (left) the valve is actuated by pressures of less than 0.1 kPa (1 cmH$_2$O) with minimal resistance to flow. A 3/4 clockwise turn of the dial takes the valve through a range of pressure-limiting positions to the closed position (centre). In the closed position, the breathing system pressure, and therefore the intrapulmonary pressure, is protected by a pressure relief mechanism (right) actuated at 6 kPa (60 cmH$_2$O). This safety relief mechanism cannot be overridden.

It serves as a very inaccurate guide to the patient's tidal volume.

3. It can be used to assist or control ventilation.
4. When employed in conjunction with the T-piece (Mapleson F), a 0.5 litre double-ended bag is used. The distal hole acts as an expiratory port (Fig. 4.4).

Problems in practice and safety features

1. Because of its compliance, the reservoir bag can accommodate rises in pressure in the breathing system better than other parts. When grossly overinflated, the rubber reservoir bag can limit the pressure in the breathing system to about 40 cmH$_2$O. This is due to the law of Laplace dictating that the pressure (P) will fall as the bag's radius (r) increases: P = 2(tension)/r.
2. The size of the bag depends on the breathing system and the

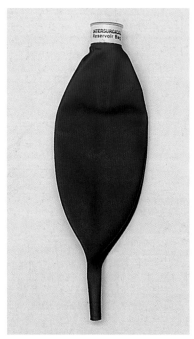

Fig. 4.4 A 0.5 litre double-ended reservoir.

patient. A small bag may not be large enough to provide a sufficient reservoir for a large tidal volume.

3. Too large a reservoir bag makes it difficult for it to act as a respiratory monitor.

> **Reservoir bag**
>
> - Made of rubber or plastic.
> - 2 litre size commonly used for adults. Bigger sizes can be used for inhalational induction in adults.
> - Accommodates fresh gas flow.
> - Can assist or control ventilation.
> - Limits pressure build-up in the breathing system.

TUBING

Specific configurations are described below.

Magill system (Mapleson A)

This breathing system is popular and widely used in the UK.

Components

1. Corrugated rubber or plastic tubing (usually 110–180 cm in length).
2. A reservoir bag, mounted at the machine end.
3. APL valve situated at the patient end.

Mechanism of action

As the patient exhales (Fig. 4.5C), initially the gases from the anatomical dead space are channelled through the tubing back towards the reservoir bag which is filled continuously with fresh gas flow.

Pressure builds up opening the APL valve and expelling the alveolar gases first (Fig. 4.5D). By that time the patient inspires again (Fig. 4.5B), getting a mixture of fresh gas flow and the rebreathed anatomical dead space gases.

It is a very efficient system for spontaneous breathing. Because there is no gas exchange in the anatomical dead space, the fresh gas flow requirements to prevent rebreathing of alveolar gases are theoretically equal to the patient's alveolar minute volume (about 70 mL/kg/min).

The Magill system is not an efficient system for controlled ventilation. A fresh gas flow rate of three times the alveolar minute volume is required to prevent rebreathing.

Problems in practice and safety features

It is not suitable for use with children of less than 25–30 kg body weight. This is because of the increased dead space caused by the system's geometry at the patient end. Dead space is further increased by the angle piece and face mask.

One of its disadvantages is the heaviness of the APL valve at the patient's end, especially if connected to a scavenging system. This places a lot of drag on the connections at the patient end.

> **Magill (Mapleson A) breathing system**
>
> - Efficient for spontaneous ventilation. Fresh gas flow required is equal to alveolar minute volume (about 70 mL/kg/min).
> - Inefficient for controlled ventilation. Fresh gas flow three times alveolar minute volume.
> - APL valve is at the patient's end.
> - Not suitable for paediatric practice.

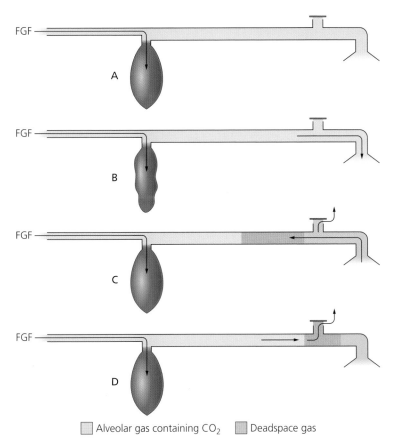

Alveolar gas containing CO_2 Deadspace gas

Fig. 4.5 Mechanism of action of the Magill breathing system during spontaneous ventilation; see text for details (FGF: fresh gas flow) (reproduced with permission from Aitkenhead R, Smith G. Textbook of Anaesthesia, 3rd edn. Churchill Livingstone, 1996).

2. A fresh gas flow rate of about 70 mL/kg/min is required in order to prevent rebreathing. This makes it an efficient breathing system for spontaneous ventilation.
3. Since it is based on the Magill system, it is not suitable for controlled ventilation.

Instead of the coaxial design, a parallel tubing version of the system exists (Fig. 4.6B). This has separate inspiratory and expiratory tubing, and retains the same flow characteristics as the coaxial version.

Lack breathing system

- Coaxial version of Mapleson A, making it efficient for spontaneous ventilation. Fresh gas flow rate of about 70 mL/kg/min is required.
- Fresh gas flow is delivered along the outside tube and the exhaled gases flow along the inner tube.
- APL valve is at the machine end.
- Not suitable for controlled ventilation.

Lack system (Mapleson A)

This is a coaxial modification of the Magill Mapleson A system.

Components

1. 1.8 m length coaxial tubing (tube inside a tube). The fresh gas flows through the outside tube, and the exhaled gases flow through the inside tube (Fig. 4.6A).
2. The inside tube is wide in diameter (14 mm) to reduce resistance to expiration. The outer tube's diameter is 30 mm.
3. The reservoir bag is mounted at the machine end.
4. The APL valve is mounted at the machine end eliminating the drag on the connections at the patient end, which is a problem with the Magill system.

Mechanism of action

1. A similar mechanism to the Magill system except the Lack system is a coaxial version. The fresh gas flows through the outside tube whereas the exhaled gases flow through the inside tube.

Mapleson B and C systems (Fig. 4.1)

Components

1. A reservoir bag. In the B system, corrugated tubing is attached to the bag and both act as a reservoir.
2. An APL valve at the patient's end.
3. Fresh gas flow is added just proximal to the APL.

Mechanism of action

Both systems are not efficient during spontaneous ventilation. A fresh gas flow of 1.5–2 times the minute volume is required to prevent rebreathing.

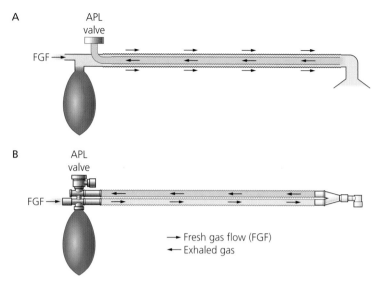

Fig. 4.6 (A) The coaxial Lack breathing system. (B) The parallel Lack breathing system.

During controlled ventilation, the B system is more efficient due to the corrugated tubing acting as a reservoir. A fresh gas flow of more than 50% of the minute ventilation is still required to prevent rebreathing.

> **Mapleson B and C breathing systems**
>
> - B system has a tubing and bag reservoir.
> - Both B and C systems are not efficient for spontaneous and controlled ventilation.
> - B system is more efficient than A system during controlled ventilation.

Bain system (Mapleson D)

The Bain system is a coaxial version of the Mapleson D system (Fig. 4.7). It is lightweight and compact at the patient end. It is useful where access to the patient is limited, such as during head and neck surgery.

A Manley ventilator which has been switched to spontaneous ventilation mode is an example of a non-coaxial Mapleson D system.

Components

1. A length of coaxial tubing (tube inside a tube). The usual length is 180 cm, but it can be supplied at 270 cm (for dental or ophthalmic surgery) and 540 cm (for MRI scans where the anaesthetic machine needs to be kept outside the scanner's magnetic field). Increasing the length of the tubing does not affect the physical properties of the breathing system.
2. The fresh gas flows through the inner tube while the exhaled gases flow through the outside tube. The internal lumen has a swivel mount at the patient end. This ensures that the internal tube cannot kink, so ensuring delivery of fresh gas to the patient.
3. The reservoir bag is mounted at the machine end.
4. The APL valve is mounted at the machine end.

Mechanism of action

1. During spontaneous ventilation, the patient's exhaled gases are channelled back to the reservoir bag and become mixed with fresh gas (Fig. 4.8B). Pressure build-up within the system will open the APL valve allowing the venting of the mixture of the exhaled gases and fresh gas (Fig. 4.8C).
2. The fresh gas flow required to prevent rebreathing (as seen in Fig. 4.8D) during spontaneous ventilation is about 1.5–2 times the alveolar minute volume. A flow rate of 150–200 mL/kg/min is required. This makes it an inefficient and uneconomical system for use during spontaneous ventilation.
3. It is a more efficient system for controlled ventilation. A flow of

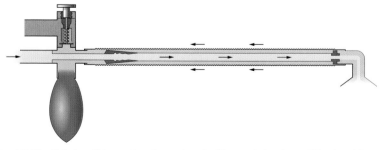

Fig. 4.7 The Bain breathing system (reproduced with permission from Aitkenhead R, Smith G. Textbook of Anaesthesia, 3rd edn. Churchill Livingstone, 1996).

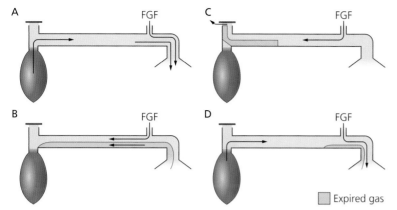

Fig. 4.8 Mechanism of action of the Mapleson D breathing system during spontaneous ventilation (reproduced with permission from Aitkenhead R, Smith G. Textbook of Anaesthesia, 3rd edn. Churchill Livingstone, 1996).

hypoxaemia and hypercapnia. Movement of the reservoir bag during spontaneous ventilation is not therefore an indication that the fresh gas is being delivered to the patient.

Bain breathing system

- Coaxial version of Mapleson D. A parallel version exits.
- Fresh gas flows along the inner tube and the exhaled gases flow along the outer tube.
- Not efficient for spontaneous ventilation. Fresh gas flow rate required is 150–200 mL/kg/min.
- Efficient during controlled ventilation. Fresh gas flow rate required is 70–100 mL/kg/min.

70–100 mL/kg/min will maintain normocapnia. A flow of 100 mL/kg/min will cause moderate hypocapnia during controlled ventilation.
4. Connection to a ventilator is possible (Fig. 4.9). By removing the reservoir bag, a ventilator such as the Penlon Nuffield 200 can be connected to the bag mount using a 1 m length of corrugated tubing (the volume of tubing must exceed 500 mL if the driving gas from the ventilator is not to enter the breathing

system). The APL valve must be fully closed.
5. A parallel version of the D system is available.

Problems in practice and safety features

1. The internal tube can kink, preventing fresh gas being delivered to the patient.
2. The internal tube can become disconnected at the machine end causing a large increase in the dead space, resulting in

T-piece system (Mapleson E and F)

This is a valveless breathing system used in anaesthesia for children up to 25–30 kg body weight (Fig. 4.10). It is suitable for both spontaneous and controlled ventilation.

Components

1. A T-shaped tubing with three open ports (Fig. 4.11).

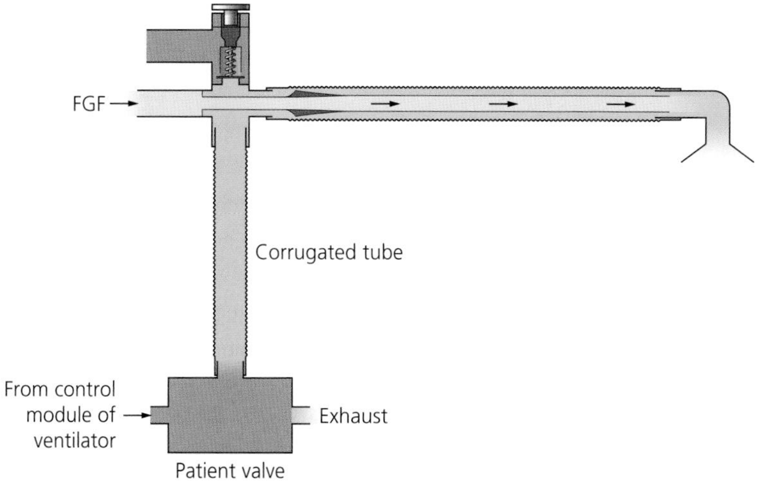

Fig. 4.9 The Bain breathing system connected to a ventilator (e.g. Penlon Nuffield 200) via tubing connected to the bag mount (reproduced with permission from Aitkenhead R, Smith G. Textbook of Anaesthesia, 2nd edn. Churchill Livingstone, 1990).

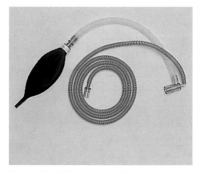

Fig. 4.10 A T-piece breathing system.

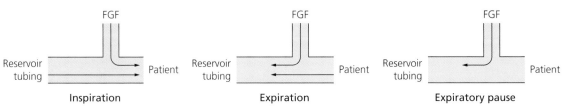

Fig. 4.11 Mechanism of action of the T-piece breathing system.

2. Fresh gas from the anaesthetic machine is delivered via a tube to one port.
3. The second port leads to the patient's mask or tracheal tube. The connection should be as short as possible to reduce dead space.
4. The third port leads to reservoir tubing. Jackson-Rees added a double-ended bag to the end of the reservoir tubing (making it Mapleson F).
5. A recent modification exists where an APL valve is included before a closed ended 500 mL reservoir bag. A pressure relief safety mechanism in the APL valve is actuated at a pressure of 30 cmH$_2$O (Fig. 4.12). This design allows effective scavenging.

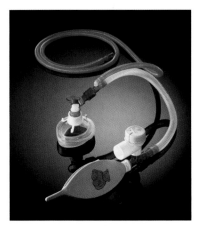

Fig. 4.12 Intersurgical T-piece incorporating an APL valve and closed reservoir bag to enable effective scavenging.

Mechanism of action

1. The system requires a fresh gas flow of 2.5–3 times the minute volume to prevent rebreathing with a minimal flow of 4 L/min.
2. The double-ended bag acts as a visual monitor during spontaneous ventilation. In addition, the bag can be used for assisted or controlled ventilation.
3. The bag can provide a degree of CPAP during spontaneous ventilation.
4. Controlled ventilation is performed either by manual squeezing of the double-ended bag (intermittent occlusion of the reservoir tubing in the Mapleson E) or by removing the bag and connecting the reservoir tubing to a ventilator such as the Penlon Nuffield 200.
5. The volume of the reservoir tubing determines the degree of rebreathing (too large a tube) or entrainment of ambient air (too small a tube). The volume of the reservoir tubing should approximate to the patient's tidal volume.

Problems in practice and safety features

1. Since there is no APL valve used in this breathing system, scavenging is a problem.
2. Patients under 6 years of age have a low functional residual capacity (FRC). Mapleson E was designed before the advantages of CPAP were recognized for increasing the FRC. This problem

can be partially overcome in the Mapleson F with the addition of the double-ended bag.

T-Piece E and F breathing system

- Used in paediatric practice up to 25–30 kg body weight.
- Requires a high fresh gas flow during spontaneous ventilation.
- Offers minimal resistance to expiration.
- Valveless breathing system.
- Scavenging is difficult.
- A recent design with an APL valve and a closed-ended reservoir allows effective scavenging.

The Humphrey ADE breathing system

This is a very versatile breathing system which combines the advantages of Mapleson A, D and E systems. It can therefore be used efficiently for spontaneous and controlled ventilation in both adults and children. The mode of use is determined by the position of one lever which is mounted on the Humphrey block (Fig. 4.13). Both parallel and coaxial versions exist with similar efficiency. The parallel version will be considered here.

Components

1. Two lengths of 15 mm smooth bore tubing (corrugated tubing is

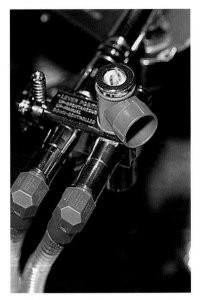

Fig. 4.13 The parallel Humphrey ADE breathing system.

not recommended). One delivers the fresh gas and the other carries away the exhaled gas. Distally they are connected to a Y-connection leading to the patient. Proximally they are connected to the Humphrey block.

2. The Humphrey block is at the machine end and consists of:
   a) an APL valve featuring a visible indicator of valve performance (Fig. 4.14)
   b) a 2 litre reservoir bag
   c) a lever to select either spontaneous or controlled ventilation
   d) a port to which a ventilator can be connected, e.g. Penlon Nuffield 200
   e) a safety pressure relief valve which opens at pressure in excess of 60 cmH$_2$O
   f) a new design incorporating a soda lime canister.

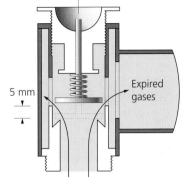

Fig. 4.14 The Humphrey ADE breathing system's APL valve (reproduced with permission from Dr D. Humphrey).

Mechanism of action

1. With the lever up (Fig. 4.15A) in the spontaneous mode, the reservoir bag and APL valve are connected to the breathing system as in the Magill system.

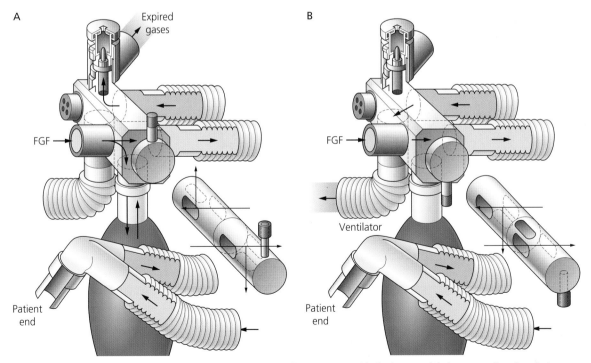

Fig. 4.15 Mechanism of action of the parallel Humphrey ADE breathing system. With the lever up (A) the system functions in its Mapleson A mode for spontaneous ventilation. For mechanical ventilation the lever is down (B) and the system functions in its Mapleson E mode (reproduced with permission from Dr D. Humphrey).

2. With the lever down (Fig. 4.15B) in the ventilator mode, the reservoir bag and the APL valve are isolated from the breathing system as in the Mapleson E system. The expiratory tubing channels the exhaled gas via the ventilator port. Scavenging occurs at the ventilator's expiratory valve.

3. The system is suitable for paediatric and adult use. The tubing is rather narrow, with a low internal volume. Because of its smooth bore, there is no significant increase in resistance to flow compared to 22 mm corrugated tubing used in other systems. Small tidal volumes are possible during controlled ventilation and less energy is needed to overcome the inertia of gases during spontaneous ventilation.

4. The presence of an APL valve in the breathing system offers a physiological advantage during paediatric anaesthesia, since it is designed to offer a small amount of PEEP (1 cmH$_2$O).

5. During spontaneous ventilation:
   a) a fresh gas flow of about 50–60 mL/kg/min is needed in adults;
   b) the recommended initial fresh gas flow for children weighing less than 25 kg body weight is 3 L/min. This offers a considerable margin for safety.

6. During controlled ventilation:
   a) a fresh gas flow of 70 mL/kg is needed in adults;
   b) the recommended initial fresh gas flow for children weighing less than 25 kg body weight is 3 L/min. However, adjustment may be necessary to maintain normocarbia.

Humphrey ADE breathing system

- Can be used efficiently for spontaneous and controlled ventilation.
- Can be used in both adult and paediatric anaesthetic practice.
- Both parallel and coaxial versions exist.
- A ventilator can be connected.

Soda lime and circle breathing system

In this breathing system, soda lime is used to absorb the patient's exhaled carbon dioxide (Fig. 4.16). Fresh gas flow requirements are low, making the circle system very efficient and causing minimal pollution. As a result, there has been renewed interest in low flow anaesthesia due to the cost of new, expensive inhalational agents, together with the increased awareness of the pollution caused by the inhalational agents themselves (see Table 3.1).

Depending on the FGF, the system can either be:

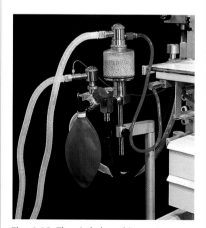

Fig. 4.16 The circle breathing system.

- **Closed circle anaesthesia.** The FGF is just sufficient to replace the volume of gas and vapour taken up by the patient. No gas leaves via the APL valve and the exhaled gases are rebreathed after carbon dioxide is absorbed. Significant leaks from the breathing system are eliminated. In practice this is possible only if the gases sampled by the gas analyser are returned back to the system.
- **Low-flow anaesthesia.** The FGF used is less than the patient's alveolar ventilation (usually below 1.5 L/min). Excess gases leave the system via the APL valve.

Components

1. A vertically positioned canister containing soda lime. The canister has;
   a) an inlet delivering fresh gas flow from the anaesthetic machine
   b) two ports, one to deliver fresh gas flow to the patient and the other to receive exhaled gases from the patient. Each port incorporates a unidirectional valve
   c) an APL valve connected to a 2 litre reservoir bag.
2. Inspiratory and expiratory tubings connected to the canister.
3. A vaporizer mounted on the anaesthetic machine back bar (*v*aporizer *o*utside *c*ircle – VOC) or a vaporizer positioned on the expiratory limb within the system (*v*aporizer *i*nside *c*ircle – VIC).
4. Soda lime consists of 94% calcium hydroxide and 5% sodium hydroxide with a small amount of potassium hydroxide (less than 0.1%). It has a pH of

13.5 and a moisture content of 14–19%. Some modern types of soda lime have no potassium hydroxide. Silica (0.2%) is added to prevent disintegration of the granules into powder. A dye is added to change the granules' colour when the soda lime is exhausted. Colour changes can be from white to violet (ethyl violet dye), from pink to white (titan yellow dye) or from green to violet. Colour changes occur when the pH is less than 10. Newer types of soda lime have a low concentration of a zeolite added. This helps to maintain the pH at a high level for longer and retains moisture so improving carbon dioxide absorption and reducing the formation of carbon monoxide and compound A.

5. The size of soda lime granules is 4–8 mesh. Strainers with 4–8 mesh have four and eight openings per inch respectively. Therefore, the higher the mesh number, the smaller the particles are. Recently produced soda lime made to a uniform shape of 3–4 mm spheres allows more even flow of gases and a reduction in channelling. This results in a longer life with lower dust content and lower resistance to flow. 1 kg can absorb more than 120 litres of CO_2.

Mechanism of action

1. High FGF of several litres per minute is needed in the initial period to denitrogenate the circle system and the functional residual capacity (FRC). This is important to avoid the build up of unacceptable levels of nitrogen in the system. In closed circle anaesthesia, a high FGF is needed for up to 15 minutes. In low-flow anaesthesia, a high FGF of up to 6 minutes is required. The FGF can be later reduced to 0.5–1 L/min. If no N_2O is used during anaesthesia (i.e. an oxygen/air mix is used), it is not necessary to eliminate nitrogen because air contains nitrogen. A short period of high flow is needed to prime the system and the patient with the inhalational agent.

2. Exhaled gases are circled back to the canister, where carbon dioxide absorption takes place and water and heat (exothermic reaction) are produced. The warmed and humidified gas joins the fresh gas flow to be delivered to the patient (Fig. 4.17).

3. **Chemical sequences for the absorption of carbon dioxide by soda lime:**

    Note how both NaOH and KOH are re-generated at the expense of $Ca(OH)_2$. This explains soda lime's mix – only a little Na(OH) and K(OH) and a lot of $Ca(OH)_2$.

$$H_2O + CO_2 \rightarrow H_2CO_3$$

then

$$H_2CO_3 + 2KOH \rightarrow K_2CO_3 + 2H_2O$$

then

$$K_2CO_3 + Ca(OH)_2 \rightarrow CaCO_3 + 2KOH$$

or

$$CO_2 + 2NaOH \rightarrow Na_2CO_3 + H_2O + heat$$

then

$$Na_2CO_3 + Ca(OH)_2 \rightarrow 2NaOH + CaCO_3$$

3. The direction of gas flow is controlled via the unidirectional disc valves. These are mounted in see-through plastic domes so that they can be seen to be working satisfactorily.

4. The canister is positioned vertically to prevent exhaled gas channelling through unfilled portions. Larger canisters are more efficient than smaller ones because of the higher litres of CO_2/kg weight capacity. Double absorbers with two cartridges used simultaneously are more efficient than single absorbers.

5. The lower the FGF used, the more rapidly soda lime granules are consumed. This is because most of the exhaled gases pass through the absorber with very little being discarded through the APL valve. For a 70–80 kg patient with a tidal volume of 500 mL, respiratory rate of 12/min and CO_2 production of 250 mL/min, using an FGF of 1

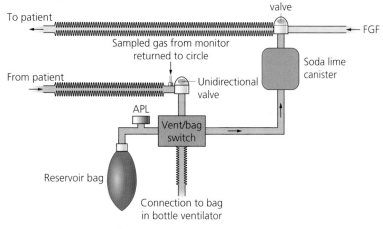

Fig. 4.17 Mechanism of action of the circle breathing system.

L/min, the soda lime will be exhausted after 5–7 hours of use. For the same patient but using an FGF of 3 L/min, the soda lime will be exhausted after 6–8 hours of use.

6. The circle system can be used for both spontaneous and controlled ventilation.

7. Disposable circle breathing systems exist. They feature coaxial inspiratory tubing. The inner tubing delivers the fresh gas flow from the anaesthetic machine and the outer tubing delivers the recircled gas flow. Both gas flows mix distally. This allows a more rapid change in the inhalational gas and vapour concentration at the patient end.

USE OF VAPORIZERS IN THE CIRCLE BREATHING SYSTEM

VOC vaporizers (Fig. 4.18) are positioned on the back bar of the anaesthetic machine. They are high efficiency vaporizers that can deliver high output concentrations at low flows. They have high internal resistance.

1. The vaporizer should be able to deliver accurate concentrations of inhalational agent with both high

and low fresh gas flows. This is easily achieved by most modern vaporizers, e.g. Tec series.

2. The volume of the circle system is large in relation to the low fresh gas flow used. Rapid changes in the concentration of the inspired vapour can be achieved by increasing the fresh gas flow to the circle system. Delivering the fresh gas flow distally, using a coaxial inspiratory tubing design, allows faster changes in inspired vapour concentration compared to conventional circle systems at low flows.

VIC vaporizers (Fig. 4.18) are designed to offer minimal resistance to gas flow and have no wicks on which water vapour might condense (e.g. Goldman vaporizer). The VIC is a low efficiency vaporizer adding only small amounts of vapour to the gas recirculating through it.

1. Fresh gas flow will be vapour free and thus dilutes the inspired vapour concentration.

2. During spontaneous ventilation, respiration is depressed with deepening of anaesthesia. Uptake of the anaesthetic agent is therefore reduced. This is an example of a feedback safety mechanism. The

safety mechanism is lost during controlled ventilation.

Problems in practice and safety features

1. Adequate monitoring of inspired oxygen, end-tidal carbon dioxide and inhalational agent concentrations is essential.

2. The unidirectional valves may stick and fail to close because of water vapour condensation. This leads to an enormous increase in dead space.

3. The resistance to breathing is increased especially during spontaneous ventilation. Dust formation can increase resistance to breathing further. It can also lead to clogging and channelling, so reducing efficiency. Newer soda lime designs claim less dust formation.

4. Compound A (a penta-fluoro-isoproprenyl fluoro-methyl ether, which is nephrotoxic in rats) is produced when sevoflurane is used in conjunction with soda lime. This is due to the degradation of sevoflurane (de-hydrohalogenation) as a result of the alkali metal hydroxide present in soda lime. The amount produced is proportional to the sevoflurane concentration and the temperature of the absorber. The latter is higher with lower FGF. Newer designs of soda lime, being non-caustic (no KOH and only very low levels of NaOH), claim less or no production of compound A.

5. Carbon monoxide production can occur when volatile agents containing the CHF_2 moiety (enflurane/isoflurane) are used with totally dry soda lime. More recent designs of soda lime claim less or no production of carbon monoxide.

6. Uneven filling of the canister with soda lime leads to channelling of gases and decreased efficiency.

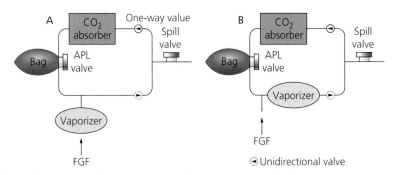

Fig. 4.18 Diagrammatic representation of the circle system with (A) vaporizer outside the circle (VOC) and (B) vaporizer inside the circle (VIC) (reproduced with permission from Aitkenhead R, Rowbotham DJ, Smith G. Textbook of Anaesthesia, 4th edn. Churchill Livingstone, 2001.)

7. The circle system is bulkier, less portable and more difficult to clean.
8. Soda lime is corrosive. Protective clothing, gloves and eye/face protection can be used.
9. Because of the many connections, there is an increased potential for leaks and disconnection.

The circle breathing system

- Soda lime canister with two unidirectional valves attached to inspiratory and expiratory tubings. An APL valve and a reservoir bag are connected to the canister.
- Soda lime consists of 94% calcium hydroxide, 5% sodium hydroxide and a small amount of potassium hydroxide.
- Soda lime absorbs the exhaled carbon dioxide and produces water and heat (so humidifies and warms inspired gases).
- Very efficient breathing system using low fresh gas flow and reducing pollution.
- A high initial flow is required.
- Vaporizers can be VIC or VOC.

Waters canister ('to-and-fro') breathing system

Currently, this system is not widely used in anaesthetic practice. It consists of a Mapleson C system with a soda lime canister positioned between the APL valve and the reservoir. A filter is positioned in the canister to prevent the soda lime granules 'entering' the breathing system and the risk of inhaling them. It is not an efficient system as the granules nearest to the patient are exhausted first, so increasing the dead space. It is also a cumbersome system as the canister has to be positioned horizontally and packed tightly with the soda lime granules to prevent channelling of the gases (Fig. 4.19).

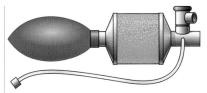

Fig. 4.19 The Waters canister breathing system.

FURTHER READING

Miller DM. Breathing systems for use in anaethesia. Evaluation using a physical lung model. British Journal of Anaesthesia 1988;60:555–564.

Protecting the breathing circuit in anaesthesia. London: Department of Health, 2004.

Shelgaonkar JR, Al-Shaikh B. Closed-circle anaesthesia. In: Pollard B, ed. Handbook of Anaesthesia, 2nd edn. London: Churchill Livingstone, 2004, pp. 700–703.

MCQs

In the following lists, which of the statements (a) to (e) are true?

1. APL valve in a breathing system.
   a) In the open position, a pressure of less than $1\,cmH_2O$ (0.1 kPa) is needed to actuate the valve.
   b) A pressure relief mechanism is activated at a pressure of $60\,cmH_2O$.
   c) Is incorporated in the T-piece breathing system.
   d) The dead space of the breathing system is reduced during spontaneous ventilation when excessive negative pressure from the scavenging system is applied through the APL valve.
   e) Should be closed during controlled ventilation using a Bain breathing system and an intermittent blower ventilator.

2. Breathing systems
   a) The fresh gas flow rate required to prevent rebreathing of alveolar gas in the breathing system is a measure of the efficiency of a breathing system.
   b) The reservoir bag limits the pressure build-up in a breathing system to about $40\,cmH_2O$.
   c) A fresh gas flow of $150\,mL/kg/min$ is needed in the Mapleson A system during spontaneous ventilation.
   d) The inner tube in the Bain system delivers the fresh gas flow.
   e) The Humphrey ADE system can be used for spontaneous ventilation only.

3. Dead space
   a) The face mask in the Mapleson A breathing system has no effect on the dead space.
   b) Disconnection of the inner tube at the patient's end in the Bain system results in an increase in dead space.
   c) Failure of the unidirectional valves to close in the circle system has no effect on the system's dead space.
   d) The anatomic dead space is about 150 mL.
   e) Bohr's equation is used to measure the physiological dead space.

4. Concerning soda lime
   a) 20% volume for volume of soda lime is sodium hydroxide.
   b) 90% is calcium carbonate.
   c) 1 kg of soda lime can absorb about 120 mL of CO_2.
   d) The reaction with carbon dioxide is exothermic.
   e) Soda lime fills half of the canister.

5. The Bain breathing system
   a) Is an example of a Mapleson A system.
   b) Requires a fresh gas flow of $70\,mL/kg$ during spontaneous ventilation.
   c) Is made of standard corrugated tubing.
   d) Can be used in a T-piece system.
   e) Can be used for both spontaneous and controlled ventilation.

6. T-piece breathing system
   a) Can be used in paediatric practice only.
   b) Mapleson F system is the E system plus an open ended reservoir bag.
   c) Is an efficient system.
   d) With a constant FGF, a too small reservoir has no effect on the performance of the system.
   e) The reservoir bag in Mapleson F provides a degree of CPAP during spontaneous ventilation.

7. Which of the following are true
   and which are false?
   a) The Magill classification is
      used to describe anaesthetic
      breathing systems.
   b) Modern anaesthetic breathing
      systems are constructed using
      antistatic materials.
   c) Efficiency of a breathing
      system is determined by the
      mode of ventilation of the
      patient.
   d) As long as the valve is present
      in a breathing system, its
      position is not important.
   e) Circle systems must only be
      used with very low fresh gas
      flows.

8. The circle breathing system
   a) With low flow rates, substance
      A can be produced when
      sevoflurane is used.
   b) The Goldman vaporizer is an
      example of a VOC.
   c) Failure of the unidirectional
      valves to close leads to an
      enormous increase in the dead
      space.
   d) Patients should not be allowed
      to breathe spontaneously,
      because of the high resistance
      caused by the soda lime.
   e) Exhaustion of the soda lime
      can be detected by an end-tidal
      CO_2 rebreathing waveform.

9. Regarding the circle system
   a) A high FGF is needed in the
      first 15 minutes to wash out
      any CO_2 remaining in the
      breathing system.
   b) The pH of soda lime is highly
      acidic.
   c) The lower the FGF, the slower
      the exhaustion of soda lime
      granules.
   d) The Waters to-and-fro system
      is very efficient.
   e) Partially harmful substances
      can be produced when using
      soda lime.

Answers

1. APL valve in a breathing system
   a) *True.* The valve is designed to offer minimal resistance to exhalation and to prevent build up of positive pressure in the breathing system in cases of malfunction or obstruction. A very low pressure of less than $1\,cmH_2O$ is needed to actuate it. This is designed for the safety of the patient.
   b) *True.* This is a safety feature in the design of the APL valve. If the APL valve is closed, a build up of pressure within the breathing system puts the patient at the risk of barotrauma. A pressure relief mechanism is activated at a pressure of $60\,cmH_2O$, allowing the reduction of pressure within the system.
   c) *False.* There are no valves in the standard T-piece system. This is to keep resistance to a minimum. A recent modification exists where an APL valve is included before a closed ended 500 mL reservoir bag. A pressure relief safety mechanism in the APL valve is actuated at a pressure of $30\,cmH_2O$. This design allows effective scavenging.
   d) *False.* There is a huge increase in the dead space resulting in rebreathing. This is because excessive negative pressure can lead the APL valve to remain open throughout breathing.
   e) *True.* When ventilation is controlled using a Bain breathing system and an intermittent blower ventilator, the APL valve must be closed completely. This is to prevent the escape of inhaled gases through the APL valve leading to inadequate ventilation.

2. Breathing systems
   a) *True.* The fresh gas flow rate required to prevent rebreathing is a measure of the efficiency of a breathing system; e.g. in spontaneous breathing, the circle system is the most efficient system whereas the Bain system is the least efficient.
   b) *True.* This is a safety feature to protect the patient from overpressure. Because of its high compliance, the reservoir bag can accommodate rises in pressure within the system better than other parts. Due to the law of Laplace (pressure = 2 tension/radius), when the reservoir is overinflated, it can limit the pressure in the breathing system to about $40\,cmH_2O$.
   c) *False.* Mapleson A system is an efficient system during spontaneous breathing needing a fresh gas flow of about 70 mL/kg/min. Mapleson D needs an FGF of 150–200 mL/ kg/min.
   d) *True.* The inner tube delivers the FGF as close as possible to the patient. The outer tube, which is connected to the reservoir bag, takes the exhaled gases.
   e) *False.* The Humphrey ADE system is a very versatile system and can be used for both spontaneous and controlled ventilation both for adults and in paediatrics.

3. Dead space
   a) *False.* The face mask increases the dead space in the Mapleson A breathing system. The dead space can increase up to 200 mL in adults.
   b) *True.* Disconnection of the inner tube, which delivers the FGF, at the patient's end in the Bain system leads to an increase in dead space and rebreathing.
   c) *False.* The unidirectional valves are essential for the performance of the circle system. Failure to close leads to a significant increase in the dead space.
   d) *True.* The anatomic dead space is that part of the respiratory system which takes no part in the gas exchange.
   e) *True.*

$$V_D/V_T = P_A CO_2 - P_E CO_2/P_A CO_2$$

where V_D is dead space; V_T is tidal volume; $P_A CO_2$ is alveolar CO_2 tension; $P_E CO_2$ is mixed expired CO_2 tension. Normally $V_D/V_T = 0.25–0.35$

4. Concerning soda lime
   a) *False*. *Sodium hydroxide constitutes about 5% of the soda lime.*
   b) *False*. *Calcium carbonate is a product of the reaction between soda lime and carbon dioxide.*

   $$CO_2 + 2NaOH \rightarrow Na_2CO_3 + H_2O + heat$$

   $$Na_2CO_3 + Ca(OH)_2 \rightarrow 2NaOH + CaCO_3$$

   c) *False*. *1 kg of soda lime can absorb 120 L of CO_2.*
   d) *True*. *Heat is produced as a by-product of the reaction between CO_2 and sodium hydroxide.*
   e) *False*. *In order to achieve adequate CO_2 absorption, the canister should be well packed to avoid channelling and incomplete CO_2 absorption.*

5. The Bain breathing system
   a) *False*. *The Bain breathing system is an example of a Mapleson D system.*
   b) *False*. *A fresh gas flow of about 150–200 mL/kg/min is required to prevent rebreathing in the Bain system during spontaneous ventilation. This makes it an inefficient breathing system.*
   c) *False*. *The Bain system is usually made of a coaxial tubing. A more recent design, a pair of parallel corrugated tubings, is also available.*
   d) *False*. *The Bain breathing system is a Mapleson D whereas the T-piece system is an E system. The Bain system has an APL valve whereas the T-piece is a valveless system.*
   e) *True*. *The Bain system can be used for spontaneous ventilation requiring an FGF of 150–200 mL/kg. It can also be used for controlled ventilation requiring an FGF of 70–100 mL/kg. During controlled ventilation, the APL valve is fully closed, the reservoir bag is removed and a ventilator like the Penlon Nuffield 200 with a 1 m length of tubing is connected instead.*

6. T-piece breathing system
   a) *False*. *Although the T-piece breathing system is mainly used in paediatrics, it can be used in adults with a suitable FGF and reservoir volume. An FGF of 2.5–3 times the minute volume and a reservoir approximating the tidal volume are needed. Such a system is usually used in recovery and for ITU patients.*
   b) *True*. *Jackson-Rees added a double-ended bag to the reservoir tubing of the Mapleson E thus converting it to a Mapleson F. The bag acts as a visual monitor during spontaneous ventilation and can be used for assisted or controlled ventilation.*
   c) *False*. *The T-piece system is not an efficient system as it requires an FGF of 2.5–3 times the minute volume to prevent rebreathing.*
   d) *False*. *If the reservoir is too small, entrainment of ambient air will occur resulting in dilution of the FGF.*
   e) *True*. *Patients under the age of 6 years have a small FRC. General anaesthesia causes a further decrease in the FRC. The reservoir bag in the Mapleson F provides a degree of CPAP during spontaneous ventilation, helping to improve the FRC.*

7. Which of the following are true or false?
   a) *False. Mapleson classification is used. The Mapleson A breathing system was described by Magill.*
   b) *False. As modern anaesthetic agents are not flammable, modern breathing systems are not constructed using antistatic materials. They are normally made of plastic.*
   c) *True. Efficiency of a breathing system differs during spontaneous and controlled ventilation; e.g. the Mapleson A system is more efficient during spontaneous than controlled ventilation whereas the opposite is true of the D system.*
   d) *False. The position of the valve in the breathing system is crucial in the function and efficiency of a breathing system.*
   e) *False. The circle system can be used with low flows (e.g. 2–3 L/min) as well as very low flows (e.g. 0.5–1.5 L/min). This can be achieved safely with adequate monitoring of the inspired and exhaled concentration of the gases and vapours used.*

8. The circle breathing system
   a) *True. Substance A can be produced when sevoflurane is used with soda lime under low flow rates. Newer designs of soda lime claim lesser production of substance A.*
   b) *False. The Goldman vaporizer is a VIC. It is positioned on the expiratory limb with minimal resistance to flow and no wicks.*
   c) *True. The function of the unidirectional valves in the circle system is crucial for its function. Failure of the valve to close causes rebreathing resulting from the huge increase in the dead space of the system. This usually happens because of water vapour condensing on the valve.*
   d) *False. The circle system can be used for both spontaneous and controlled ventilation. Soda lime increases the resistance to flow but is clinically insignificant.*
   e) *True. As the soda lime gets exhausted, a rebreathing end-tidal CO_2 waveform can be detected. A dye is added that changes the granules' colour as they become exhausted.*

9. Regarding circle system
   a) *False. High FGF (several litres per minute) is needed initially to denitrogenate the system and the functional residual capacity (FRC) to avoid the build up of unacceptable levels of nitrogen in the system. In closed circle anaesthesia, a high FGF for up to 15 minutes and in low-flow anaesthesia, a high FGF of up to 6 minutes are required and these can be later reduced to 0.5–1 L/min. If no N_2O is used during anaesthesia, it is not necessary to eliminate nitrogen. A short period of high flow is needed to prime the system and the patient with the inhalational agent.*
   b) *False. The pH of soda lime is highly alkaline, 13.5, because of the presence of calcium hydroxide, sodium hydroxide and small amounts, if any, of potassium hydroxide. This makes the soda lime a corrosive substance. Colour changes occur when the ph is less than 10.*

c) **False.** The lower the FGF, the more rapidly soda lime granules are exhausted because most of the exhaled gases pass through the absorber with very little being discarded through the APL valve. For a 70–80 kg patient with a tidal volume of 500 mL, respiratory rate of 12/min and CO_2 production of 250 mL/min, using an FGF of 1 L/min, the soda lime will be exhausted in 5–7 h of use. For the same patient but using an FGF of 3 litres/min, the soda lime will be exhausted in 6–8 hours of use.

d) **False.** It is not an efficient system as the granules nearest to the patient are exhausted first so increasing the dead space.

e) **True.** Substance A, nephrotoxic in rats, can be produced when sevoflurane is used with soda lime although newer designs claim less or no substance A production. Carbon monoxide can occur when dry soda lime is used. Newer designs claim less or no carbon monoxide production.

Chapter 5

Tracheal and tracheostomy tubes and airways

Tracheal tubes

Tracheal tubes provide a means of securing the patient's airway. These can be made of either plastic (disposable) or rubber (reusable after cleaning and autoclaving). The plastic disposable tracheal tubes are made of polyvinyl chloride (PVC) which could be clear, ivory or siliconized. The plastic tubes have a radio-opaque line running along their length, which enables their position to be determined on chest X-rays. The siliconized PVC aids the passage of suction catheters through the tube.

FEATURES OF TRACHEAL TUBES (FIGS 5.1 AND 5.2)

Size

1. The **internal diameter** is marked on the outside of the tube in millimetres. Narrower tubes increase the resistance to gas flow, therefore the largest possible internal diameter should be used. This is especially important during spontaneous ventilation where the patient's own respiratory effort must overcome the tube's resistance. Usually, a size 8.5–9 mm internal diameter tube is selected for an average size adult male and a size 7.5–8 mm internal diameter tube for an average size adult female. Paediatric sizes are determined on the basis of the age and weight (Table 5.1).

2. The **length** (taken from the tip of the tube) is marked in centimetres on the outside of the tube. The tube can be cut down to size to suit the individual patient. If the tube is cut too long, there is a significant risk of it advancing into one of the main bronchi (usually the right one, see Fig. 5.3). A black Intubation Depth Marker located 3 cm proximal to the cuff can be seen in some designs (Fig. 5.2, bottom). This assists the accurate placement of the tracheal tube tip within the trachea.

The bevel

1. The bevel is left-facing and oval in shape in most tube designs. A left-facing bevel improves the view of the vocal cords during intubation.

2. Some designs have a side hole just above and opposite the bevel, called a Murphy eye. This enables ventilation to occur should the bevel become occluded by secretions, blood or the wall of the trachea.

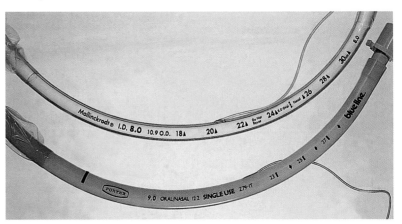

Fig. 5.2 Markings on a Mallinckrodt 8 mm ID tracheal tube (top) and Portex 9 mm ID tracheal tube (bottom). (IT stands for implantation tested. Z-79 stands for the Z-79 Committee of the American National Standards Institute.)

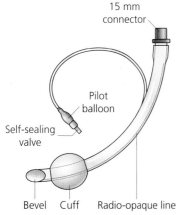

Fig. 5.1 Features of a tracheal tube.

Table 5.1 A guide to the size and length of oral tracheal tubes used in paediatric practice

Age	Weight (kg)	Size (ID mm)	Length (cm)
Neonate	2–4	2.5–3.5	10–12
1–6 months	4–6	4.0–4.5	12–14
6–12 months	6–10	4.5–5.0	14–16
1–3 years	10–15	5.0–5.5	16–18
4–6 years	15–20	5.5–6.5	18–20
7–10 years	25–35	6.5–7.0	20–22
10–14 years	40–50	7.0–7.5	22–24

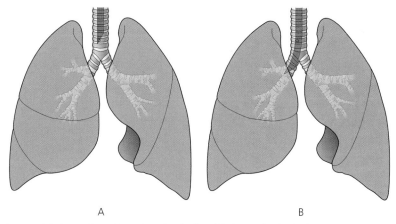

Fig. 5.3 (A) Correctly positioned tracheal tube. (B) The tracheal tube has been advanced too far, into the right main bronchus.

The cuff

Tracheal (oral or nasal) tubes can be either cuffed or uncuffed. The cuff, when inflated, provides an airtight seal between the tube and the tracheal wall (Fig. 5.4). This airtight seal protects the patient's airway from aspiration and allows efficient ventilation during IPPV.

1. The cuff is connected to its pilot balloon which has a self-sealing valve for injecting air. The pilot balloon also indicates whether the cuff is inflated or not. After intubation, the cuff is inflated until no gas leak can be heard during IPPV.
2. The narrowest point in the adult's airway is the glottis (which is hexagonal). In order to achieve an airtight seal, cuffed tubes are used in adults.
3. The narrowest point in a child's airway is the cricoid cartilage. Since this is essentially circular, a correctly sized uncuffed tube will fit well. Because of the narrow upper airway in children, post-extubation sub-glottic oedema can be a problem. In order to minimize the risk, the presence of a small leak around the tube at an airway pressure of $15\,cmH_2O$ is desirable.
4. Cuffs can either be:
   a) high pressure/low volume
   b) low pressure/high volume.

High pressure/low volume cuffs

1. These can prevent the passing of vomitus, secretions or blood into the lungs.
2. At the same time, they exert a high pressure on the tracheal wall. If left in position for long periods they may cause necrosis of the tracheal mucosa (Fig. 5.5).

Low pressure/high volume cuffs

1. These exert minimal pressure on the tracheal wall as the pressure equilibrates over a wider area (Fig. 5.6). This allows the cuff

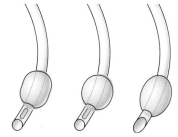

Fig. 5.4 Different sizes of tracheal tube cuffs. High volume (left), intermediate volume (centre), low volume (right).

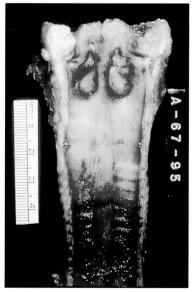

Fig. 5.5 A post mortem tracheal specimen. Note the black necrotic area which was caused by long-term intubation with a high pressure cuffed tube.

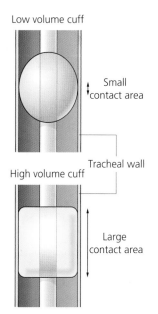

Fig. 5.6 Diagram illustrating how a low volume cuff (top) maintains a seal against a relatively small area of tracheal wall compared to a high volume cuff (bottom).

to remain inflated for longer periods.

2. They are less capable of preventing the aspiration of vomitus or secretions. This is due to the possibility of wrinkles forming in the cuff.

The pressure in the cuff should be checked at frequent and regular intervals (Fig. 5.7). The pressure may increase mainly because of diffusion of nitrous oxide into the cuff. Expansion of the air inside the cuff due to the increase in its temperature from room to body temperature and the diffusion of oxygen from the anaesthetic mixture (about 33%) into the air (21%) in the cuff can also lead to increase in the intra-cuff pressure. An increase in pressure of about 10–12 mmHg is expected after 30 minutes of anaesthesia with 66% nitrous oxide. A new design cuff material (Soft Seal, Portex) allows minimum diffusion of nitrous oxide into the cuff with a pressure increase of 1–2 mmHg only. The pressure may decrease because of a leak in the cuff or pilot balloon's valve.

Route of insertion

1. Tubes can be inserted orally or nasally (Fig. 5.8).
2. The indications for nasal intubation include

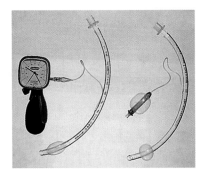

Fig. 5.7 A cuff pressure gauge (left). The Brandt system (right) which uses an oversized pilot balloon to facilitate diffusion of nitrous oxide, limiting rises in cuff pressure.

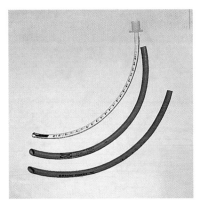

Fig. 5.8 A selection of uncuffed tracheal tubes. Plastic oral/nasal tube (top), oral red rubber tube (middle), nasal red rubber tube (bottom). Note the increased angle of curvature in the oral compared to the nasal red rubber tube.

a) surgery where access via the mouth is necessary, e.g. ENT, or dental operations
b) long-term ventilated patients on intensive care units. Patients tolerate a nasal tube better, and cannot bite on the tube. However, long-term nasal intubation may cause sinus infection.

3. Nasal intubation is usually avoided, if possible, in children up to the age of 8–11 years. Hypertrophy of the adenoids in this age group increases the risk of profuse bleeding if nasal intubation is performed.
4. Ivory PVC naso-tracheal tubes cause less trauma to the nasal mucosa.

Connectors

These connect the tracheal tubes to the breathing system (or catheter mount). There are various designs and modifications (Fig. 5.9). They are made of plastic or metal and should have an adequate internal diameter to reduce the resistance to gas flow.

The British Standard connector has a 15 mm diameter at the

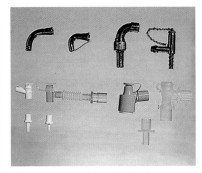

Fig. 5.9 A range of tracheal tube connectors. Top row from left to right: Magill oral, Magill nasal, Nosworthy, Cobb suction. (Note the Magill nasal connector has been supplied with a piece of wire threaded through it to demonstrate its patency.) Bottom row: Paediatric 8.5 mm connectors (left), standard 15 mm connectors (right).

proximal end. An 8.5 mm diameter version exists for neonatal use. Connectors designed for use with nasal tracheal tubes have a more acute angle than the oral ones (e.g. Magill's connector). Some designs have an extra port for suction.

Problems in practice and safety features

1. Obstruction of the tracheal tube by kinking, herniation of the cuff, occlusion by secretions, foreign body or the bevel lying against the wall of the trachea.
2. Oesophageal or bronchial intubation.
3. Trauma and injury to the various tissues and structures during and after intubation.

Tracheal tubes

- Made of plastic or rubber.
- Oral or nasal (avoid nasal intubation in children).
- Cuffed or uncuffed.
- The cuff can be low pressure/high volume, high pressure/low volume.

Specially designed tracheal tubes

OXFORD TRACHEAL TUBE

This anatomically L-shaped tracheal tube is used in anaesthesia for head and neck surgery because it is non-kinking (Fig. 5.10). The tube can be made of rubber or plastic and can be cuffed or uncuffed. The bevel is oval in shape and faces posteriorly and an introducing stylet is supplied to aid the insertion of the tube. Its thick wall adds to the tube's external diameter making it wider for a given internal diameter. This is undesirable especially in paediatric anaesthesia.

The distance from the bevel to the curve of the tube is fixed. If the tube is too long, the problem can not be corrected by withdrawing the tube and shortening it because this means losing its anatomical fit.

ARMOURED TRACHEAL TUBE

Armoured tracheal tubes are made of plastic or silicone rubber (Fig. 5.10). The walls of the armoured tube are thicker than ordinary tracheal tubes because they contain a spiral of metal wire or tough nylon.

They are used in anaesthesia for head and neck surgery. The spiral helps to prevent the kinking and occlusion of the tracheal tube when the head and/or neck is rotated or flexed. An introducer stylet is used to aid intubation.

Because of the spiral, it is not possible to cut the tube to the desired length. This increases the risk of bronchial intubation. Two markers, situated just above the cuff, are present on some designs. These indicate the correct position for the vocal cords.

POLAR AND RAE TRACHEAL TUBES

The **Polar tube** is a north- or south-facing preformed nasal cuffed or uncuffed tracheal tube (Fig. 5.11). It is used mainly during anaesthesia for maxillofacial surgery as it does not impede surgical access. Because of its design and shape, it lies over the nose and the forehead. It can be converted to an ordinary tracheal tube by cutting it at the scissors mark just proximal to the pilot tube and reconnecting the 15 mm connector. An oral version of the Polar tube exists.

The **RAE (Ring, Adair and Elwyn) tube** has a preformed shape to fit the mouth or nose without kinking. It has a bend located just as the tube emerges, so the connections to the breathing system are at the level of the chin or forehead and not interfering with the surgical access. RAE tubes can be either north- or south-facing, cuffed or uncuffed (Fig. 5.11).

Because of its preformed shape, there is a higher risk of bronchial intubation than with ordinary tracheal tubes. The cuffed RAE tracheal tube has one Murphy eye whereas the uncuffed version has two eyes (Fig. 5.12). Since the uncuffed version is mainly used in paediatric practice, two Murphy eyes ensure adequate ventilation should the tube prove too long.

The tube can be temporarily straightened to insert a suction catheter.

LASER RESISTANT TRACHEAL TUBE

This tube is used in anaesthesia for laser surgery on the larynx or trachea (Fig. 5.13). It is designed to withstand the effect of carbon dioxide and KTP laser beams, avoiding the risk of fire or damage

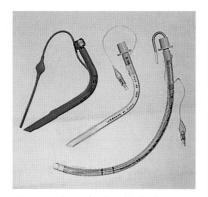

Fig. 5.10 The Oxford tracheal tube, red rubber (left) and plastic (centre), an armoured tracheal tube mounted on an introducer (right).

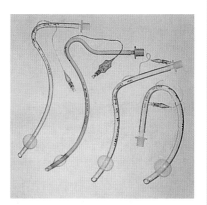

Fig. 5.11 Cuffed oral RAE tracheal tubes. Cuffed north-facing nasal RAE tube (far left), Portex polar nasal tube (centre left), north-facing oral RAE (centre right) and south-facing oral RAE (far right).

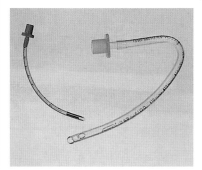

Fig. 5.12 Uncuffed paediatric tracheal tubes. A 3 mm ID tracheal tube fitted with an 8.5 mm connector (left) and a 6 mm ID south-facing RAE tracheal tube with two Murphy eyes (right).

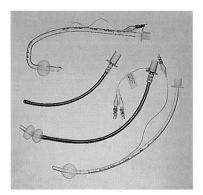

Fig. 5.13 A laryngectomy tube (top), uncuffed and double cuffed laser resistant tracheal tubes (centre) and a microlaryngeal tube (bottom).

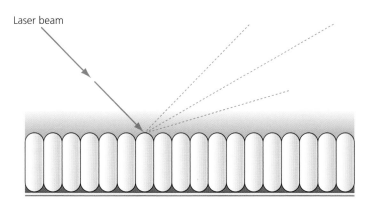

Laser beam

Fig. 5.14 The reflected laser beam is defocused.

to the tracheal tube. It has a flexible stainless steel body. Reflected beams from the tube are defocused to reduce the accidental laser strikes to healthy tissues (Fig. 5.14).

Some designs have two cuffs. This ensures a tracheal seal should the upper cuff be damaged by laser. An airfilled cuff, hit by the laser beam, may ignite and so it is recommended that the cuffs are filled with saline instead of air.

MICROLARYNGEAL TUBE

This tube allows better exposure and surgical access to the larynx. It has a small diameter (usually 5 mm ID) with an adult sized cuff (Fig. 5.13). Its length is sufficient to allow nasal intubation if required. The tube is made of ivory PVC to reduce trauma to the nasal mucosa.

Tracheostomy tracheal tubes

These are curved plastic tubes usually inserted through the second, third and fourth tracheal cartilage rings (Fig. 5.15).

Components

1. An introducer used for insertion.
2. Wings attached to the proximal part of the tube to fix it in place with a ribbon or suture. Some designs have an adjustable flange to fit the variable thickness of the subcutaneous tissues.
3. They can be cuffed or uncuffed.
4. The proximal end can have a standard 15 mm connector.
5. The tip is usually cut square, rather than bevelled. This is to decrease the risk of obstruction by lying against the tracheal wall.

6. A more recent design with an additional suctioning lumen which opens just above the cuff exists. The cuff shape is designed to allow the secretions above it to be suctioned effectively through the suctioning lumen (Fig. 5.16).
7. Some tubes have an inner cannula. Secretions can collect and dry out on the inner lumen of the tube leading to obstruction. The internal cannula can be replaced instead of changing the complete tube in such cases. The cannula leads to a slight

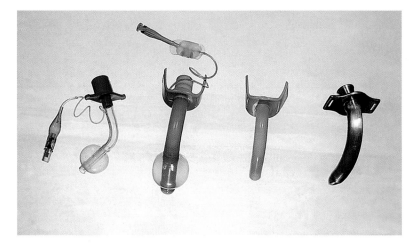

Fig. 5.15 A selection of tracheostomy tubes. Paediatric cuffed (left), adult cuffed (centre left) and uncuffed (centre right) tracheostomy tubes. A silver tracheostomy tube (right).

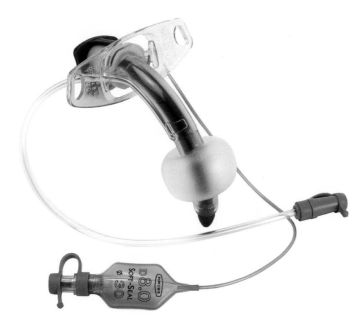

Fig. 5.16 Smith's Portex tracheostomy tube with an above-cuff suction facility.

reduction of the internal diameter of the tube.

8. There are different sizes of tracheostomy tubes to fit neonates to adults.

Tracheostomy tubes are used for the following

1. Long-term intermittent positive pressure ventilation.
2. Upper airway obstruction that cannot be bypassed with an oral/nasal tracheal tube.
3. Maintenance of an airway and to protect the lungs in patients with impaired pharyngeal or laryngeal reflexes and after major head and neck surgery (e.g. laryngectomy).
4. Long-term control of excessive bronchial secretions especially in patients with a reduced level of consciousness.
5. To facilitate weaning from a ventilator. This is due to a reduction in the sedation required, as the patients tolerate tracheostomy tubes better than tracheal tubes. Also, there is a reduction in the anatomical dead space.

> **Benefits of tracheostomy**
>
> - Increased patient comfort
> - Less need for sedation
> - Improved access for oral hygiene
> - Possibility of oral nutrition
> - Bronchial suctioning aided
> - Reduced dead space
> - Reduced airway resistance
> - Reduced risk of glottic trauma

Problems in practice and safety features

Surgical tracheostomy has a mortality rate of <1% but has a total complications rate as high as 40%. The complications rate is higher in the ICU and emergency patients.

The complications can be divided into

1. Immediate
   a) haemorrhage
   b) tube misplacement (e.g. into a main bronchus)
   c) occlusion of tube by cuff herniation
   d) occlusion of the tube tip against carina or tracheal wall
   e) pneumothorax.

2. Delayed
   a) blockage of the tube by secretions which can be sudden or gradual; this is rare with adequate humidification and suction
   b) infection of the stoma
   c) overinflation of the cuff leads to ulceration and distension of the trachea
   d) mucosal ulceration because of excessive cuff pressures, asymmetrical inflation of the cuff or tube migration.

3. Late
   a) granulomata of the trachea may cause respiratory difficulty after extubation
   b) persistent sinus at the tracheostomy site
   c) tracheal dilatation
   d) tracheal stenosis at the cuff site
   e) scar formation.

THE FENESTRATED TRACHEOSTOMY TUBE (FIG. 5.17)

1. The fenestration (window) in the greater curvature channels air to the vocal cords allowing the patient to speak.

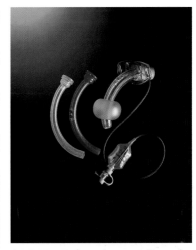

Fig. 5.17 A Portex unfenestrated inner cannula (left), fenestrated inner cannula (middle) and Blue Line Ultra fenestrated tracheostomy tube with Soft-Seal cuff (right).

2. After deflation of the cuff, the patient can breathe around the cuff and through the fenestration as well as through the stoma. This reduces airway resistance and assists in weaning from tracheostomy in spontaneously breathing patients.
3. Some tubes have a fenestrated inner cannula.

METAL TRACHEOSTOMY TUBES (FIG. 5.15)

1. These tubes are used in patients needing longer term intubation.
2. They are made of a non-irritant and bactericidal silver.
3. They are uncuffed.
4. They have an inner tube which can be removed for cleaning at regular intervals.
5. Some designs have a one-way flap valve and a window at the angle of the tube to allow the patient to speak.

LARYNGECTOMY (MONTANDON) TUBE

This is a cuffed tube inserted through a tracheostome to facilitate intermittent positive pressure ventilation during surgery (Fig. 5.13). It has the advantage of offering better surgical access by allowing the breathing system to be connected well away from the surgical field.

Tracheostomy tubes

- Can be plastic or metal, cuffed or uncuffed.
- The tip is cut horizontally.
- Used for long term intubation.
- Percutaneous tracheostomy tubes are becoming more popular and have fewer complications than the surgical technique.
- Speaking versions exist.

TRACHEOSTOMY SPEAKING VALVE (FIG. 5.18)

This is a one-way speaking valve. It is fitted to the uncuffed tracheostomy tube or to the cuffed tracheostomy tube with its cuff deflated.

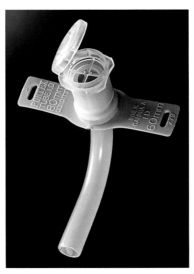

Fig. 5.18 A tracheostomy speaking valve mounted on an uncuffed tracheostomy tube.

PERCUTANEOUS TRACHEOSTOMY TUBES (FIGS 5.19 AND 5.20)

These tubes are inserted between the 1st and 2nd or 2nd and 3rd tracheal rings, usually at the bedside in ITU.

1. If the patient is intubated, the tracheal tube is withdrawn until the tip is just below the vocal cords. Then the cuff is inflated and rested on the vocal cords. A laryngeal mask can be used instead.
2. Through an introducing needle, a Seldinger guidewire is inserted into the trachea. A fibreoptic bronchoscope should be used throughout the procedure. It helps to ensure the initial puncture of the trachea is in the midline and free of the tracheal tube. It can also ensure that the posterior tracheal wall is not damaged during the procedure. Finally, it can assess the position of the tracheostomy tube relative to the carina.
3. A pair of specially designed Griggs forceps are inserted over

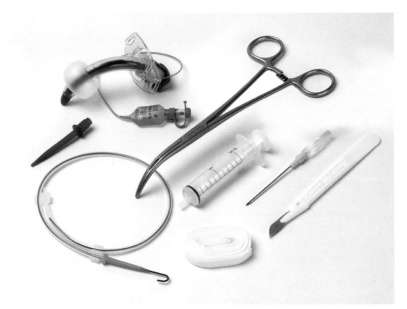

Fig. 5.19 Smith's Portex Griggs percutaneous tracheostomy set.

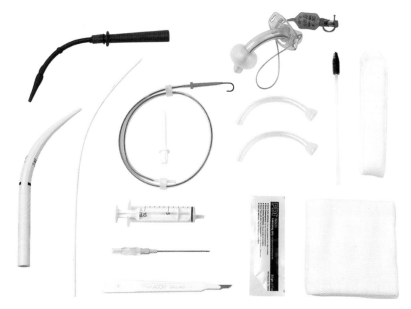

Fig. 5.20 Smith's Portex Ultraperc single dilator percutaneous tracheostomy set.

A track is formed after long-term intubation and the tracheostomy tube can be removed. In order to protect the patency of the tract, a tracheostomy button is inserted into the stoma. It also acts as a route for tracheal suction. Tracheostomy buttons are made of straight rigid plastic.

Minitracheostomy tube

This tube is inserted percutaneously into the trachea through the avascular cricothyroid membrane (Fig. 5.21).

Components

1. A siliconized PVC tube 10 cm in length with an internal diameter of 4 mm. Some designs have lengths ranging from 3.5 to 7.5 cm with internal diameters from 2 to 6 mm.
2. The proximal end of the tube has a standard 15 mm connector that allows attachment to breathing systems. The proximal end also has wings used to secure the tube with the ribbon supplied.
3. A 2 cm, 16 G needle is used to puncture the cricothyroid cartilage. A 50 cm guidewire

the guidewire. These forceps are used to dilate the trachea. A tracheostomy tube is threaded over the guidewire and advanced into the trachea. The guidewire is then removed (Fig. 5.19).
4. A series of curved dilators can be used instead of the dilating forceps. The diameter of the stoma is serially increased until the desired diameter is achieved. A single curved dilator of a graduated diameter can be used instead (Fig. 5.20). A tracheostomy tube can then be inserted.
5. An adjustable flange percutaneous tracheostomy is available. The flange can be adjusted to suit the patient's anatomy, e.g. in the obese patient. The flange can be moved away from the stoma site to aid in cleaning around the stoma.
6. The procedure can be performed in ITU with a lower incidence of complications than the conventional open surgical method (infection rate, subglottic stenosis and bleeding problems). The operative time

is about half that of a formal surgical procedure.
7. Percutaneous tracheostomy can be performed faster using the dilating forceps technique compared to the dilator technique.
8. There is an increased risk of surgical emphysema due to air leaks from the trachea to the surrounding tissues. Loss of the airway, bleeding and incorrect placement of the needle are potential difficulties during the procedure. The risk of aspiration is increased when the tracheal tube has to be withdrawn at the start of the procedure.
9. Relative contraindications include enlarged thyroid gland, non-palpable cricoid cartilage, paediatric application, previous neck surgery and PEEP of more than 15 cmH$_2$O. The latter is because of the difficulty in applying a high PEEP during the process of insertion.
10. Re-insertion of a percutaneously fashioned tube can be more difficult than the surgical one as the stoma may close immediately.

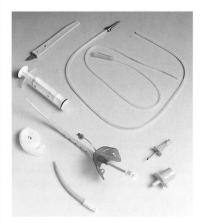

Fig. 5.21 The Portex minitracheostomy set inserted using the Seldinger technique.

is used to help in the tracheal cannulation. A 10 mL syringe is used to aspirate air to confirm the correct placement of the needle.

4. A 7 cm curved dilator and a curved introducer are used to facilitate the insertion of the cricothyrotomy tube in some designs.

Mechanism of action

1. The Seldinger technique is used to insert the tube.
2. It is an effective method to clear tracheobronchial secretions in patients with an inefficient cough.
3. In an emergency, it can be used in patients with upper airway obstruction that cannot be bypassed with a tracheal tube.

Problems in practice and safety features

Percutaneous insertion of minitracheostomy has the risk of:

1. Pneumothorax.
2. Perforation of the oesophagus.
3. Severe haemorrhage.
4. Ossification of the cricothyroid membrane.
5. Incorrect placement.

Minitracheostomy

● Tube inserted into the trachea through the cricothyroid membrane using the Seldinger technique.
● Used for clearing secretions and maintaining an airway in an emergency.

Cricothyrotomy tube (Fig. 5.22)

This tube is used to maintain the airway in emergency situations such as on the battlefield. It is inserted into the trachea through the cricothyroid cartilage.

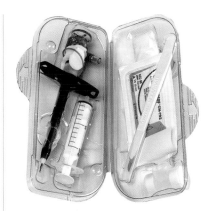

Fig. 5.22 Smith's Portex cricothyrotomy set.

Components

1. A scalpel and syringe
2. A needle with a veress design and a dilator. The needle has a 'red flag' indicator. This helps in locating the tissues.
3. 6 mm cuffed tube.

Mechanism of action

1. After a 2 cm horizontal skin incision has been made, the needle is inserted perpendicular to the skin.
2. As the needle enters the trachea, the red indicator disappears. The needle is advanced carefully until the red reappears, indicating contact with the posterior wall of the trachea.
3. As the cricothyrotomy tube is advanced into the trachea, the needle and the dilator are removed.

Problems in practice and safety features

The cricothyrotomy tube has complications similar to the minitracheostomy tube.

Cricothyrotomy

● A cuffed 6 mm tube is inserted into the trachea through the cricothyroid cartilage.
● A veress needle is designed to locate the trachea.
● Used in emergencies to establish an airway.

Double lumen endobronchial tubes

During thoracic surgery there is a need for one lung to be deflated. This offers the surgeon easier and better access within the designated hemithorax. In order to achieve this, double lumen tubes are used which allow the anaesthetist to selectively deflate one lung whilst maintaining standard ventilation of the other.

Components

1. The Mallinckrodt Bronchocath double lumen tube has two separate colour-coded lumens, each with its own bevel (Fig. 5.23). One lumen ends in the trachea and the other lumen ends in either the left or right main bronchus.
2. Each lumen has its own cuff (tracheal and bronchial cuffs) and colour-coded pilot balloons. Both lumens and pilot balloons are labelled.
3. There are two curves to the tube: the standard anterior curve to fit into the oropharyngeal laryngeal tracheal airway and the second curve, either to the right or left, to fit into the right or left bronchus respectively.
4. The proximal end of these tubes is connected to a Y-shaped catheter mount attached to the breathing system.

Mechanism of action

1. Because of the differing anatomy of the main bronchi and their branches, both right and left versions of any particular double lumen tube must exist.
2. Once the tubes are correctly positioned, the anaesthetist can selectively ventilate one lung. So, for operations requiring that the right lung is deflated, a left-sided

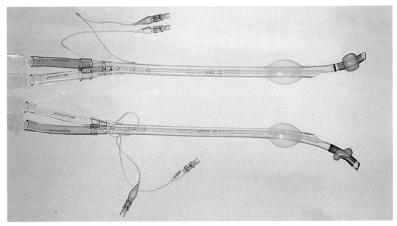

Fig. 5.23 Bronchocath double lumen tubes. Left-sided (top), right-sided (bottom).

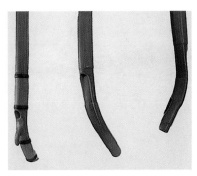

Fig. 5.24 White double lumen tube with carinal hook (left). Left and right versions of the Robertshaw double lumen tube (centre and right).

double lumen tube would be used that enabled selective ventilation of the left lung alone and vice versa.

3. It is desirable, when possible, to insert a left double lumen tube instead of a right one. This reduces the risk of upper lobe bronchus obstruction by the bronchial cuff in the right-sided version.

4. The right-sided version has an eye in the bronchial cuff to facilitate ventilation of the right upper lobe. The distance between the right upper lobe bronchus and the carina in an adult is only 2.5 cm, so there is a real risk of occluding it with the bronchial cuff. There is no eye in the left-sided version because the distance between the carina and the left upper lobe bronchus is about 5 cm, which is adequate to place the cuff.

5. The tubes come in different sizes to fit adult patients, but not in paediatric sizes.

Tube positioning

1. The position of the tube should be checked by auscultation immediately after intubation and after positioning the patient for the operation. It is also recommended to use a fibreoptic bronchoscope to confirm correct positioning of the double lumen tube.

2. The tracheal cuff is inflated first until no leak is heard. At this point, both lungs can be ventilated. Next, the tracheal limb of the Y-catheter mount is clamped and disconnected from the tracheal lumen tube. Then, the bronchial cuff is inflated with only a few millilitres of air until no leak is heard from the tracheal tube. At this stage only the lung ventilated via the bronchial lumen should be ventilated. The ability to selectively ventilate the other lung should also be checked by clamping the bronchial limb of the Y-catheter mount and disconnecting it from the bronchial lumen having already reconnected the tracheal lumen. At this stage only the lung ventilated via the tracheal lumen should be ventilated.

The commonly used double lumen bronchial tubes are:

1. **Robertshaw** (rubber) tubes (Fig. 5.24).

2. **Single use plastic** tubes. These tubes require an introducer for insertion. A more recent version of the single use has the facility of applying CPAP to the deflated lung to improve arterial oxygenation (Fig. 5.25).

3. **Carlens** (left-sided version) and **White** (right-sided version) tubes that use a carinal hook to aid final positioning of the tube (Fig. 5.24). The hook can cause trauma to the larynx or carina. Because of the relatively small lumens (6 and 8 mm), the Carlens tube causes an increase in airway resistance and difficulty in suctioning thick secretions.

Double lumen endobronchial tubes

- Two separate lumens each with its own cuff and pilot tube.
- There are two curves, anterior and lateral.
- The right-sided version has an eye in the bronchial cuff to facilitate ventilation of the right upper lobe.
- Commonly used ones are Robertshaw, Bronchocath and Carlens (and White). The latter has a carinal hook.

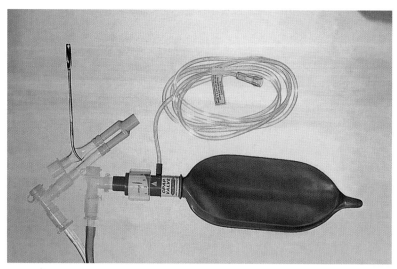

Fig. 5.25 Bronchocath double lumen tube with the bronchial lumen connected to a CPAP valve assembly. The disconnected limb of the Y-shaped catheter mount has been clamped.

Endobronchial blocker

The endobronchial blocker is an alternative means to the double lumen tube for providing one-lung ventilation (Fig. 5.26).

Components

1. The blocker catheter. This is a 9 FG, 78 cm catheter that has a distal cuff inflated via a pilot balloon. A guide loop emerges from its tip (Fig. 5.27).
2. Multiport adapter.

Mechanism of action

The patient is intubated with a standard endotracheal tube. A specially designed multiport adapter is connected to the tube's standard 15 mm connector. The blocker can be advanced over a paediatric fibreoptic bronchoscope into the desired main bronchus whilst maintaining ventilation.

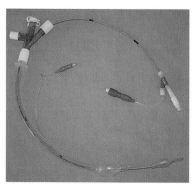

Fig. 5.26 The Arndt endobronchial blocker set.

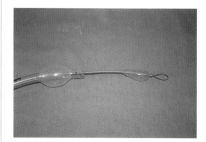

Fig. 5.27 Detail of the blocker emerging from a standard endotracheal tube. The guide loop is used to advance the blocker over a paediatric fibreoptic bronchoscope into the desired main bronchus.

When the blocker's position is satisfactory, the balloon can be inflated, sealing off the desired main bronchus. Ventilation of the contralateral lung is maintained via the tracheal tube.

Oropharyngeal airway

This anatomically shaped airway is inserted through the mouth into the oropharynx above the tongue to maintain the patency of the upper airway (Fig. 5.28).

Components

1. The curved body of the oropharyngeal airway contains the air channel. It is flattened anteroposteriorly and curved laterally.
2. There is a flange at the oral end to prevent the oropharyngeal airway from falling back into the mouth.
3. The bite portion is straight and fits between the teeth. It is made of hard plastic to prevent occlusion of the air channel should the patient bite the oropharyngeal airway.

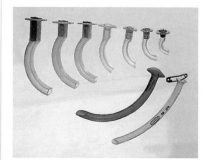

Fig. 5.28 A range of oropharyngeal (Guedel) airways (top) and nasopharyngeal airways (bottom). The safety pin is to prevent the airway from migrating into the nose.

Mechanism of action

1. The patient's airway is kept patent by preventing the tongue and epiglottis from falling backwards.
2. Oropharyngeal airways are designed in different sizes to fit the majority of patients from neonates to adults.
3. The air channel should be as large as possible in order to pass suction catheters.

Problems in practice and safety features

1. Trauma to the different tissues during insertion.
2. Trauma to the teeth, crowns/caps if the patient bites on it.
3. If inserted in a patient whose pharyngeal reflexes are not depressed enough, the gag reflex and vomiting can occur.

Oropharyngeal airway

- Anatomically shaped.
- Inserted through the mouth above the tongue into the oropharynx.
- Maintains the patency of the upper airway.
- Can cause trauma and injury to different structures.
- Risk of gag reflex stimulation and vomiting.

Nasopharyngeal airway

This airway is inserted through the nose into the nasopharynx, bypassing the mouth and the oropharynx. The distal end is just above the epiglottis and below the base of the tongue (Fig. 5.28).

Components

1. The rounded curved body of the nasopharyngeal airway.
2. The bevel is left-facing.
3. The proximal end has a flange. A 'safety pin' is provided to prevent the airway from migrating into the nose.

Mechanism of action

1. It is an alternative to the oropharyngeal airway when the mouth cannot be opened or an oral airway does not relieve the obstruction.
2. Nasotracheal suction can be performed using a catheter passed through the nasal airway.
3. It is better tolerated by semi-awake patients than the oral airway.
4. A lubricant is used to help in its insertion.

Problems in practice and safety features

1. Its use is not recommended when the patient has a bleeding disorder, is on anticoagulants, has nasal deformities or sepsis
2. Excess force should not be used during insertion as a false passage may be created.

Nasopharyngeal airway

- Inserted through the nose into the nasopharynx.
- A useful alternative to the oropharyngeal airway.
- Not recommended in coagulopathy, nasal sepsis and deformities.

Laryngeal mask

This very useful device is frequently used as an alternative to either the face mask or tracheal tube during anaesthesia (Fig. 5.29).

Components

1. A transparent tube of wide internal diameter. The proximal end is a standard 15 mm connection.
2. An elliptical cuff at the distal end. The cuff resembles a small face mask and is inflated via a pilot balloon with a self-sealing valve. A non-metallic self-sealing valve is available for use during MRI scans.
3. Some designs have two slits or bars at the junction between the tube and the cuff to prevent the epiglottis from obstructing the lumen of the laryngeal mask. Newer designs omit the bars with no adverse clinical effects.
4. A more recent design (LMA-ProSeal) has a double lumen (Fig. 5.30). One lumen leads to the cuff for ventilation (as in the conventional design). The second lumen (drain tube) ends at the distal end of the cuff. The drain tube opens at the oesophageal sphincter allowing blind passage of an oro-gastric tube and helps in the drainage of gastric air or secretions.
5. Recently low cost disposable laryngeal masks have been introduced and widely used (Fig. 5.31).

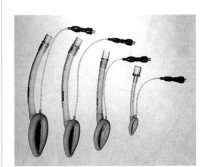

Fig. 5.29 A range of different sized laryngeal masks (non-reinforced).

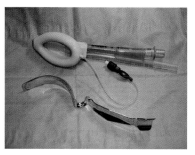

Fig. 5.30 The LMA-ProSeal. Note the additional lumen for placement of a gastric drainage tube.

Table 5.2 The recommended sizes and cuff inflation volumes

	Size of patient	Cuff inflation volume
Size 1	Neonates, infants up to 5 kg	up to 4 mL
Size 1½	Infants 5–10 kg	up to 7 mL
Size 2	Infants/children 10–20 kg	up to 10 mL
Size 2½	Children 20–30 kg	up to 14 mL
Size 3	Paediatric 30–50 kg	up to 20 mL
Size 4	Adult 50–70 kg	up to 30 mL
Size 5	Adult 70–100 kg	up to 40 mL
Size 6	Large adult over 100 kg	up to 60 mL

Mechanism of action

1. The cuff is deflated and lubricated before use. It is inserted through the mouth. The cuff lies over the larynx.
2. Once the cuff in position, it is inflated (Table 5.2).
3. Partial inflation of the cuff before insertion is used by some anaesthetists.
4. The laryngeal masks have wide internal diameters in order to reduce the flow resistance to a minimum (e.g. the internal diameters of sizes 2, 3, 4 and 5 are 7, 10, 10 and 11.5 mm respectively). This makes them suitable for long procedures using a spontaneous ventilation technique.
5. It also has a role as an aid in difficult intubation. Once in position, it can be used to introduce a bougie or a narrow lumen tracheal tube into the trachea. Alternatively, the laryngeal mask may be used to guide passage of a fibreoptic bronchoscope into the trachea, thus allowing intubation of the trachea.

The **reinforced version** of the laryngeal masks is used for head and neck surgery (Fig. 5.32).

1. The tubes, although flexible, are kink and crush resistant, because of a stainless steel wire spiral in their wall. The tube can be moved during surgery without loss of the cuff's seal against the larynx. The breathing system can easily be connected at any angle from the mouth.
2. A throat pack can be used with the reinforced version.
3. The reinforced laryngeal masks have smaller internal diameters and longer lengths than the standard versions, causing an

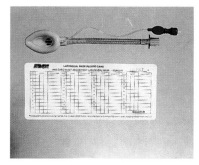

Fig. 5.32 A reinforced laryngeal mask with its autoclaving record card.

increase in flow resistance. This makes their use with spontaneous ventilation for prolonged periods less suitable.

The recommended safety checks before the use of laryngeal masks

1. Inflate the cuff and look for signs of herniation.
2. Check that the lumen of the tube is patent.
3. The tube can be bent to 180° without kinking or occlusion.

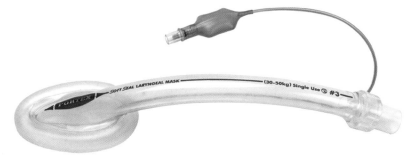

Fig. 5.31 Smith's Portex single use Soft Seal laryngeal mask.

THE INTUBATING LARYNGEAL MASK AIRWAY

This is a recent modification of the laryngeal mask designed to facilitate tracheal intubation with a tracheal tube. The specially designed laryngeal mask is inserted first (Fig. 5.33). A specially designed tracheal tube is then passed, blindly, through the laryngeal mask through the vocal cords into the trachea (Fig. 5.34).

Problems in practice and safety features

1. The laryngeal mask does not protect against the aspiration of gastric contents.
2. Despite the presence of the slits or bars, about 10% of patients develop airway obstruction because of down-folding of the epiglottis. Although clinically often insignificant, a higher proportion of obstructions by the epiglottis can be observed endoscopically.
3. The manufacturers recommend using the laryngeal masks for a maximum of 40 times. The cuff is likely to perish after autoclaving. A record card that accompanies

the laryngeal mask registers the number of autoclaving episodes.
4. Unlike the tracheal tube, rotation of the laryngeal mask may result in complete airway obstruction. In order to assess the laryngeal mask's orientation when inserted, a black line is present on the tube. This should face the upper lip of the patient when the laryngeal mask is in position.
5. Cricoid pressure may prevent correct placement of the laryngeal mask.

Currently there is a trend to use disposable single use laryngeal masks. These can be termed 'supra-glottic airway devices'. Some have similar designs to the original Classic LMA such as Portex Soft Seal, Intavent Unique and Marshall laryngeal masks. Some have different designs such as the Ambu laryngeal mask and the Cobra airway device. Their clinical performance is similar to the original Classic LMA with some achieving even better results and with less trauma. They are made of PVC apart from the Marshall airway device, which is made of silicone rubber.

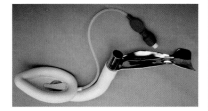

Fig. 5.33 The Intubating LMA.

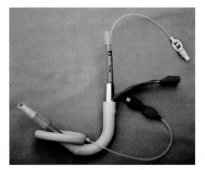

Fig 5.34 The Intubating LMA.

FURTHER READING

Brimacombe J. Laryngeal Mask Anesthesia: Principles and Practice, 2nd edn. Philadelphia: WB Saunders, 2004.

Gothard JWW. Anaesthetic equipment for thoracic surgery. Anaesthesia and Intensive Care Medicine 2005; 6(12):425–427.

Laryngeal masks

- Used instead of face masks or tracheal tubes during spontaneous and controlled ventilation.
- Can be used as an aid in difficult intubation.
- The reinforced version can be used for head and neck surgery.
- Does not protect against aspiration.
- The intubating laryngeal mask airway allows blind tracheal intubation.

MCQs

In the following lists, which of the statements (a) to (e) are true?

1. Concerning tracheal tubes
   a) The RAE tracheal tube is ideal for microlaryngeal surgery.
   b) Pre-formed tracheal tubes have a higher risk of bronchial intubation.
   c) Laryngeal masks can be used in nasal surgery.
   d) RAE tubes stand for *Reinforced Anaesthetic Endotracheal* tubes.
   e) The Oxford tracheal tube has a left-facing bevel.

2. Laryngeal masks
   a) They can prevent aspiration of gastric contents.
   b) The bars at the junction of the cuff and the tube prevent foreign bodies from entering the trachea.
   c) Because of its large internal diameter, it can be used in spontaneously breathing patients for long periods of time.
   d) It can be autoclaved used repeatedly for an unlimited number of times.
   e) The standard design can be used in MRI.

3. Double lumen endobronchial tubes
   a) Robertshaw double lumen tubes have carinal hooks.
   b) The left-sided tubes have an eye in the bronchial cuff to facilitate ventilation of the left upper lobe.
   c) Carlens double lumen tubes have relatively small lumens.
   d) CPAP can be applied to the deflated lung to improve oxygenation.
   e) Fibreoptic bronchoscopy can be used to ensure correct positioning of the tube.

4. Concerning the tracheal tube cuff during anaesthesia
   a) Low pressure/high volume cuffs prevent aspiration of gastric contents.
   b) The intra-cuff pressure can rise significantly because of the diffusion of the anaesthetic inhalational vapour.
   c) High pressure/low volume cuffs may cause necrosis of the tracheal mucosa if left in position for long periods.
   d) Low volume cuffs have a smaller contact area with the tracheal wall than high volume cuffs.
   e) The pressure in the cuff may decrease because of the diffusion of nitrous oxide.

5. Concerning tracheal tubes
   a) The ID diameter is measured in centimetres.
   b) Red rubber tubes never have cuffs.
   c) Armoured tubes need to be cut to length.
   d) Tubes should have a Murphy eye to allow suction.
   e) The tip is cut square.

Answers

1. Concerning tracheal tubes
   a) *False. A RAE tube is a normal size preformed tracheal tube. It does not allow good visibility of the larynx because of its large diameter. A microlaryngeal tracheal tube of 5–6 mm ID is more suitable for microlaryngeal surgery, allowing good visibility and access to the larynx.*
   b) *True. Because the shape of these tubes is fixed, they might not fit all patients of different sizes and shapes; e.g. a small, short-necked patient having a RAE tube inserted is at risk of an endobronchial tube position.*
   c) *True. Some anaesthetists use the laryngeal mask in nasal surgery with a throat pack. This technique has a higher risk of aspiration.*
   d) *False. RAE stands for the initials of the designers (Ring, Adair and Elwyn).*
   e) *False. The Oxford tube is one of the few tracheal tubes with a front-facing bevel. This might make intubation more difficult as it obscures the larynx.*

2. Laryngeal masks
   a) *False. Laryngeal masks do not protect the airway from the risks of aspiration.*
   b) *False. The bars in the cuff are designed to prevent the epiglottis from blocking the lumen of the tube.*
   c) *True. The laryngeal mask has a large internal diameter, in comparison with a tracheal tube. This reduces the resistance to breathing which is of more importance during spontaneous breathing. This makes the laryngeal mask more suitable for use in spontaneously breathing patients for long periods of time.*
   d) *False. The laryngeal mask can be autoclaved up to forty times. The cuff is likely to perish after repeated autoclaving. A record should be kept of the number of autoclaves.*
   e) *False. The standard laryngeal mask has a metal component in the one-way inflating valve. This makes it unsuitable for use in MRI. A specially designed laryngeal mask with no metal parts is available for MRI use.*

3. Double lumen endobronchial tubes
   a) *False. The Robertshaw double lumen tube does not have a carinal hook. The Carlens double lumen tube has a carinal hook.*
   b) *False. Left-sided tubes do not have an eye in the bronchial cuff to facilitate ventilation of the left upper lobe. This is because the distance between the carina and the upper lobe bronchus is about 5 cm, which is enough for the bronchial cuff. Right-sided tubes have an eye to facilitate ventilation of the right upper lobe because the distance between the carina and the upper lobe bronchus is only 2.5 cm.*
   c) *True. Carlens double lumen tubes have relatively small lumens in comparison to the Robertshaw double lumen tube.*
   d) *True. CPAP can be applied to the deflated lung to improve oxygenation during one lung anaesthesia.*
   e) *True. It is sometimes difficult to ensure correct positioning of the double lumen endobronchial tube. By using a fibreoptic bronchoscope, the position of the tube can be adjusted to ensure correct positioning.*

4. Concerning the tracheal tube cuff during anaesthesia

   a) *False. The design of the low pressure high volume cuff allows wrinkles to be formed around the tracheal wall. The presence of the wrinkles allows aspiration of gastric contents to occur.*

   b) *False. The rise in the intra-cuff pressure is mainly due to the diffusion of N_2O. Minimal changes are due to diffusion of oxygen (from 21% to say 33%) and because of increase in the temperature of the air in the cuff (from 21° to 37°C). The diffusion of inhalational agents causes minimal changes in pressure due to the low concentrations used (1–2%). New design material cuffs prevent the diffusion of gases thus preventing significant changes in pressure.*

   c) *True. The high pressures achieved by the high pressure/low volume cuffs, especially during nitrous oxide anaesthesia, can cause necrosis to the mucosa of the trachea if left in position for a long period.*

   d) *True. Because of the design of the low volume cuffs, a seal can be maintained against a relatively small area of the tracheal wall. In the case of the high volume/low pressure cuffs, a large contact area on the tracheal wall is achieved.*

   e) *False. The pressure in the cuff may decrease because of a leak in the cuff or pilot balloon's valve.*

5. Concerning tracheal tubes

   a) *False. The ID is measured in millimetres.*

   b) *False.*

   c) *False. An armoured tube should not be cut, as that will cut the spiral present in its wall. This increases the risk of tube kinking.*

   d) *False. A Murphy eye allows pulmonary ventilation in the situation where the bevel of the tube is occluded.*

   e) *False. The bevel of the tube is usually left-facing to allow easier visualization of the vocal cords. The tracheostomy tube has a square-cut tip.*

Chapter 6

Masks and oxygen delivery devices

Face masks and angle pieces

The face mask is designed to fit the face anatomically. It comes in different sizes to fit patients of different age groups (from neonates to adults). It is connected to the breathing system via the angle piece.

Components

1. The body of the mask which rests on an airfilled cuff (Fig. 6.1). Some paediatric designs do not have a cuff, e.g. Rendell–Baker (Fig. 6.2).
2. The proximal end of the mask has a 22 mm inlet connection to the angle piece.
3. Some designs have clamps for a harness to be attached.
4. The angle piece has a 90° bend with a 22 mm end to fit into a catheter mount or a breathing system.

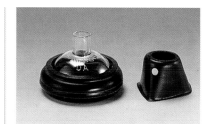

Fig. 6.2 Paediatric face masks. Ambu design (left) and Rendell–Baker design (right).

Mechanism of action

1. They can be made of silicon rubber or transparent plastic. The latter allows the detection of vomitus or secretions. It is also more acceptable to the patient during inhalational induction. Some masks are 'flavoured', e.g. strawberry flavour.
2. The air-filled cuff helps to ensure a snug fit over the face. It also helps to minimize the mask's pressure on the face.
3. The design of the interior of the mask determines the size of

its contribution to apparatus dead space. The dead space may increase by up to 200 mL in adults.

Problems in practice and safety features

1. Excessive pressure by the mask may cause injury to the branches of the trigeminal or facial nerves.
2. Sometimes it is difficult to achieve an air-tight seal over the face. Edentulous patients and those with nasogastric tubes pose particular problems.

F.

- ... licone rubber or plastic.
- Their design ensures a snug fit over the face of the patient.
- Cause an increase in dead space (up to 200 mL in adults).

Nasal masks (inhalers)

1. These masks are used during dental chair anaesthesia.
2. An example is the Goldman inhaler (Fig. 6.3) which has an inflatable cuff to fit the face and an APL valve at the proximal end. The mask is connected to tubing which delivers the fresh gas flow.
3. Other designs have an inlet for delivering the inspired fresh gas flow and an outlet connected to tubing with a unidirectional valve for expired gases.

Catheter mount

This is the flexible link between the breathing system tubing and the tracheal tube, face mask, laryngeal mask or tracheostomy tube

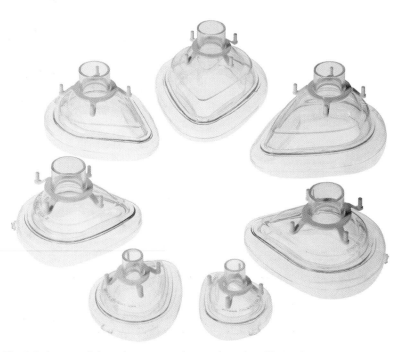

Fig. 6.1 A range of sizes of transparent face masks with airfilled cuffs.

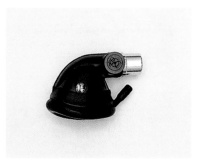

Fig. 6.3 The Goldman nasal inhaler.

(Fig. 6.4). The length of the catheter mount varies from 45 to 170 mm.

Components

1. A corrugated disposable plastic or rubber tubing. Some catheter mounts have a concertina design allowing their length to be adjusted.
2. The distal end is connected to either a 15 mm standard tracheal tube connector, usually in the shape of an angle piece, or a 22 mm mask fitting.
3. The proximal end has a 22 mm connector for attachment to the breathing system.
4. Some designs have a condenser humidifier built into them.
5. A gas sampling port is found in some designs.

Mechanism of action

1. The mount minimizes the transmission of accidental

movements of the breathing system to the tracheal tube. Repeated movements of the tracheal tube can cause injury to the tracheal mucosa.
2. Some designs allow for suction or the introduction of a fibreoptic bronchoscope. This is done via a special port.

Problems in practice and safety features

1. The catheter mount contributes to the apparatus dead space. This is of particular importance in paediatric anaesthesia. The concertina design allows adjustment of the dead space from 25 to 60 mL.
2. Foreign bodies can lodge inside the catheter mount causing an unnoticed blockage of the breathing system. To minimize this risk, the catheter mount should remain wrapped in its sterile packaging until needed.

Catheter mount

- Acts as an adapter between the tracheal tube and breathing system in addition to stabilizing the tracheal tube.
- Can be made of rubber or plastic with different lengths.
- Some have a condenser humidifier built in.
- Its length contributes to the apparatus dead space.
- Can be blocked by a foreign body.

Oxygen delivery devices

Currently, a variety of delivery devices are used. These devices differ in their ability to deliver a set fractional inspired oxygen concentration (FiO_2). The delivery devices can be divided into variable and fixed performance devices. The former devices deliver a fluctuating FiO_2 whereas the latter devices deliver a more constant and predictable FiO_2 (Table 6.1). The FiO_2 delivered to the patient is dependent on device and patient related factors. The FiO_2 delivered can be calculated by measuring the end-tidal oxygen fraction in the nasopharynx using oxygraphy.

Variable performance masks (medium concentration MC)

These masks are used to deliver oxygen-enriched air to the patient (Fig. 6.5). They are also called *Low-Flow Delivery Devices*. They are widely used in the hospital because of greater patient comfort,

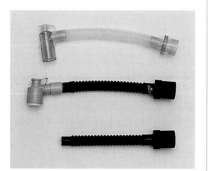

Fig. 6.4 A range of catheter mounts.

Table 6.1 Classification of the oxygen delivery systems

Variable performance devices	Fixed performance devices
Hudson face masks and partial re-breathing masks Nasal cannulae (prongs or spectacles) Nasal catheters	Venturi-operated devices Anaesthetic breathing systems with a suitably large reservoir

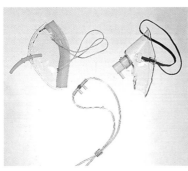

Fig. 6.5 Variable performance masks (top) and nasal cannulae (bottom).

low cost, simplicity and the ability to manipulate the FiO$_2$ without changing the appliance. Their performance varies between patients and from breath to breath within the same patients. These systems have a limited reservoir capacity, so in order to function appropriately the patient must inhale some ambient air to meet the inspiratory demands. The ⌐ is determined by the oxygen the size of the oxygen ˙he respiratory pattern

Compon˙

1. The plastic b˙ ˙f the mask with side holes on both sides.
2. A port connected to an oxygen supply.
3. Elastic band(s) to fix the mask to the patient's face.

Mechanism of action

1. Ambient air is entrained through the holes on both sides

of the mask. The holes also allow exhaled gases to be vented out.

2. During the expiratory pause, the fresh oxygen supplied helps in venting the exhaled gases through the side holes. The body of the mask (acting as a reservoir) is filled with fresh oxygen supply and is available for the start of the next inspiration.
3. The final concentration of inspired oxygen depends on
   a) the oxygen supply flow rate
   b) the pattern of ventilation. If there is a pause between expiration and inspiration, the mask fills with oxygen and a high concentration is available at the start of inspiration
   c) the patient's inspiratory flow rate. During inspiration, oxygen is diluted by the air drawn in through the holes when the inspiratory flow rate exceeds the flow of oxygen supply. During normal tidal ventilation, the peak inspiratory flow rate is 20–30 L/min, which is higher than the oxygen supplied to the patient and the oxygen that is contained in the body of the mask, so some ambient air is inhaled to meet the demands thus diluting the fresh oxygen supply. The peak inspiratory flow rate increases further during deep inspiration and during hyperventilation
   d) how tight the mask's fit is on the face.

4. If there is no expiratory pause, alveolar gases may be rebreathed from the mask at the start of inspiration.
5. The rebreathing of carbon dioxide from the body of the mask (apparatus dead space of about 100 mL) is usually of little clinical significance in adults but may be a problem in some patients who are not able to compensate by increasing their alveolar ventilation. Carbon dioxide elimination can be improved by increasing the fresh oxygen flow and is inversely related to the minute ventilation. The rebreathing is also increased when the mask body is large and when the resistance to flow from the side holes is high (when the mask is a good fit). The patients may experience a sense of warmth and humidity, indicating significant rebreathing.
6. A typical example of 4 L/min of oxygen flow delivers an FiO$_2$ of about 0.35–0.4 providing there is a normal respiratory pattern.
7. Adding a 600–800 mL bag to the mask will act as an extra reservoir. Such masks are known as 'partial rebreathing masks'. The inspired oxygen is derived from the continuous fresh oxygen supply, oxygen present in the reservoir (a mixture of the fresh oxygen and exhaled oxygen) and ambient air. Higher variable FiO$_2$ can be achieved with such masks.

Problems in practice and safety features

These devices are used only when delivering a fixed oxygen concentration is not critical. Patients whose ventilation is dependent on a hypoxic drive must not receive oxygen from a variable performance mask.

Table 6.2 Factors that affect the delivered FiO$_2$ in the variable performance masks

High FiO$_2$ delivered	Low FiO$_2$ delivered
Low peak inspiratory flow rate	High peak inspiratory flow rate
Slow respiratory rate	Fast respiratory rate
High fresh oxygen flow rate	Low fresh oxygen flow rate
Tightly fitting face mask	Less tightly fitting face mask

Nasal cannulae

Nasal cannulae are ideal for patients on long term oxygen therapy (Fig. 6.5). A flow rate of 2–4 L/min delivers an FiO_2 of 0.28–0.36 respectively. Higher flow rates are uncomfortable.

Components

1. Two prongs which protrude about 1 cm into the nose.
2. These are held in place by an adjustable head strap.

Mechanism of action

1. There is entrainment of ambient air through the nostrils. The nasopharynx acts as a reservoir.
2. The FiO_2 achieved is proportional to
   a) the flow rate of oxygen
   b) the patient's tidal volume, inspiratory flow and respiratory rate
   c) the volume of the nasopharynx.
3. Mouth breathing causes inspiratory air flow. This produces a Venturi effect in the posterior pharynx entraining oxygen from the nose.
4. There is increased patient compliance with nasal cannulae compared to facial oxygen masks.

The patient is able to speak, eat and drink.

Problems in practice and safety features

The cannulae and the dry gas flow cause trauma and irritation to the nasal mucosa. They are not appropriate in patients with blocked nasal passages.

Nasal catheters

Nasal catheters comprise a single lumen catheter, which is lodged into the anterior naris (nostril) by a foam collar (Fig. 6.6). The catheter can be secured to the patient's face by using tape. It should not be used when a nasal mucosal tear is suspected because of the risk of surgical emphysema.

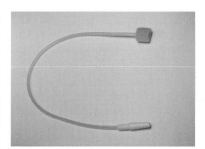

Fig 6.6 Nasal catheter.

Fixed performance devices

VENTURI MASK

These masks are fixed performance devices (sometimes called *h*igh *a*ir *f*low *o*xygen *e*nrichment, HAFOE).

Components

1. The plastic body of the mask with holes on both sides.
2. The proximal end of the mask consists of a Venturi device. The Venturi devices are colour-coded and marked with the recommended oxygen flow rate to provide the desired oxygen concentration (Figs 6.7 and 6.8).
3. Alternatively, a calibrated variable Venturi device can be used to deliver the desired FiO_2.

Mechanism of action

1. The Venturi mask uses the Bernoulli principle, described in 1778, in delivering a predetermined and fixed concentration of oxygen to the patient. The size of the constriction determines the final concentration of oxygen for a given gas flow. This is achieved in spite of the patient's respiratory pattern by providing a higher gas flow than the peak inspiratory flow rate.
2. As the flow of oxygen passes through the constriction, a negative pressure is created. This causes the ambient air to be entrained and mixed with the oxygen flow (Fig. 6.9). The oxygen concentration can be 0.24, 0.28, 0.31, 0.35, 0.4 or 0.6.
3. The Bernoulli effect can be written as:

$$P + \tfrac{1}{2}\rho v^2 = \kappa$$

where ρ is the density, v is the velocity, P is the pressure.

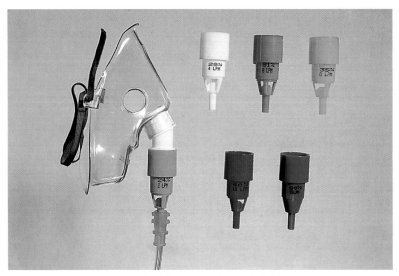

Fig. 6.7 Fixed performance mask with a range of Venturi devices.

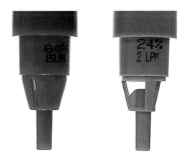

Fig. 6.8 Detail of the Venturi device. Design for administering 60% oxygen (left) and 24% (right). Note the difference in recommended oxygen flow rates and air entrainment apertures.

4. The total energy during a fluid (gas or liquid) flow consists of the sum of kinetic and potential energy. The kinetic energy is related to the velocity of the flow whereas the potential energy is related to the pressure. As the flow of fresh oxygen passes through the constricted orifice into the larger chamber, the velocity of the gas increases distal to the orifice causing the kinetic energy to increase. As the total energy is constant, there

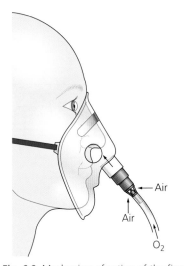

Fig. 6.9 Mechanism of action of the fixed performance Venturi mask.

is a decrease in the potential energy so a negative pressure is created. This causes the ambient air to be entrained and mixed with the oxygen flow. The FiO_2 is dependent on the degree of air entrainment. Less entrainment ensures higher FiO_2 is delivered and smaller entrainment apertures are one

method of achieving this (Fig. 6.8). The devices must be driven by the correct oxygen flow rate, calibrated for the aperture size if a predictable FiO_2 is to be achieved.

4. Because of the high fresh gas flow rate, the expired gases are rapidly flushed from the mask, via its holes. Therefore there is no rebreathing and no increase in dead space.

5. These masks are recommended when a fixed oxygen concentration is desired in patients whose ventilation is dependent on the hypoxic drive.

6. For example, a 24% oxygen Venturi mask has an air:oxygen entrainment ratio of 23:1. This means an oxygen flow of 2 L/min delivers a total flow of 48 L/min, well above the peak inspiratory flow rate.

Problems in practice and safety features

1. These masks are recommended when a fixed oxygen concentration is desired in patients whose ventilation is dependent on their hypoxic drive, such as those with chronic obstructive pulmonary disease. However, caution should be exercised as it has been shown that the average FiO_2 delivered in such masks is up to 5% above the expected value.

2. The Venturi mask with its Venturi device and the oxygen delivery tubing is often not well tolerated by patients because it is noisy and bulky.

Anaesthetic breathing systems are other examples of the fixed performance devices. The reservoir bag acts to deliver a fresh gas flow that is greater than the patient's peak inspiratory flow rate.

Venturi mask

- Fixed performance device (HAFOE).
- Uses the Venturi principle to entrain ambient air.
- No rebreathing or increase in dead space.
- Changes in kinetic and potential energy during gas flow lead to negative pressure and air entrainment.

FURTHER READING

Agusti AG, Carrera M, Barbe F et al. Oxygen therapy during exacerbations of chronic obstructive pulmonary disease. European Respiratory Journal 1999;14:934–939.

Khakhar M, Heah T, Al-Shaikh B. Oxygen delivery systems for the spontaneously breathing patient. CPD Anaesthesia 2002;4(1):27–30.

Stausholm K, Rosenberg-Adamsen S, Skriver M et al. Comparison of three devices for oxygen administration in the late postoperative period. British Journal of Anaesthesia 1995; 74(5): 607–609.

Waldau T, Larsen VH, Bonde J. Evaluation of five oxygen delivery devices in spontaneously breathing subjects by oxygraphy. Anaesthesia 1998;53:256–263.

MCQs

In the following lists, which of the statements (a) to (e) are true?

1. Concerning the Venturi mask
   a) Gas flow produced should be more than 20 L/min.
   b) Reducing the flow of oxygen from 12 to 8 L/min results in a reduction in oxygen concentration.
   c) With a constant oxygen supply flow, widening the orifice in the Venturi device increases the oxygen concentration delivered to the patient.
   d) There is rebreathing in the mask.
   e) The mask is a fixed performance device.

2. High air flow oxygen enrichment face masks
   a) Use the Venturi principle to deliver a fixed O_2 concentration to the patient.
   b) The size of the constriction of the Venturi has no effect on the final O_2 concentration delivered to the patient.
   c) The holes on the side of the mask are used to entrain ambient air.
   d) The gas flow delivered to the patient is more than the peak inspiratory flow rate.
   e) There is significant rebreathing.

3. Face masks used during anaesthesia
   a) The rubber mask is covered by carbon particles which act as an anti-static measure.
   b) Masks have no effect on the apparatus dead space.
   c) The mask's cuff has to be checked and inflated before use.
   d) The dental nasal masks are also known as nasal inhalers.
   e) Masks have a 15 mm end to fit the catheter mount.

4. Concerning the oxygen nasal cannula
   a) Is a fixed performance device.
   b) Is a variable performance device.
   c) There is a Venturi effect in the posterior pharynx.
   d) An oxygen flow of 8 L/min is usually used in an adult.
   e) Has increased patient compliance.

5. Variable performance masks
   a) During slow and deep breathing, a higher FiO_2 can be achieved.
   b) Ambient air is not entrained into the mask.
   c) Alveolar gas rebreathing is not possible.
   d) Normal inspiratory peak flow rate is 20–30 L/min for an adult.
   e) Can be used safely on all patients.

6. Regarding variable performance devices
   a) They can offer greater patient compliance.
   b) They can deliver an FiO_2 that can vary from breath to breath in the same patient.
   c) The size of the medium concentration oxygen face mask has no effect on rebreathing and CO_2 elimination.
   d) Capnography can be used to measure the FiO_2 delivered to the patient.
   e) With a variable performance mask, the FiO_2 is higher when the face mask is a tight fit.

7. Concerning fixed performance devices
   a) Anaesthetic breathing systems with reservoirs are fixed performance devices.
   b) Distal to the constriction of a Venturi, there an increase in potential energy.
   c) In a Venturi mask, the higher the entrainment ratio, the higher the FiO_2.
   d) A nasal oxygen catheter is a fixed performance device.
   e) Venturi masks are very well tolerated by patients.

Answers

1. Concerning the Venturi mask
   a) *True. The Venturi mask is a fixed performance device. In order to achieve this, the flow delivered to the patient should be more than the peak inspiratory flow rate. A flow of more than 20 L/min is adequate.*
   b) *True. It is the flow rate of oxygen through the orifice that determines the final FiO_2 the patient receives. With a constant orifice, the amount of air entrained remains constant. So by reducing the oxygen flow rate from 12 to 8 L/min, there will be less oxygen in the final mixture.*
   c) *True. The wider the orifice, the less the drop in pressure across the orifice and the less the entrainment of the ambient air, hence the less the dilution of the O_2, resulting in an increase in oxygen concentration delivered to the patient. The opposite is also correct.*
   d) *False. There is no rebreathing in the mask because of the high fresh gas flow rates causing the exhaled gases to be flushed from the mask through the side holes.*
   e) *True. The Venturi mask is a fixed performance device that delivers a constant concentration of oxygen in spite of the patient's respiratory pattern, by providing a higher gas flow than the peak inspiratory flow rate.*

2. High air flow oxygen enrichment face masks
   a) *True. Laminar flow through a constriction causes a decrease in pressure at the constriction. This leads to entrainment of ambient air leading to mixture of fixed oxygen concentration.*
   b) *False. It is the size of the orifice that determines the degree of decrease in pressure at the constriction. This determines the amount of ambient air being entrained, hence the final concentration of oxygen.*
   c) *False. In such a mask, the holes are used to expel the exhaled gases. There is no entrainment of ambient air in such a mask because of the high gas flows. The holes in a variable performance mask are used to entrain ambient air.*
   d) *True. The gas flow generated is higher than the peak inspiratory flow rate. This allows the delivery of a fixed oxygen concentration to the patient regardless of the inspiratory flow rate. It also prevents rebreathing.*
   e) *False. There is no rebreathing because of the high flows delivered to the patient. The exhaled gases are expelled through the holes in the mask.*

3. Face masks used during anaesthesia
   a) *True. Carbon particles prevent the build up of static electricity. The rubber face masks and the rubber tubings used in anaesthesia are covered with carbon. With modern anaesthetic practice where no flammable drugs are used, its significance has all but disappeared.*
   b) *False. Face masks can have a significant effect on the apparatus dead space if the wrong size is chosen. In an adult, the dead space can increase by about 200 mL. It is of more importance in paediatric practice.*
   c) *True. The cuff of the face mask is designed to ensure a snug fit over the patient's face and also to minimize the mask's pressure on the face. Ensuring that the cuff is inflated before use is therefore important.*
   d) *True. Nasal inhalers are nasal masks used during dental anaesthesia allowing good surgical access to the mouth. The Goldman nasal inhaler is an example.*
   e) *False. The face masks have a 22 mm end to fit the angle piece or catheter mount.*

4. Concerning the oxygen nasal cannula

   a) *False. It is not a fixed performance device. The final FiO_2 depends on the flow rate of oxygen, tidal volume, inspiratory flow, respiratory rate and the volume of the nasopharynx.*

   b) *True. See above.*

   c) *True. During mouth breathing, the inspiratory air flow produces a Venturi effect in the posterior pharynx entraining oxygen from the nose.*

   d) *False. It is uncomfortable for the patient to have higher flows than 2–4 L/min.*

   e) *True. Patients tolerate the nasal cannula for much longer periods than a face mask. Patients are capable of eating, drinking and speaking despite the cannula.*

5. Variable performance masks

   a) *True. This allows FGF during the expiratory pause to fill the mask ready for the following inspiration. In tachypnoea (fast and shallow breathing) the opposite occurs where there is not enough time for the FGF to fill the mask.*

   b) *False. The maximum inspiratory flow rate is much higher than the FGF, so ambient air is entrained into the mask through the side holes.*

   c) *False. During tachypnoea, there is not enough time for the FGF to fill the mask and expel the exhaled gases. This leads to rebreathing of the exhaled gases.*

   d) *True.*

   e) *False. As their performance is variable, the FiO_2 the patient is getting is uncertain. Patients who are dependent on their hypoxic drive require a fixed performance mask.*

6. Regarding variable performance devices

   a) *True. These devices are better tolerated by patients because they are more comfortable. They also offer simplicity, low cost and the ability to manipulate the FiO_2 without changing the appliance.*

   b) *True. The FiO_2 delivered can vary from one breath to another in the same patient. This is because of changes in the inspiratory flow rate and respiratory pattern. These lead to changes in the amount of air entrained so altering the FiO_2.*

   c) *False. Rebreathing is increased when the mask body is large. In addition, the high inspiratory resistance of the side holes increases the rebreathing. CO_2 elimination can be improved by increasing the fresh oxygen flow and is inversely related to the minute ventilation.*

   d) *False. Oxygraphy can be used to measure the FiO_2 by measuring the end-tidal oxygen fraction in the nasopharynx.*

   e) *True. The tighter the fit of the face mask, the higher the FiO_2. Low peak inspiratory flow rate, slow respiratory rate and a higher oxygen flow rate can also increase the FiO_2.*

7. Concerning fixed performance devices
   a) *True. Anaesthetic breathing systems are fixed performance devices. The reservoir bag acts to deliver an FGF that is greater than the patient's peak inspiratory flow rate.*
   b) *False. The potential energy is related to the pressure, whereas the kinetic energy is related to the velocity of the flow. As the flow of fresh oxygen supply passes through the constricted orifice into the larger chamber, the velocity of the gas increases distal to the orifice causing the kinetic energy to increase. As the total energy is constant, there is a decrease in the potential energy so a negative pressure is created. This causes the ambient air to be entrained and mixed with the oxygen flow.*
   c) *False. The higher the entrainment ratio, the lower the FiO_2 delivered. This is because of the 'dilution' of the 100% oxygen fresh flow by ambient air.*
   d) *False. Nasal catheters are variable performance devices.*
   e) *False. Venturi masks are not very well tolerated by patients because of the noise and bulkiness of the masks and the attachments.*

Chapter 7

Laryngoscopes and tracheal intubation equipment

Laryngoscopes

These devices are used to perform direct laryngoscopy and to aid in tracheal intubation (Fig. 7.1).

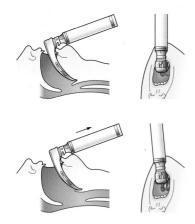

Fig. 7.1 Performing direct laryngoscopy. The vocal cords are visualized by lifting the laryngoscope in an upwards and forwards direction (see arrow).

Components

1. The handle houses the power source (batteries) and is designed in different sizes.
2. The blade is fitted to the handle and can be either curved or straight. There is a wide range of designs for both curved and straight blades (Figs 7.2 and 7.3).

Mechanism of action

1. Usually the straight blade is used for intubating neonates and infants. The blade is advanced over the posterior border of the relatively large, floppy V-shaped epiglottis which is then lifted directly in order to view the larynx (Fig. 7.4b). There are larger size straight blades that can be used in adults.
2. The curved blade (**Macintosh blade**) is designed to fit into the oral and oropharyngeal cavity. It is inserted through the right angle of the mouth and advanced gradually, pushing the tongue to the left and

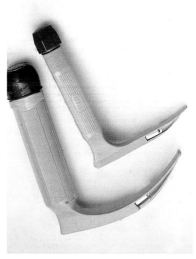

Fig. 7.3 Plastic laryngoscopes.

away from the view until the tip of the blade reaches the valleculla. The blade has a small bulbous tip to help lift the larynx (Fig 7.4a). The laryngoscope is lifted upwards elevating the larynx and allowing the vocal cords to be seen. The Macintosh blade is made in four sizes.

3. The light source is a bulb screwed on to the blade and an electrical connection is made when the blade is opened ready for use. Some designs place the bulb in the handle and the light is transmitted to the blade by means of fibreoptics.
4. A left-sided Macintosh blade is available. It is used in patients with right-sided facial deformities making the use of the right-sided blade difficult.
5. The **McCoy laryngoscope** is based on the standard Macintosh blade. It has a hinged tip which is operated by the lever mechanism present on the back of the handle. It is suited for both routine use and in cases of difficult intubation (Figs 7.5 and 7.6). A more recent McCoy design has a straight blade with a hinged tip. Both the curved and the straight McCoy laryngoscopes use either

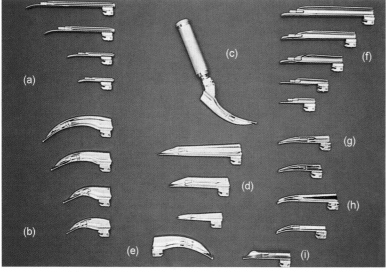

Fig. 7.2 A wide range of laryngoscope blades. (a) Miller blades (large, adult, infant, premature); (b) Macintosh blades (large, adult, child, baby); (c) Macintosh polio blade; (d) Soper blades (adult, child, baby); (e) left-handed Macintosh blade; (f) Wisconsin blades (large, adult, child, baby); (g) Robertshaw's blades (infant, neonatal); (h) Seward blades (child, baby); (i) Oxford infant blade.

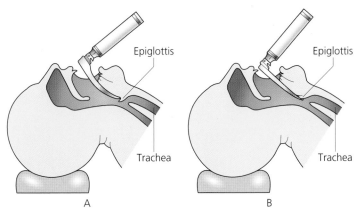

Fig. 7.4 Use of the laryngoscope (reproduced with permission from Aitkenhead R, Smith G. Textbook of Anaesthesia, 2nd edn. Churchill Livingstone, 1990).

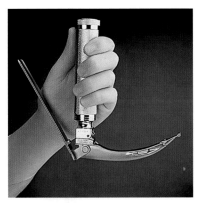

Fig. 7.5 The McCoy laryngoscope, based on a standard Macintosh blade.

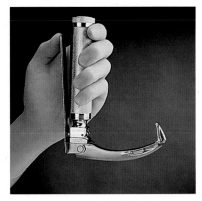

Fig. 7.6 Demonstrating the McCoy laryngoscope's hinged blade tip.

a traditional bulb in the blade or a lamp mounted in the handle which fibreoptically transmits the light to the blade.

6. A more recent design called the Flexiblade exists, where the whole distal half of the blade can be manoeuvered rather than just the tip, as in the McCoy. This can be achieved using a lever on the front of the handle.

Problems in practice and safety features

1. The risk of trauma and bruising to the different structures (e.g. epiglottis) is higher with the straight blade.
2. It is of vital importance to check the function of the laryngoscope before anaesthesia is commenced. Reduction in power or total failure due to the corrosion at the electrical contact point is possible.
3. Patients with large amounts of breast tissue present difficulty during intubation. Insertion of the blade into the mouth is restricted by the breast tissue impinging on the handle. To overcome this problem, specially designed blades are used such as the polio blade.

The polio blade is at about 120° to the handle allowing laryngoscopy without restriction. The polio blade was first designed to intubate patients ventilated in the iron lung during the poliomyelitis epidemic in the 1950s. A Macintosh laryngoscope blade attached to a short handle can be also useful in this situation.

4. To prevent cross infection between patients, a disposable PVC sheath, the Penlon Larygard, can be put on the blade of the laryngoscope. The sheath has low light impedance allowing good visibility.

Laryngoscopes

- Consists of a handle and a blade. The latter can be straight or curved.
- The bulb is either in the blade or in the handle.
- Different designs and shapes exist.

Fibreoptic intubating laryngoscope

These devices have revolutionized airway management in anaesthesia and intensive care (Fig. 7.7). They are used to perform oral or nasal tracheal intubation (Figs 7.8 and 7.9), to evaluate

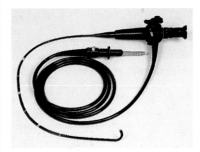

Fig. 7.7 A fibreoptic intubating laryngoscope.

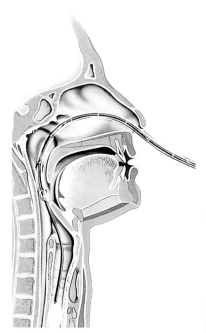

Fig. 7.8 Performing fibreoptic nasal intubation.

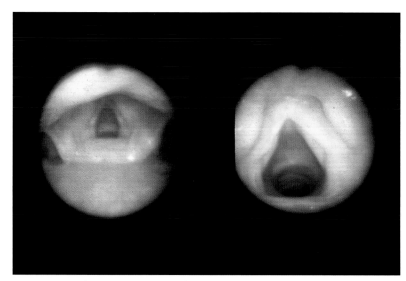

Fig. 7.9 Views of the vocal cords as seen through a fibreoptic laryngoscope.

the airway in trauma, tumour, infection and inhalational injury, to confirm tube placement (tracheal, endobronchial, double lumen or tracheostomy tubes) and to perform tracheobronchial toilet.

Components

1. Control unit which consists of the following:
   a) tip deflection control knob (the bending angle range is 60–180° in the vertical plane)
   b) eye piece
   c) diopter adjustment ring (focusing)
   d) suction channel which can also be used to insufflate oxygen and administer local anaesthetic solutions.
2. The flexible insertion cord consists of bundles of glass fibres. Each bundle consists of 10 000–15 000 fibres nearly identical in diameter and optical characteristics.

3. Light transmitting cable to transmit light from an external source.
4. Other equipment may be needed, e.g. endoscopic face mask, oral airway, bite block, defogging agent.

Mechanism of action

1. The fibreoptic laryngoscope uses light transmitted through glass fibres. The fibres used have diameters of 5–20 μm, making them capable of transmitting light and being flexible at the same time.
2. The fibres are coated with a thin external layer of glass (of lower refractive index) thus providing optical insulation of each fibre in the bundle.
3. Light enters the fibre at a specific angle of incidence. It travels down the fibre, repeatedly striking and being reflected from the external layer of glass at a similar angle of incidence until it emerges from the opposite end.
4. The insertion cords vary in length and diameter. The latter determines the size of the tracheal tube that can be used. Smaller scopes are available for intubating children. The outer diameter ranges from 1.8

to 6.4 mm allowing the use of tracheal tubes of 3.0–7.0 mm internal diameter.

Problems in practice and safety features

1. The intubating fibreoptic laryngoscope is a delicate instrument that can easily be damaged by careless handling. Damage to the fibre bundles results in loss of the image and light in individual fibres which can not be repaired.
2. The laryngoscope should be cleaned and dried thoroughly as soon as possible after use.

Fibreoptic intubating laryngoscope

- The insertion cord consists of glass fibres arranged in bundles.
- Light is transmitted through the glass fibres.
- Used for tracheal intubation, airway evaluation and tracheobronchial toilet.
- Damage to the fibres causes loss of image.

Magill forceps

These forceps are designed for ease of use within the mouth and oropharynx. Magill forceps come in small or large sizes (Fig. 7.10). During tracheal intubation, they can be used to direct the tracheal tube towards the larynx and vocal cords.

Care should be taken to protect the tracheal tube cuff from being damaged by the forceps.

Other uses include the insertion and removal of throat packs and removal of foreign bodies in the oropharynx and larynx.

Introducer, bougie, bite guard, local anaesthetic spray, Endotrol tube and Nosworthy airway

1. A **local anaesthetic spray** is used to coat the laryngeal and tracheal mucosa, usually with lignocaine. This decreases the stimulus of intubation.
2. A **bite guard** protects the front upper teeth during direct laryngoscopy.
3. The **Endotrol tube** has a ring-pull on its inner curvature connected to the distal end of the tube. During intubation, the ring-pull can be used to adjust the curvature of the tube.
4. An **introducer** is used to adjust the curvature of a tracheal tube to help direct it through the vocal cords.
5. A gum elastic **bougie** is used when it is difficult to visualize the vocal cords. First, the bougie is inserted through the vocal cords, then the tracheal tube is railroaded over it. Single use bougies are currently available (Fig. 7.11).
6. The **Nosworthy** airway is an example of the many modifications that exist in oropharyngeal airway design. This airway allows the connection of a catheter mount.

Cook retrograde intubation set (Fig. 7.12)

This set is used to assist in placement of a tracheal tube when a difficult intubation is encountered.

Components

1. An introducer needle (18 G and 5 cm in length).
2. A guidewire with a J-shaped end.
3. A 14 G 70 cm hollow guiding catheter with distal sideports. The proximal end has a 15 mm connector.

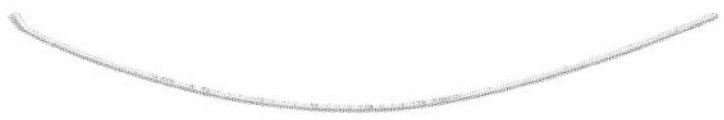

Fig. 7.11 Smith's Portex single use intubating bougie.

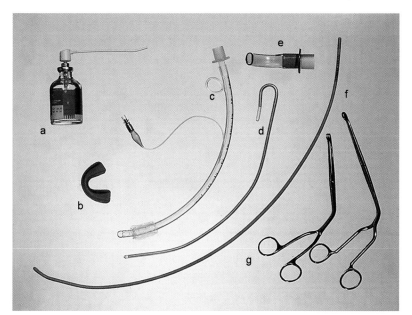

Fig. 7.10 Intubation aids. (a) Local anaesthetic spray; (b) bite guard; (c) Endotrol tube; (d) introducer; (e) Nosworthy airway; (f) gum elastic bougie; (g) Magill forceps.

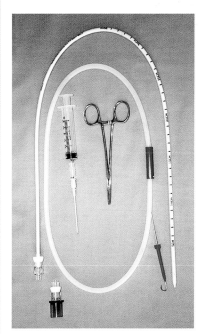

Fig. 7.12 The Cook retrograde intubation set.

Mechanism of action

1. The introducer needle is inserted through the cricothyroid membrane.
2. The guidewire is advanced in a retrograde (cephalic) direction to exit orally or nasally.
3. The hollow guiding catheter is then introduced in an antegrade direction into the trachea. The proximal end of the catheter can be connected to an oxygen supply.
4. A tracheal tube (5 mm or larger) can be introduced over the guiding catheter into the trachea.

Problems in practice and safety features

1. Pneumothorax.
2. Haemorrhage.
3. Failure.

Retrograde intubation kit

- The introducer needle is inserted through the cricothyroid.
- The guidewire is advanced in a cephalic direction.
- Pneumothorax and haemorrhage are potential complications.

FURTHER READING

Hendersen JJ. Development of the 'gum-elastic bougie'. Anaesthesia 2003;58:103–104.

Popat M. Practical Fiberoptic Intubation. Oxford: Butterworth-Heinemann, 2001.

Hendersen JJ. The use of paraglossal straight blade laryngoscopy in difficult tracheal intubation. Anaesthesia 1997;52:552–560.

MCQs

In the following lists, which of the statements (a) to (e) are true?

1. Laryngoscopes
   a) Straight blade laryngoscopes are only used in neonates and infants.
   b) The left-sided Macintosh blade is designed for a left-handed anaesthetist.
   c) The Macintosh blade is designed to elevate the larynx.
   d) The Macintosh polio blade can be used in patients with large breasts.
   e) The McCoy laryngoscope can improve the view of the larynx.

2. Light failure during laryngoscopy can be caused by
   a) Battery failure.
   b) A loose bulb.
   c) The wrong-sized blade has been used.
   d) A blown bulb.
   e) Inadequate connection due to corrosion.

3. Concerning retrograde intubation
   a) The introducer needle is inserted at the level of second and third tracheal cartilages.
   b) It is a very safe procedure with no complications.
   c) A guidewire is inserted in a cephalic direction.
   d) Supplemental oxygen can be administered.
   e) A tracheal tube (5 mm or larger) can be introduced over the guiding catheter into the trachea.

Answers

1. Laryngoscopes
   a) *False. Straight blade laryngoscopes can be used for adults, neonates and infants. Because of the shape and size of the larynx in small children, it is usually easier to intubate with a straight blade laryngoscope. The latter can be used in adults, but the curved blade laryngoscope is usually used.*
   b) *False. The left-sided Macintosh blade is designed to be used in cases of difficult access to the right side of the mouth or tongue, e.g. trauma or tumour.*
   c) *True. The Macintosh curved blade is designed to elevate the larynx thus allowing better visualization of the vocal cords.*
   d) *True. The polio blade was designed during the polio epidemic in the 1950s to overcome the problem of intubating patients who were in an 'iron lung'. In current practice, it can be used in patients with large breasts where the breasts do not get in the way of the handle.*
   e) *True. By using the hinged blade tip, the larynx is further elevated. This improves the view of the larynx.*

2. Light failure during laryngoscopy can be caused by
   a) *True.*
   b) *True.*
   c) *False. This should not cause light failure. It may, however, cause a worse view of the larynx.*
   d) *True.*
   e) *True. This usually happens in the traditional laryngoscope design where the handle needs good contact with the blade for the current to flow from the batteries to the bulb in the blade. Corrosion at that junction can cause light failure. Laryngoscopes using fibreoptics do not suffer from this problem as the bulb is situated in the handle.*

3. Concerning retrograde intubation
   a) *False. The needle is inserted through the cricothyroid membrane.*
   b) *False. Retrograde intubation can cause haemorrhage or pneumothorax.*
   c) *True. The guidewire is inserted in a retrograde cephalic direction to exit through the mouth or nose.*
   d) *True. Oxygen can be given through the proximal end of the guiding catheter.*
   e) *True.*

Chapter 8

Ventilators

Ventilators are used to provide controlled ventilation (IPPV). Some have the facilities to provide other ventilatory modes. They can be used in the operating theatre, intensive care unit, during transport of critically ill patients and also at home (e.g. for patients requiring nocturnal respiratory assistance).

Classification of ventilators

There are many ways of classifying ventilators (Table 8.1).

1. The **method of cycling** is used to change over from inspiration to exhalation and vice versa.
   a) **Volume cycling:** when the predetermined tidal volume is reached during inspiration, the ventilator changes to exhalation.
   b) **Time cycling:** when the predetermined inspiratory duration is reached, the ventilator changes to exhalation. The cycling is not affected by the compliance of the patient's lungs. Time cycling is the most common method used.
   c) **Pressure cycling:** when the predetermined pressure is reached during inspiration, the ventilator changes over to exhalation. The duration needed to achieve the critical pressure depends on the compliance of the lungs. The stiffer the lungs are, the quicker the pressure is achieved and vice versa. The ventilator delivers a different tidal volume if compliance or resistance changes.
   d) **Flow cycling:** when the predetermined flow is reached during inspiration, the ventilator changes over to exhalation. This method is used in older design ventilators.

2. **Inspiratory phase gas control**
   a) **Volume:** a preset volume is delivered.
   b) **Pressure:** a preset pressure is not exceeded.

3. **Source of power** – can be electric or pneumatic.

4. **Suitability for use in theatre** and/or intensive care.

5. **Suitability for paediatric practice.**

6. **Method of operation** (pattern of gas flow during inspiration)
   a) **Pressure generator:** the ventilator produces inspiration by generating a constant and predetermined pressure. Bellows or a moderate weight produce the pressure. The inspiratory flow changes with changes in lung compliance (Table 8.2).
   b) **Flow generator:** the ventilator produces inspiration by delivering a predetermined flow of gas. A piston, heavy weight or compressed gas produce the flow. The flow remains unchanged by changes in lung compliance, although pressures will change (Table 8.2). These ventilators have a high internal resistance to protect the patient from high working pressures.

7. **Sophistication:** new ventilators can function in many of the above modes. They have other modes, e.g. SIMV, PS and CPAP (see pp 111–112).

8. **Function**
   a) **Minute volume dividers:** FGF powers the ventilator. The minute volume equals the FGF divided into preset tidal volumes thus determining the frequency.
   b) **Bag squeezers** replace the hand ventilation of a Mapleson D or circle system. They need an external source of power.
   c) **Lightweight portable:** powered by compressed gas and consists of the control unit and patient valve.

Table 8.1 Summary of the methods used in classifying ventilators

Method of cycling	Volume cycling
	Time cycling
	Pressure cycling
	Flow cycling
Inspiratory phase gas control	Volume
	Pressure
Source of power	Electric
	Pneumatic
Suitability for use	Operating theatre
	ICU
	Both
Paediatrics use	Yes/no
Method of operation	Pressure generator
	Flow generator
Sophistication	SIMV, PS, CPAP
Function	Minute volume divider
	Bag squeezer
	Lightweight portable

Characteristics of the ideal ventilator

1. The ventilator should be simple, portable, robust and economical to purchase and use. If compressed gas is used to drive the ventilator,

Table 8.2 Differences between the pressure generator and flow generator ventilators

	Changes in lung compliance	Leak in the system
Pressure generator	can not compensate	can compensate (to a degree)
Flow generator	can compensate (to a degree)	can not compensate

a significant wastage of the compressed gas is expected. Some ventilators use a Venturi to drive the bellows, to reduce the use of compressed oxygen.

2. It should be versatile and supply tidal volumes up to 1500 mL with a respiratory rate of up to 60/min and variable I:E ratio. It can be used with different breathing systems. It can deliver any gas or vapour mixture. The addition of PEEP should be possible.

3. It should monitor the airway pressure, inspired and exhaled minute and tidal volume, respiratory rate and inspired oxygen concentration.

4. There should be facilities to provide humidification. Drugs can be nebulized through it.

5. Disconnection, high airway pressure and power failure alarms should be present.

6. There should be the facility to provide other ventilatory modes, e.g. SIMV, CPAP and pressure support.

7. It should be easy to clean and sterilize.

Some of the commonly used ventilators are described below.

Manley MP3 ventilator

This is a minute volume divider (time cycled, pressure generator). All the fresh gas flow (the minute volume) is delivered to the patient divided into readily set tidal volumes (Figs 8.1 and 8.2).

Components

1. Rubber tubing delivers the fresh gas flow from the anaesthetic machine to the ventilator.
2. Two sets of bellows (Fig. 8.3). The smaller time-cycling bellows (B1) receives the fresh gas flow

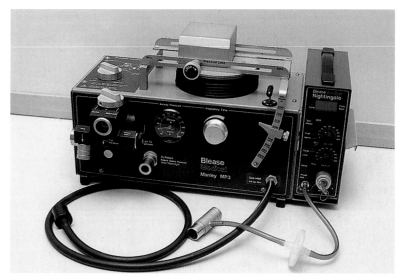
Fig. 8.1 The Blease Manley MP3 with ventilator alarm (right).

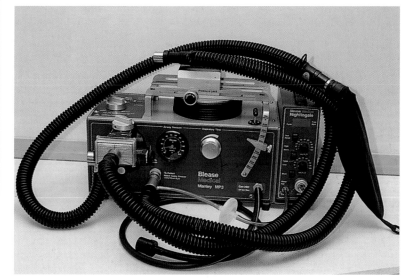
Fig. 8.2 The Blease Manley MP3 with tubing fitted.

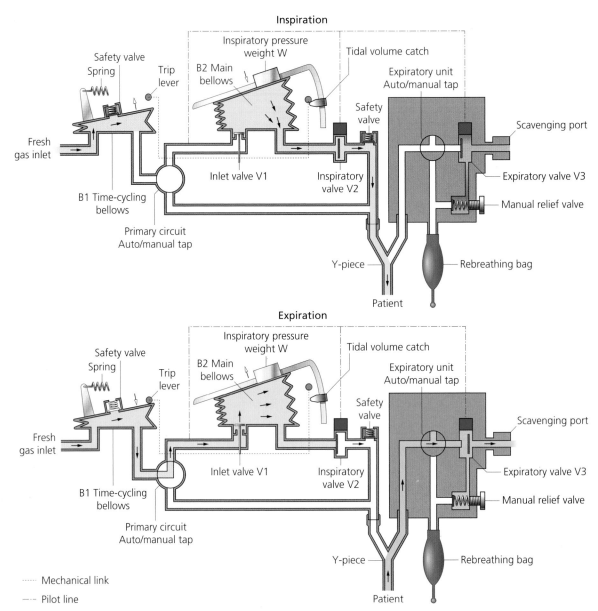

Fig. 8.3 Components and mechanism of action of the Manley MP3 ventilator. See text for details. (Reproduced with permission from Blease Medical Equipment Ltd.)

directly from the gas source and then empties into the main bellows (B2).

3. Three unidirectional valves
   a) The first (V1) is between the two sets of bellows (closes during inspiration)

b) The second (V2) is between the main bellows and the patient (closes during expiration)

c) The third (V3) is between the patient and the APL valve (opens during expiration).

4. An APL valve with tubing and a reservoir bag used during spontaneous or manually controlled ventilation.

5. The ventilator has a pressure gauge (up to 100 cmH$_2$O), inspiratory time dial, tidal

volume adjuster (up to 1000 mL), two knobs to change the mode of ventilation from and to controlled and spontaneous (or manually controlled) ventilation. The inflation pressure is adjusted by sliding the weight to an appropriate position along its rail. The expiratory block is easily removed for autoclaving.

Mechanism of action

1. The fresh gas flow drives the ventilator.
2. During inspiration, the smaller bellows receives the fresh gas flow, while the main bellows delivers its contents to the patient. The inspiratory time dial controls the extent of filling of the smaller bellows before it empties into the main bellows.
3. During expiration, the smaller bellows delivers its contents to the main bellows until the predetermined tidal volume is reached to start inspiration again.
4. Using the ventilator in the spontaneous (manual) ventilation mode changes it to a Mapleson D breathing system.
5. Earlier models (MN2) incorporated a negative end-expiratory pressure mode which is not widely used.

Problems in practice and safety features

1. The ventilator ceases to cycle and function when the fresh gas flow is disconnected. This allows rapid detection of gas supply failure.
2. Ventilating patients with poor pulmonary compliance is not easily achieved.
3. It generates back pressure in the back bar as it cycles.
4. The emergency oxygen flush in the anaesthetic machine should not be activated while ventilating a patient with the Manley.

> Manely MP3 ventilator
>
> - It is a minute volume divider.
> - Consists of two sets of bellows, three unidirectional valves, an APL valve and a reservoir bag.
> - Acts as a Mapleson D breathing system during spontaneous ventilation.

Penlon Anaesthesia Nuffield Ventilator Series 200

This is an intermittent blower ventilator. It is small, compact, versatile and easy to use with patients of different sizes, ages and lung compliances. It can be used with different breathing systems (Fig. 8.4). It is a volume preset, time cycled, flow generator in adult use. In paediatric use, it is a pressure preset, time cycled, flow generator.

Components

1. The control module, consisting of an airway pressure gauge

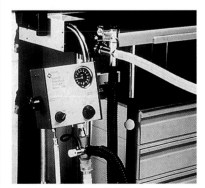

Fig. 8.4 The Penlon Nuffield 200 ventilator ready for use. Note that the APL valve of the Bain breathing system is fully closed.

(cmH_2O), inspiratory and expiratory time dials (seconds), inspiratory flow rate dial (L/s) and an on/off switch. Underneath the control module there are connections for the driving gas supply and the valve block. Tubing connects the valve block to the airway pressure gauge.
2. The valve block has three ports:
   a) a port for tubing to connect to the breathing system reservoir bag mount
   b) an exhaust port which can be connected to the scavenging system
   c) a pressure relief valve which opens at 60 cmH_2O.
3. The valve block can be changed to a paediatric (Newton) valve.

Mechanism of action

1. The ventilator is powered by a driving gas independent from the fresh gas flow (Fig. 8.5). The commonly used driving gas is oxygen (at about 400 kPa) supplied from the compressed oxygen outlets on the anaesthetic machine. The driving gas should not reach the patient as it dilutes the fresh gas flow, lightening the depth of anaesthesia.
2. It can be used with different breathing systems such as Bain, Humphrey ADE, T-piece and the circle. In the Bain and circle systems, the reservoir bag is replaced by the tubing delivering the driving gas from the ventilator. The APL valve of the breathing system must be fully closed during ventilation.
3. The inspiratory and expiratory times can be adjusted to the desired I/E ratio. Adjusting the inspiratory time and inspiratory flow rate controls determines the tidal volume. The inflation pressure is adjusted by the inspiratory flow rate control.

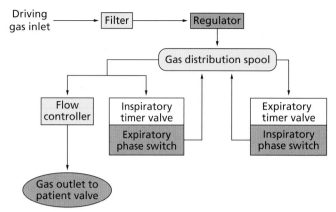

Fig. 8.5 A schematic diagram of the working principles of the Penlon Nuffield 200 ventilator. The driving gas passes through a filter and pressure regulator before entering the gas distribution spool. During the inspiratory phase, it is directed initially to the gas outlet via the flow controller and simultaneously to the inspiratory timer valve. At the end of inspiration the expiratory phase switch causes the driving gas to be redirected by the distribution spool to the expiratory timer valve. At the end of expiration the inspiratory phase switch causes the distribution spool to redirect the driving gas for the next inspiratory phase.

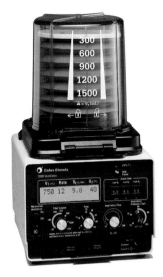

Fig. 8.6 A bag in bottle ventilator.

4. With its standard valve, the ventilator acts as a time-cycled flow generator to deliver a minimal tidal volume of 50 mL. When the valve is changed to a paediatric (Newton) valve, the ventilator changes to a time-cycled pressure generator capable of delivering tidal volumes between 10 and 300 mL. This makes it capable of ventilating premature babies and neonates. It is recommended that the Newton valve is used for children of less than 20 kg body weight.
5. A PEEP valve may be fitted to the exhaust port.

Problems in practice and safety features

1. The ventilator continues to cycle despite breathing system disconnection.
2. Requires high flows of driving gas.

> Penlon Nuffield Anaesthesia Ventilator Series 200
>
> - An intermittent blower with a pressure gauge, inspiratory and expiratory time and flow controls.
> - Powered by a driving gas.
> - Can be used for both adults and paediatric patients.
> - Can be used with different breathing systems.

Bag in bottle ventilator

Modern anaesthetic machines often incorporate a bag in bottle ventilator.

Components

1. A driving unit consisting of:
   a) a chamber (Fig. 8.6) with a tidal volume range of 0–1500 mL

(a paediatric version with a range of 0–400 mL exists)
   b) an ascending bellows accommodating the fresh gas flow.
2. A control unit with a variety of controls, displays and alarms: the tidal volume, respiratory rate (6–40/min), I/E ratio, airway pressure and power supply (Fig. 8.7).

Mechanism of action

1. It is a time-cycled ventilator.
2. Compressed air is used as the driving gas (Fig. 8.8). On entering the chamber, the compressed

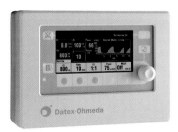

Fig. 8.7 Control panel of the Datex-Ohmeda 7900 ventilator.

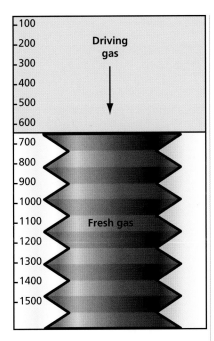

Fig. 8.8 Mechanism of action of the bag in bottle ventilator.

air forces the bellows down, delivering the fresh gas to the patient (the fresh gas is accommodated in the bellows).
3. The driving gas and the fresh gas remain separate.
4. The volume of the driving gas reaching the chamber is equal to the tidal volume.
5. Some designs feature a descending bellows instead.

Problems in practice and safety features

1. Positive pressure in the standing bellows causes a PEEP of 2–4 cmH$_2$O.
2. The ascending bellows collapses to an empty position and remains stationary in cases of disconnection or leak.

3. The descending bellows hangs down to a fully expanded position in case of disconnection and may continue to move almost normally in cases of leak.

> **Bag in bottle ventilator**
> ● It is a time-cycled ventilator.
> ● Consists of driving and control units.
> ● Fresh gas is within the bellows whereas the driving gas is within the chamber.

Servo-*i* ventilator

The Servo-*i* is a versatile intensive care ventilator, capable of being used for paediatric and adult patients. It is fully transportable, utilizing 12 V battery power when mains electricity is not available. It is not intended for use with inhalational anaesthetics, however it can be used with intravenous anaesthetics in the theatre setting if required. It can be used to 'non-invasively' ventilate patients with a tight fitting nasal mask or face mask instead of an endotracheal tube or tracheostomy.

Components (see Fig. 8.9)

1. 'Patient unit' where gases are mixed and administered.
2. 'Graphical user interface' where settings are made and ventilation monitored.

Mechanism of action

1. Gas flow from the oxygen and air inlets is regulated by their respective gas modules.

2. Oxygen concentration is measured by an oxygen cell.
3. The pressure of the delivered gas mixture is measured by the inspiratory pressure transducer.
4. The patient's expiratory gas flow is measured by ultrasonic transducers and the pressure measured by the expiratory pressure transducer.
5. PEEP in the patient system is regulated by the expiratory valve.

There are various modes of ventilation available.

1. **Synchronized intermittent mandatory ventilation (SIMV).** The ventilator provides

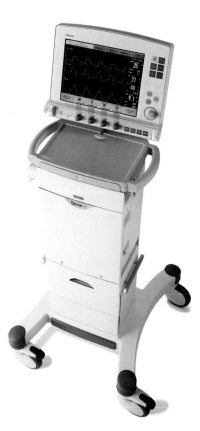

Fig. 8.9 Servo-*i* ventilator.

mandatory breaths, which are synchronized with the patient's respiratory effort (if present). The type of mandatory breath supplied depends on the setting selected. Usually one of the following is selected.

a) **Pressure regulated volume control (PRVC):** A preset tidal volume is delivered but limited to $5\,cmH_2O$ below the set upper pressure limit. This automatically limits barotrauma if the upper pressure limit is appropriately set. The flow during inspiration is decelerating. The patient can trigger extra breaths.

b) **Volume control:** A preset tidal volume and respiratory rate are selected. The breath is delivered with constant flow during a preset inspiratory time. The set tidal volume will always be delivered despite high airway pressures if the patient's lungs are not compliant. To prevent excessive pressures being generated in this situation, the upper pressure limit must be set to a suitable level to prevent barotrauma.

c) **Pressure control:** A pressure control level above PEEP is selected. The delivered tidal volume is dependent upon the patient's lung compliance and airways resistance together with the tubing and endotracheal tube's resistance. Pressure control ventilation is preferred when there is a leak in the breathing system (e.g. uncuffed endotracheal tube) or where barotrauma is to be avoided (e.g. acute lung injury). If the resistance or compliance improves quickly there is a risk of excessive tidal volumes being delivered (volutrauma) unless the pressure control setting is reduced.

2. **Supported ventilation modes.** Once the patient has enough respiratory drive to trigger the ventilator, usually one of the following modes is selected in addition to the PEEP setting.

a) **Volume support:** Assures a set tidal volume by supplying the required pressure support needed to achieve that tidal volume. It allows patients to wean from ventilatory support themselves as their lungs' compliance and inspiratory muscle strength improves. This is shown by a gradual reduction in the peak airway pressure measured by the ventilator. Once the support is minimal, extubation can be considered.

b) **Pressure support (PS):** The patient's breath is supported with a set constant pressure above PEEP. This will give a tidal volume that is dependent on the lung compliance and patient's inspiratory muscle strength. The pressure support setting needs reviewing regularly to allow the patient to wean from respiratory support.

c) **Continuous positive airway pressure (CPAP):** A continuous positive pressure is maintained in the airways similar to that developed with a conventional CPAP flow generator (see Chapter 13). This differs from the conventional CPAP flow generator by allowing measurement of tidal volume, minute volume and respiratory rate, and trends can be observed also.

Problems in practice and safety features

1. A comprehensive alarm system is featured.
2. A mainstream carbon dioxide analyzer is available which allows continuous inspiratory and expiratory monitoring of CO_2 to be displayed if required.
3. A single battery module offers 30 minutes of ventilator use. Multiple battery modules (up to 6) can be loaded on the ventilator if a long transport journey is anticipated, allowing extended use. It is recommended at least two battery modules are loaded for even the shortest transport.
4. The ventilator is heavier (20 kg) than a dedicated transport ventilator.

Servo-*i* ventilator

- Versatile intensive care ventilator suitable for both paediatric and adult use.
- Wide range of controls, displays and alarms.
- Portable with battery power.

High frequency jet ventilator

This ventilator reduces the extent of the side-effects of conventional IPPV. There are lower peak airway pressures with better maintenance of the cardiac output and less anti-diuretic hormone production and fluid retention. It is better tolerated by alert patients than conventional IPPV (Figs 8.10 and 8.11).

Components

1. A Venturi injector is used: a cannula positioned in a tracheal tube (Fig. 8.12B), a cannula positioned in the trachea via the cricothyroid membrane, or a modified tracheal tube with two additional small lumens opening distally (Figs 8.12A & 8.13).
2. Solenoid valves are used to deliver the jet gas.

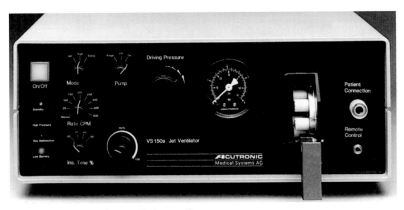

Fig. 8.10 The Acutronic VS 150s jet ventilator.

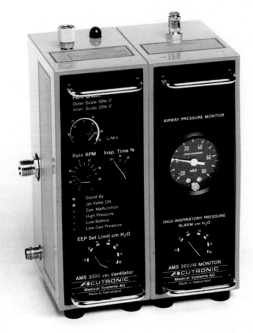

Fig. 8.11 The portable Acutronic AMS 3000M jet ventilator, which also features airway pressure monitoring.

3. The fresh gas leaving the narrow injector at a very high velocity causes entrainment of gas. The amount of entrained gas is uncertain making measurement of tidal volume and FiO_2 difficult.
4. The jet and entrained gases impact into the much larger volume of relatively immobile gases in the airway, causing them to move forward.
5. Expiration is passive. PEEP occurs automatically at a respiratory rate of over 100/min. Additional PEEP can be added by means of a PEEP valve.

Problems in practice and safety features

1. Barotrauma can still occur as expiration is dependent on passive lung and chest wall recoil driving the gas out through the tracheal tube.
2. High pressure ($35–40\,cmH_2O$) and system malfunction alarms are featured.

High frequency jet ventilator

- Time-cycled ventilator.
- A Venturi injector is used.
- Built-in peristaltic pump for humidification.
- Frequencies of 20–500 cycles/min. Minute volumes of 5–60 L/min.

---

3. Dials and display for driving pressure, frequency and inspiratory time.
4. Built-in peristaltic pump for nebulizing drugs or distilled water for humidifying the jet gas.
5. High flow air/oxygen or nitrous oxide/oxygen blender determines the mix of the jet gas.

Mechanism of action

1. Frequencies of 20–500 cycles/min can be selected, with minute volumes ranging from 5 to 60 L/min.
2. It is a time-cycled ventilator delivering gas in small jet pulsations. The inspiratory time is adjustable from 20% to 50% of the cycle.

VentiPAC

This is a portable ventilator used during the transport of critically ill patients (Fig. 8.14). It is a flow generator, time cycled, volume preset and pressure limited. It also acts as a pressure generator at flows below 0.25 L/sec in air mix setting. ParaPAC ventilator allows

A

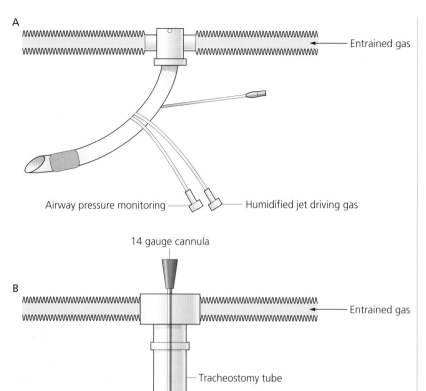

Entrained gas

Airway pressure monitoring

Humidified jet driving gas

14 gauge cannula

B

Entrained gas

Tracheostomy tube

Fig. 8.12 (A) The Mallinckrodt jet tube which offers two additional lumens for the jet driving gas and airway pressure monitoring. (B) A 14 gauge cannula positioned within a tracheostomy tube, through which the jet driving gas can be administered.

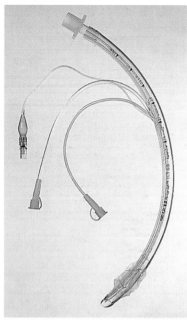

Fig. 8.13 The Mallinckrodt Hi-Lo Jet cuffed tracheal tube. An uncuffed version also exists.

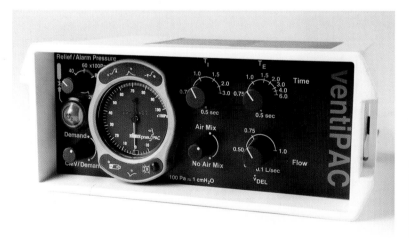

Fig. 8.14 The VentiPAC ventilator.

synchronization of ventilation with external cardiac massage during CPR. A neonatal/paediatric version exists.

Components

1. A variety of controls including:
   a) inspiratory flow (6–60 L/min)
   b) inspiratory time (0.5–3.0 sec)
   c) expiratory time (0.5–6.0 sec)
   d) adjustable inspiratory relief pressure with an audible alarm (20–80 cmH$_2$O)
   e) air mix/no air mix control
   f) a 'demand' and 'CMV/ demand' control.
2. Inflation pressure monitor to measure the airway pressure.
3. 120 cm polyester or silicone 15 mm tubing with a one-way valve to deliver gases to the patient.
4. Tubing to deliver the oxygen to the ventilator.

Mechanism of action

1. The source of power is dry, oil-free pressurized gas (270 to 600 kPa) at 60 L/min. Using air mix mode reduces gas consumption by the ventilator by almost 70%.
2. The frequency is set by adjusting the inspiratory and expiratory times.

3. The tidal volume is set by the adjustment of the flow and inspiratory time.
4. A choice of an FiO_2 of 1.0 (no air mix) or 0.45 (air mix).
5. The demand mode provides 100% oxygen to a spontaneously breathing patient. A visual indicator flashes when a spontaneous breath is detected.
6. CMV/demand mode provides continuous mandatory ventilation. If the patient makes a spontaneous breath, this causes the ventilator to operate in a synchronized minimum mandatory ventilation (SMMV) mode. Any superimposed mandatory ventilatory attempts are synchronized with the breathing pattern.
7. A PEEP valve can be added generating a PEEP of up to $20\,cmH_2O$.

Problems in practice and safety features

1. There is an adjustable inspiratory pressure relief mechanism with a range of $20–80\,cmH_2O$ to reduce the risk of overpressure and barotrauma.
2. There are audible and visual low pressure (disconnection) and high pressure (obstruction) alarms.
3. A supply gas failure alarm.
4. The ventilator is MRI compatible.

VentiPAC

- Portable ventilator powered by pressurized gas.
- Controls include flow rate, inspiratory time and expiratory time.
- An FiO_2 of 0.45 or 1.0 can be delivered.
- It has a demand valve.
- MRI compatible.

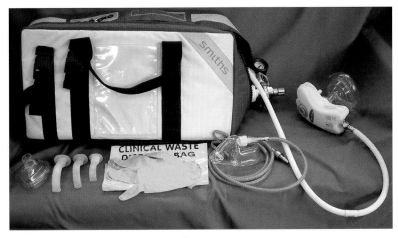

Fig. 8.15 Pneupac VR1 Emergency Ventilator.

Pneupac VR1 Emergency Ventilator (see Fig. 8.15)

This is a lightweight hand-held, time cycled, gas powered, flow generator ventilator. It is designed for use in emergency and during transport. It is MRI compatible up to 3 Tesla.

Components

1. Tidal volume/frequency control.
2. Auto/manual control with a manual trigger and push button.
3. Air mix switch allowing the delivery of oxygen at 100% or 50% concentrations.
4. Patient valve connecting to catheter mount/filter or face mask.
5. Gas supply input.

Mechanism of action

1. The source of power is pressurized oxygen (280–1034 kPa). Using air mix prolongs the duration of use from an oxygen cylinder.

2. A constant I:E ratio of 1:2 with flow rates of 11–32 L/min.
3. An optional patient demand facility is incorporated allowing synchronization between patient and ventilator.
4. The linked manual controls allow the manual triggering of a single controlled ventilation. This allows the ventilator to be used in a variety of chest compression/ventilation options in cardiac life support.
5. Suitable for children (above 10 kg body weight) and adults.

Problems in practice and safety features

1. Pressure relief valve designed to operate at $40\,cmH_2O$.
2. The manual control triggers a single ventilation equivalent to the volume of ventilation delivered in automatic ventilation. It is not a purge action so it cannot stack breaths and is therefore inherently much safer for the patient.

Pneupac VR1 Emergency Ventilator

- Hand-held, time cycled, gas powered, flow generator ventilator.
- Used in emergency and transport.
- MRI compatible up to 3 Tesla.
- Various controls.
- Can be used in children and adults.

Venturi injector device

A manually controlled Venturi ventilation device used during rigid bronchoscopy (Fig. 8.16). The anaesthetist and the operator share the airway. General anaesthesia is maintained intravenously.

Components

1. A high pressure oxygen source at about 400 kPa (from the anaesthetic machine or direct from a pipeline).
2. An on/off trigger.

3. Connection tubing that can withstand high pressures.
4. A needle of suitable gauge, which allows good air entrainment without creating excessive airway pressures.

Mechanism of action

1. The high pressure oxygen is injected intermittently through the needle placed at the proximal end of the bronchoscope.
2. This creates a Venturi effect, entraining atmospheric air and inflating the lungs with oxygen enriched air.
3. Oxygenation and carbon dioxide elimination are achieved with airway pressures of 25–30 cmH_2O.

Problems in practice and safety features

1. Barotrauma is possible. Airway pressure monitoring is not available.

2. Gastric distension can occur should ventilation commence before the distal end of the bronchoscope is beyond the larynx.

Venturi injector device

- Manually controlled Venturi used during rigid bronchoscopy.
- High pressure oxygen injected through a needle entraining air.

Self-inflating bag and mask

This is a means of providing manual IPPV. It is portable and is used during resuscitation, transport and short-term ventilation (Fig. 8.17).

Components

1. Self-inflating bag with a connection for added oxygen.

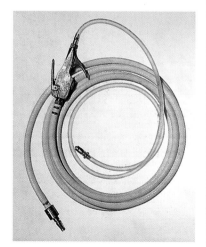

Fig. 8.16 The manually controlled injector. In practice this is connected to a rigid bronchoscope.

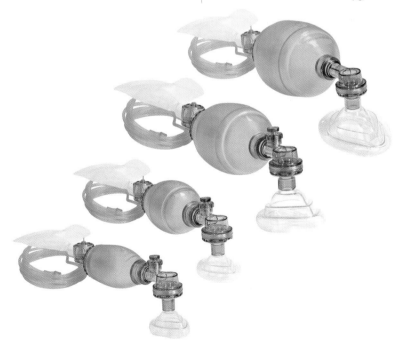

Fig. 8.17 A range of self-inflating resuscitation bags with oxygen reservoirs.

2. A one-way valve with three ports:
   a) inspiratory inlet allowing the entry of fresh gas during inspiration
   b) expiratory outlet allowing the exit of exhaled gas
   c) connection to the face mask or tracheal tube, and marked 'patient'.
3. A reservoir for oxygen to increase the FiO_2 delivered to the patient.

Mechanism of action

1. The non-rebreathing valve (Ambu valve) incorporates a silicone rubber membrane (Fig. 8.18). It has a small dead space and low resistance to flow. At a flow of 25 L/min, an inspiratory resistance of $0.4\,cmH_2O$ and an expiratory resistance of $0.6\,cmH_2O$ are achieved. The valve can be easily dismantled for cleaning and sterilization.
2. The valve acts as a spillover valve allowing excess inspiratory gas to be channelled directly to the expiratory outlet, bypassing the patient port.
3. The valve is suitable for both IPPV and spontaneous ventilation.
4. The shape of the self-inflating bag is automatically restored after compression. This allows fresh gas to be drawn from the reservoir.

5. A paediatric version exists with a smaller inflating bag and a pressure relief valve.
6. Disposable designs for both the adult and paediatric versions exist.

> Self-inflating bag
>
> - Compact, portable self-inflating bag with a one-way valve.
> - Oxygen reservoir can be added to increase FiO_2.
> - Paediatric version exists.

PEEP valve

This valve is used during IPPV to increase the FRC to improve the patient's oxygenation.

It is a spring-loaded unidirectional valve positioned on the expiratory side of the ventilator breathing system with a standard 22 mm connector. By adjusting the valve knob, a PEEP of between 0 and $20\,cmH_2O$ can be achieved (Fig. 8.19).

The valve provides almost constant expiratory resistance over a very wide range of flow rates.

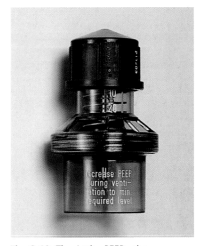

Fig. 8.19 The Ambu PEEP valve.

FURTHER READING

Bersten AD. Mechanical ventilation. In: Bersten A, Soni N, Oh TE (eds). Oh's Intensive Care Manual, 5th edn. London: Butterworth-Heinemann, 2003.

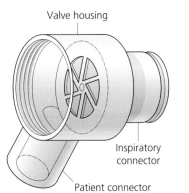

Valve housing

Expiratory connector

Valve membrane

Inspiratory connector

Patient connector

Fig. 8.18 An Ambu valve disassembled (reproduced with permission from AMBU International (UK) Ltd).

MCQs

In the following lists, which of the following statements (a) to (e) are true?

1. Bag in bottle ventilator
   a) The fresh gas flow is the driving gas at the same time.
   b) Is a minute volume divider.
   c) The bellows can be either ascending or descending.
   d) With a leak, the ascending bellows may continue to move almost normally.
   e) Can be used only for adult patients.

2. Manley ventilator
   a) Is a minute volume divider.
   b) Has one set of bellows.
   c) During controlled ventilation, it is safe to activate the emergency oxygen flush device of the anaesthetic machine.
   d) A pressure-monitoring ventilator alarm is attached to the expiratory limb.
   e) It acts as a Mapleson D system during spontaneous ventilation mode.

3. Bag in bottle ventilator
   a) It is a time-cycled ventilator.
   b) There is some mixing of the fresh gas and driving gas.
   c) For safety reasons, the descending bellows design is preferred.
   d) A small PEEP is expected.
   e) The driving gas volume in the chamber equals the tidal volume.

4. Regarding classification of ventilators
   a) A pressure generator ventilator can compensate for changes in lung compliance.
   b) A flow generator ventilator can not compensate for leaks in the system.
   c) A time-cycling ventilator is affected by the lung compliance.
   d) The duration of inspiration in a pressure-cycling ventilator is not affected by the compliance of the lungs.
   e) A pressure generator ventilator can compensate, to a degree, for leaks in the system.

5. High frequency jet ventilation
   a) The FiO_2 can be easily measured.
   b) Frequencies of up to 500 Hz can be achieved.
   c) The cardiac output is better maintained than conventional IPPV.
   d) Can be used both in anaesthesia and intensive care.
   e) Because of the lower peak airway pressures, there is no risk of barotrauma.

Answers

1. Bag in bottle ventilator
   a) *False.* The driving gas is separate from the fresh gas flow. The driving gas is usually either oxygen or, more economically, air. There is no mixing between the driving gas and the fresh gas flow. The volume of the driving gas reaching the chamber is equal to the tidal volume.
   b) *False.* The tidal volume and respiratory rate can be adjusted separately in a bag in bottle ventilator.
   c) *True.* Most of the bag in bottle ventilators use ascending bellows. This adds to the safety of the system as the bellows will collapse if there is a leak.
   d) *False.* See 'c'.
   e) *False.* The ventilator can be used for both adults and children. A different size bellows can be used for different age groups.

2. Manley ventilator
   a) *True.* The tidal volume can be set in a Manley ventilator. The whole fresh gas flow (minute volume) is delivered to the patient according to the set tidal volume, thus dividing the minute volume.
   b) *False.* There are two sets of bellows in a Manley ventilator, the time-cycling bellows and the main bellows.
   c) *False.* As it is a minute volume divider and the fresh gas flow is the driving gas (see 'a'), activating the emergency oxygen flush will lead to considerable increase in the minute volume.
   d) *False.* The pressure-monitoring alarm should be attached to the inspiratory limb and not the expiratory limb. A Wright spirometer can be attached to the expiratory limb to measure the tidal volume.
   e) *True.* During the spontaneous (manual) breathing mode, the Manley ventilator acts as a Mapleson D system.

3. Bag in bottle ventilator
   a) *True.* The inspiratory and expiratory periods can be determined by adjusting the I:E ratio and the respiratory rate. So, for example, with a rate of 10 breaths/min and an I:E ratio of 1:2 each breath lasts for 6 sec with an inspiration of 2 sec and expiration of 4 sec.
   b) *False.* There is no mixing between the fresh gas and the driving gas as they are completely separate.
   c) *False.* In case of a leak in the system, the descending bellows will not collapse. The opposite occurs with the ascending bellows.
   d) *True.* A PEEP of 2–4 cmH$_2$O is expected due to the compliance of the bellows.
   e) *True.*

4. Regarding classification of ventilators

a) *False. A pressure generator ventilator can not compensate for changes in lung compliance. It cycles when the set pressure has been reached. This can be a larger or smaller tidal volume depending on the lung compliance.*

b) *True. It will deliver the set flow whether there is a leak or not.*

c) *False. The ventilator will cycle with time regardless of the compliance.*

d) *False. In a lung with low compliance, the inspiration will be shorter because the pressure will be reached more quickly leading the ventilator to cycle and vice versa.*

e) *True. The ventilator will continue to deliver gases, despite the leak, until a pre-set pressure has been reached.*

5. High frequency jet ventilation

a) *False. The ventilator uses the Venturi principle to entrain ambient air. The amount of entrainment is uncertain, making the measurement of the FiO_2 difficult.*

b) *False. Frequencies of up to 500 per minute (not Hz; i.e. per second) can be achieved with a high frequency jet ventilator.*

c) *True. Because of the lower intrathoracic pressures generated during high frequency jet ventilation, causing a lesser effect on the venous return, the cardiac output is better maintained.*

d) *True. It can be used both in anaesthesia and intensive care, e.g. in the management of broncho-pleural fistula.*

e) *False. Although the risk is reduced, there is still a risk of barotrauma.*

Chapter 9

Humidification and filtration

Dry anaesthetic gases can cause damage to the cells lining the respiratory tract, impairing ciliary function. This increases the patient's susceptibility to respiratory tract infection. A decrease in body temperature (due to the loss of the latent heat of vaporization) occurs as the respiratory tract humidifies the dry gases.

Air fully saturated with water vapour has an absolute humidity of about 44 mg/L at 37°C. During nasal breathing at rest, inspired gases become heated to 36°C with a relative humidity of about 80–90% by the time they reach the carina, largely because of heat transfer in the nose. Mouth breathing reduces this to 60–70% relative humidity. The humidifying property of soda lime can achieve an absolute humidity of 29 mg/L when used with the circle breathing system.

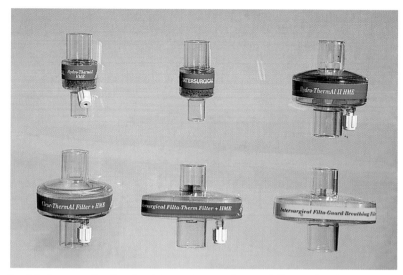

Fig. 9.1 A range of heat and moisture exchangers (top row). Heat and moisture exchangers with filtration properties (bottom left and centre). Breathing system filter with no humidification properties (bottom right).

Characteristics of the ideal humidifier

- Capable of providing adequate levels of humidification.
- Has low resistance to flow and low dead space.
- Provides microbiological protection to the patient.
- Maintenance of body temperature.
- Safe and convenient to use.
- Economical.

Heat and moisture exchanger (HME) humidifiers

These are compact, inexpensive and effective humidifiers for most clinical situations (Fig. 9.1).

The efficiency of an HME is gauged by the proportion of heat and moisture it returns to the patient. Adequate humidification is

achieved with a relative humidity of 60–70%. Inspired gases are warmed to temperatures of between 29° and 34°C. HMEs should be able to deliver an absolute humidity of a minimum of 30 g water vapour at 30°C. HMEs are easy and convenient to use with no need for an external power source.

Components

1. Two ports, designed to accept 15 and 22 mm size tubings and connections. Some designs have provision for connection of a sampling tube for gas and vapour concentration monitoring.
2. The head which contains a medium with hygrophobic properties (Fig. 9.2). It can be made of ceramic fibre, corrugated aluminium or paper, cellulose, metalized polyurethane foam or stainless-steel fibres.

Mechanism of action

1. Warm humidified exhaled gases pass through the humidifier, causing water vapour to condense

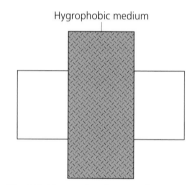

Hygrophobic medium

Fig. 9.2 Heat and moisture exchanger.

on the cooler HME medium. The condensed water is evaporated and returned to the patient with the next inspiration of dry and cold gases, humidifying them. There is no addition of water over and above that previously exhaled.
2. The greater the temperature difference between each side of the HME, the greater the potential for heat and moisture to be transferred during exhalation and inspiration.
3. The HME humidifier requires about 5–20 minutes before it reaches its optimal ability to humidify dry gases.

4. Some designs with a pore size of about 0.2 μm, can filter out bacteria, viruses and particles from the gas flow in either direction, as discussed later. They are called Heat and Moisture Exchanging Filters, HMEF.
5. Their volumes range from 7.8 mL (paediatric practice) to 100 mL. This increases the apparatus dead space.
6. The performance of the HME is affected by:
   a) water vapour content and temperature of the inspired and exhaled gases
   b) inspiratory and expiratory flow rates affecting the time the gas is in contact with the HME medium hence the heat and moisture exchange
   c) the volume and efficiency of the HME medium – the larger the medium, the greater the performance. Low thermal conductivity, i.e. poor heat conduction, helps to maintain a greater temperature difference across the HME increasing the potential performance.

Problems in practice and safety features

1. The estimated increase in resistance to flow due to these humidifiers ranges from 0.1 to 2.0 cmH$_2$O depending on the flow rate and the device used. Obstruction of the HME with mucus or because of the expansion of saturated heat exchanging material may occur and can result in dangerous increases in resistance.
2. It is recommended that they are used for a maximum of 24 hours and for single patient use only. There is a risk of increased airway resistance because of the accumulation of water in the filter housing if used for longer periods.
3. The humidifying efficiency decreases when large tidal volumes are used.
4. For the HME to function adequately, a 2-way gas flow is required.

Heat and moisture exchanger (HME) humidifier

- Water vapour present in the exhaled gases is condensed on the medium. It is evaporated and returned to the patient with the following inspiration.
- A relative humidity of 60–70 % can be achieved.
- Some designs incorporate a filter.
- There is an increase in apparatus dead space and airway resistance.
- The water vapour content and temperature of gases, flow rate of gases and the volume of the medium affect performance of HME.

Hot water bath humidifier

This humidifier is used to deliver relative humidities higher than the heat moisture exchange humidifier. It is usually used in intensive care units (Fig. 9.3).

Components

1. A container with an inlet and outlet for inspired gases. Heated sterile water partly fills the container.
2. A thermostatically controlled heating element.

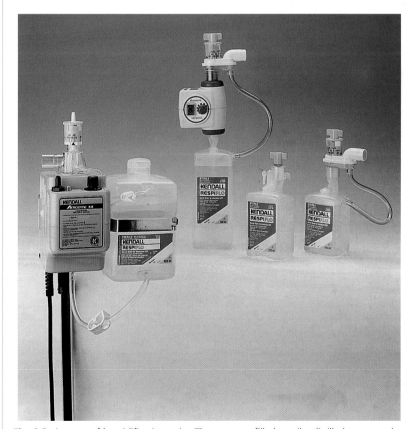

Fig. 9.3 A range of humidification units. These use prefilled, sterile, distilled water packs to avoid bacterial growth. Heated units producing warmed humidified gas (far left and centre left).

3. Tubing is used to deliver the humidified and warm gases to the patient. It should be as short as possible. A water trap is positioned between the patient and the humidifier along the tubing. The trap is positioned lower than the level of the patient.

Mechanism of action

1. The water is heated to the desired temperature (Fig. 9.4).
2. Dry cold gas enters the container where some passes close to the water surface, gaining maximum saturation. Some gas passes far from the water surface, gaining minimal saturation and heat.
3. The container has a large surface area for vaporization. This is to ensure that the gas is fully saturated at the temperature of the water bath. The amount of gas effectively bypassing the water surface should be minimal.
4. The tubing has poor thermal insulation properties causing a decrease in the temperature of inspired gases. This is partly compensated for by the release of the heat of condensation.
5. By raising the temperature in the humidifier above body temperature, it is possible to deliver gases at 37°C and fully saturated. The temperature of gases at the patient's end is measured by a thermistor. Via a feedback mechanism, the thermistor controls the temperature of water in the container.
6. The temperature of gases at the patient's end depends on the surface area available for vaporization, the flow rate and the amount of cooling and condensation taking place in the inspiratory tubing.

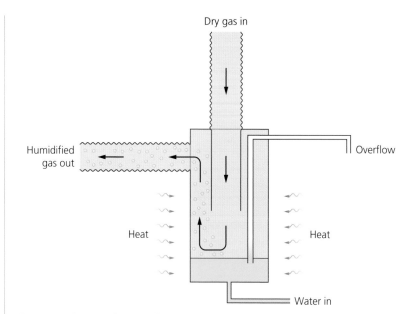

Fig. 9.4 Mechanism of action of the hot water bath humidifier.

Problems in practice and safety features

1. The humidifier, which is electrically powered, should be safe to use with no risk of scalding, overhydration and electric shock. A second back-up thermostat cuts in should there be malfunction of the first thermostat.
2. The humidifier and water trap(s) should be positioned below the level of the tracheal tube to prevent flooding of the airway by condensed water.
3. Colonization of the water by bacteria can be prevented by increasing the temperature to 60°C. This poses greater risk of scalding.
4. The humidifier is large, expensive and can be awkward to use.
5. There are more connections in a ventilator set up and so the risk of disconnections or leak increases.

Hot water bath humidifier

- Consists of a container with a thermostatically controlled heating element and tubing with water traps.
- The temperature of water in the container, via a feedback mechanism, is controlled by a thermistor at the patient's end.
- Full saturation at 37°C can be achieved.
- Colonization by bacteria is a problem.

Nebulizers (Fig. 9.5)

These produce a mist of microdroplets of water suspended in a gaseous medium. The quantity of water droplets delivered is not limited by gas temperature (as is the case with vapour). The smaller the droplets, the more stable they are. Droplets of 2–5 μm deposit in

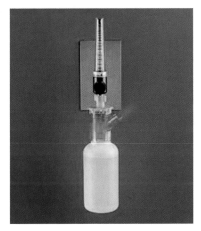

Fig. 9.5 Smith's medical gas-driven nebulizer.

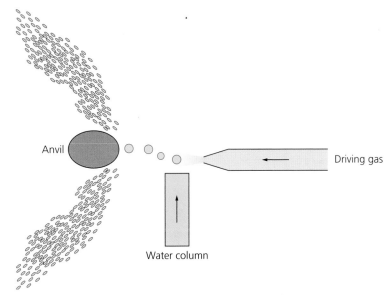

Fig. 9.6 Mechanism of action of a gas-driven nebulizer humidifier.

the tracheo-bronchial tree, whereas 0.5–1 μm droplets deposit in the alveoli. In addition to delivering water, nebulizers are used to deliver medications to peripheral airways and radio-active isotopes in diagnostic lung ventilation imaging.

There are three types: gas-driven, spinning disc and ultrasonic.

GAS-DRIVEN (JET) NEBULIZER

Components

1. A capillary tube with the bottom end immersed in a water container.
2. The top end of the capillary tube is close to a Venturi constriction (Fig. 9.6).

Mechanism of action

1. A high pressure gas flows through the Venturi, creating a negative pressure.
2. Water is drawn up through the capillary tube and broken into a fine spray. Even smaller droplets

can be achieved as the spray hits an anvil or a baffle.

3. The majority of the droplets are in the range of 2–4 μm. These droplets tend to deposit on the pharynx and upper airway with a small amount reaching the bronchial level. This nebulizer is also capable of producing larger droplets of up to 20 μm in size. Droplets with diameters of 5 μm or more fall back into the container leaving droplets of 4 μm or less to float out with the fresh gas flow.
4. The device is compact, making it easy to place close to the patient.

SPINNING DISC NEBULIZER

This is motor-driven spinning disc throwing out microdroplets of water by centrifugal force. The water impinges onto the disc after being drawn from a reservoir via a tube over which the disc is mounted.

ULTRASONIC NEBULIZER

A transducer head vibrates at an ultrasonic frequency (e.g. 3 MHz). The transducer can be immersed into water or water can be dropped on to it, producing droplets less than 1–2 μm in size. Droplets of 1 μm or less are deposited in alveoli and lower airways. There is a risk of overhydration especially in children.

Nebulizers

- Produce microdroplets of water of different sizes, 1–20 μm.
- The quantity of water droplets is not limited by the temperature of the carrier gas.
- They can be gas-driven, spinning disc or ultrasonic.

Bacterial and viral filters

These minimize the risk of cross transmission of bacteria and/or viruses between patients using the same anaesthetic breathing systems. It is thought that the incidence of bleeding after oro-tracheal intubation is 86%. The filter should be positioned as close to the patient as possible, e.g. on the disposable catheter mount, to protect the rest of the breathing system, ventilator and anaesthetic machine. It is recommended that a new filter should be used for each patient. A humidification element can be added producing a Heat and Moisture Exchanging Filter (HMEF).

Characteristics of the ideal filter

1. Efficient – the filter should be effective against both air- and liquid-borne micro-organisms. A filtration action of 99.99–99.999% should be achieved. This allows between 100 and 10 micro-organisms to pass the through the filter, respectively, after a 10^6 micro-organism challenge. The filter should be effective bi-directionally.
2. Minimal dead space, particularly for paediatric practice.
3. Minimum resistance, especially when wet.
4. Not affected by anaesthetic agents and does not affect the anaesthetic agents.
5. Effective when either wet or dry. It should completely prevent the passage of contaminated body liquids (blood, saliva and other liquids) which may be present or generated in the breathing system.
6. User friendly, lightweight, not bulky and non-traumatic to the patient.
7. Disposable.
8. Provide some humidification if no other methods being used. Adequate humidification can usually be achieved by the addition of a hygroscopic element to the device.
9. Transparent.
10. Cost effective.

Size of micro-organisms

Hepatitis virus	0.02 μm
Adenovirus	0.07 μm
HIV	0.08 μm
Mycobacterium tuberculosis	0.3 μm
Staphylococcus aureus	1.0 μm
Cytomegalovirus	0.1 μm

Components

1. Two ports designed to accept 15 and 22 mm size tubings and connections.
2. A sampling port to measure the gases'/agents' concentrations positioned on the anaesthetic breathing system side.
3. The filtration element can be either a felt-like electrostatic material or a pleated hydrophobic material.

Mechanism of action

There are five main mechanisms by which filtration can be achieved on a fibre.

1. **Direct interception:** large particles ($\geq 1\,\mu m$), such as dust and large bacteria, are physically prevented from passing through the pores of the filter because of their large size.
2. **Inertial impaction:** smaller particles (0.5–1 μm) collide with the filter medium because of their inertia. They tend to continue in straight lines, carried along by their own momentum rather than following the path of least resistance taken by the gas. The particles are held by Van der Waal's electrostatic forces.
3. **Diffusional interception:** very small particles (<0.5 μm), such as viruses, are captured because they undergo considerable Brownian motion (i.e. random movement) because of their very small mass. This movement increases their apparent diameter so that they are more likely to be captured by the filter element.
4. **Electrostatic attraction:** this can be very important but it is difficult to measure as it requires knowing the charge on the particles and on the fibres. Increasing the charge on either the particles or the fibres increases the filtration efficiency. Charged particles are attracted to oppositely charged fibres by coulombic attraction.
5. **Gravitational settling:** this affects large particles (>5 μm). The rate of settling depends on the balance between the effect of gravity on the particle and the buoyancy of the particle. In filters used in anaesthesia, it has minimal effect as most of the settling occurs before the particles reach the filter.

ELECTROSTATIC FILTERS (FIG. 9.7)

1. The element used is subjected to an electric field producing a felt-like material with high polarity. Usually two polymer fibres (modacrylic and polyprolyne) are used.
2. These filters rely on the electrical charge to attract oppositely charged particles from the gas flow. They have a filtration efficiency of 99.99%.
3. The electrical charge increases the efficiency of the filter when the element dry but can deteriorate rapidly when it is wet. The resistance to flow increases when the element is wet.
4. The electrical charge on the filter fibres decays with time so it has a limited life.
5. A hygroscopic layer can be added to the filter in order to provide humidification. In such an HMEF, the pressure drop across the element and thus the resistance to breathing will also increase with gradual absorption of water.

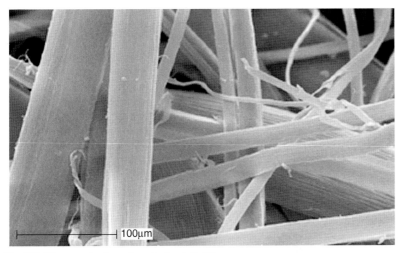

Fig. 9.7 Microscopic view of an electrostatic filter.

3. The forces between individual liquid water molecules are stronger than those between the water molecules and the hydrophobic membrane. This leads to the collection of water on the surface of the membrane with no absorption. Such a filter can successfully prevent the passage of water under pressures as high as $60\,cmH_2O$.
4. Although hydrophobic filters provide some humidification, a hygroscopic element can be added to improve humidification.

Currently there is no evidence showing any type of filter is clinically superior to another.

HYDROPHOBIC FILTERS (FIG. 9.8)

1. The very small pore size filter membrane provides adequate filtration over longer periods of time. These filters rely on the naturally occurring electrostatic interactions to remove the particles. A filtration efficiency of 99.999% can be achieved.
2. To achieve minimal pressure drop across the device with such a small pore size, so allowing high gas flows while retaining low resistance, a large surface area is required. Pleated paper filters made of inorganic fibres are used to achieve this.

Bacterial and viral filters

- Can achieve a filtration efficiency of 99.99–99.999%.
- Electrostatic filters rely on an electrical charge to attract oppositely charged particles. Their efficiency is reduced when wet and the have a limited life span.
- Hydrophobic pleated filters can repel water even under high pressures. They have a longer time span.

FURTHER READING

Medical Devices Agency. Heat and moisture exchangers (HMEs) including those intended for use as breathing system filters. UK Market-Product review. Medical Devices Agency, London, Jan 1998; No. 347.
Turnbull D, Fisher PC, Mills GH et al. Performance of breathing filters under wet conditions: a laboratory evaluation. British Journal of Anaesthesia 2005;94:675–682.
Wilkis AR, Stevens J. Association of Anaesthetists recommendations on filters to prevent cross infection in anaesthetic breathing systems. Anaesthesia 1996;51:1080–1081.

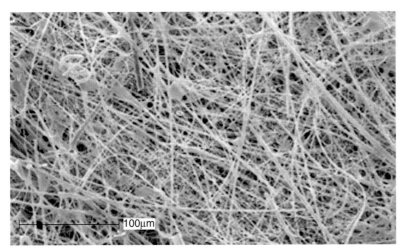

Fig. 9.8 Microscopic view of a hydrophobic filter.

MCQs

In the following lists, which of the statements (a) to (e) are true?

1. Nebulizers
   a) The gas-driven nebulizer can deliver much smaller droplets than the ultrasonic nebulizer.
   b) There is a risk of drowning.
   c) The temperature of the gas determines the amount of water delivered.
   d) The smaller the droplets are, the more stable they are.
   e) Droplets of 1 μm or less are deposited in the alveoli and lower airways.

2. Humidity
   a) Humidity is measured using a hair hygrometer.
   b) Air fully saturated with water vapour has a relative humidity of about 44 mg/L at 37°C.
   c) Using the circle breathing system, some humidification can be achieved despite using dry fresh gas flow.
   d) Relative humidity is the ratio of the mass of water vapour in a given volume of air to the mass of water vapour required to saturate the same volume at the same temperature.
   e) The ideal relative humidity in the operating theatre is about 45–55%.

3. Bacterial and viral filters
   a) Particles of less than 0.5 μm can be captured by direct interception.
   b) They can achieve a filtration action of 99.999%.
   c) They should be effective when either wet or dry.
   d) The filtration element used can be either an electrostatic or a pleated hydrophobic material.
   e) The hydrophobic filter has a more limited life span than the electrostatic filter.

4. Hot water bath humidifiers
   a) Heating the water improves the performance.
   b) Because of its efficiency, the surface area for vaporization does not have to be large.
   c) There is a risk of scalding to the patient.
   d) Temperature in the humidifier is usually kept below body temperature.
   e) The temperature of water in the container is controlled by a feedback mechanism using a thermistor which measures the temperature of the gases at the patient's end.

5. Heat exchange humidifiers
   a) Inspired gases are warmed to 29–34°C.
   b) Performance is improved by increasing the volume of the medium.
   c) An absolute humidity of 60–70% can be achieved.
   d) At high flows, the performance is reduced.
   e) Performance is affected by the temperature of the inspired and exhaled gases.

6. The following statements are true
   a) Mucus can cause obstruction of the heat and moisture exchanger (HME).
   b) 2–5 μm sized nebulized droplets are deposited in the alveoli.
   c) HMEs should deliver a minimum of 300 g water vapour at 30°C.
   d) A relative humidity of 80% at the carina can be achieved during normal breathing.
   e) HME requires some time before it reaches its optimal ability to humidify dry gases.

Answers

1. Nebulizers
   a) *False*. The ultrasonic nebulizer can deliver very much smaller droplets. 2–4 (μm droplets can be delivered by the gas-driven nebulizer. Droplets of less than 1–2 (μm in size can be delivered by the ultrasonic nebulizer.
   b) *True*. This is especially so in children using the ultrasonic nebulizer.
   c) *False*. The temperature of the gas has no effect on the quantity of water droplets delivered. The temperature of the gas is of more importance in the humidifier.
   d) *True*. Very small droplets generated by the ultrasonic nebulizer are very stable and can be deposited in the alveoli and lower airways.
   e) *True*. See 'd'.

2. Humidity
   a) *True*. The hair hygrometer is used to measure relative humidity between 15 and 85%. It is commonly used in the operating theatre. The length of the hair increases with the increase in ambient humidity. This causes a pointer to move over a chart measuring the relative humidity.
   b) *False*. It should be absolute humidity and not relative humidity. Relative humidity is measured as a percentage.
   c) *True*. Water is produced as a product of the reaction between CO_2 and NaOH. An absolute humidity of 29 mg/L at 37°C can be achieved.
   d) *True*.
   e) *True*. A high relative humidity is uncomfortable for the staff in the operating theatre. Too low a relative humidity can lead to the build up of static electricity increasing the risk of ignition.

3. Bacterial and viral filters
   a) *False*. Such small particles are captured by diffusional interception. Direct interception can capture particles with sizes equal or more than 1 μm.
   b) *True*. Hydrophobic filters can achieve a filtration action of 99.999%. Electrostatic filters can achieve 99.99% which is thought to be adequate for routine use during anaesthesia.
   c) *True*. Hydrophobic filters are effective both when dry and wet. Electrostatic filters become less effective when wet.
   d) *True*.
   e) *False*. The electrostatic filter has a more limited life span than the hydrophobic filter. The efficacy of the electrostatic filter decreases as the electrical charge on the filter fibres decays.

4. Hot water bath humidifiers
   a) *True. This is due to the loss of latent heat of vaporization as more water changes into vapour. The lower the water temperature, the less vapour is produced.*
   b) *False. A large surface area is needed to improve efficiency.*
   c) *True. A faulty thermostat can cause over-heating of the water. There is usually a second thermostat to prevent this.*
   d) *False. The temperature of the humidifier is usually kept above body temperature. A large amount of heat is lost as the vapour and gases pass through the plastic tubings.*
   e) *True.*

5. Heat exchange humidifiers
   a) *True.*
   b) *True. The larger the volume of the medium, the better the performance of the HME. This is because of the larger surface area of contact between the gas and the medium.*
   c) *False. A relative, not absolute, humidity of 60–70% can be achieved.*
   d) *True. At high flows, the time the gas is in contact with the medium is reduced so decreasing the performance of the HME. The opposite is also correct.*
   e) *True. The higher the temperature of the gases, the better the performance of the HME.*

6. The following statements are true
   a) *True. Mucus can cause obstruction of the HME resulting in dangerous increases in resistance.*
   b) *False. 2–5 µm nebulized droplets are deposited in the tracheo-bronchial tree. Smaller droplets of 0.5–1 µm are deposited in the alveoli.*
   c) *False. HME should deliver a minimum of 30 g water vapour at 30°C.*
   d) *True.*
   e) *True. HME requires 5–20 minutes before it reaches its optimal ability to humidify dry gases.*

Chapter 10

Non-invasive monitoring

Clinical observation provides vital information regarding the patient. Observations gained from the use of the various monitors should augment that information; skin perfusion, capillary refill, cyanosis, pallor, skin temperature and turgor, chest movement and heart auscultation are just a few examples. The equipment used to monitor the patient is becoming more sophisticated. It is vital that the clinician using these monitors is aware of their limitations and the potential causes of error. Errors can be due to patient, equipment and/or sampling factors.

Monitoring equipment can be invasive or non-invasive. The latter is discussed in this chapter, whereas the former is discussed in Chapter 11.

Integrated monitoring

Until recently, it was common to see the anaesthetic machine adorned with discrete, bulky monitoring devices. Significant advances in information technology have allowed an integrated monitoring approach to occur. Plug-in monitoring modules feed a single visual display on which selected values and waveforms can be arranged and colour-coded (Figs 10.1, 10.2 and 10.3).

Although some would argue that such monitoring systems are complex and potentially confusing, their benefits in term of flexibility and ergonomics are undisputed.

Electrocardiogram (ECG)

This monitors the electrical activity of the heart with electrical potentials of 0.5–2 mV at the skin surface. It

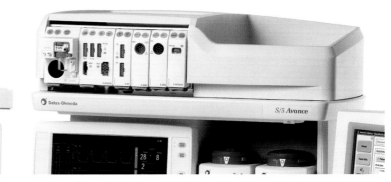

Fig. 10.1 Datex-Ohmeda plug-in monitoring modules mounted on the S/5 Advance anaesthetic machine.

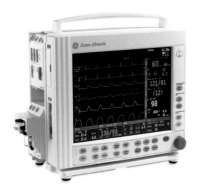

Fig. 10.2 Datex-Ohmeda compact monitor.

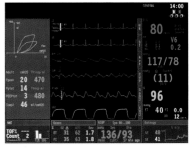

Fig. 10.3 Colour-coded values and waveforms displayed on the Datex-Ohmeda monitor.

is useful in determining the heart rate, ischaemia, the presence of arrhythmias and conduction defects. It should be emphasized that it gives no assessment of cardiac output.

The bipolar leads (I, II, III, AVR, AVL and AVF) measure voltage difference between two electrodes. The unipolar leads (V1–6) measure voltage at different electrodes relative to a zero point.

Components

1. Skin electrodes detect the electrical activity of the heart (Fig. 10.4). Silver and silver chloride form a stable electrode combination. Both are held in a cup and separated from the skin by a foam pad soaked in conducting gel.
2. The ECG signal is then boosted using an amplifier. The amplifier

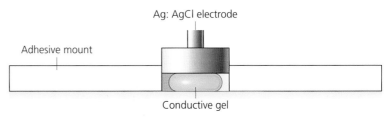

Fig. 10.4 An ECG electrode.

covers a frequency range of 0.05–100 Hz. It also filters out some of the frequencies considered to be noise.

3. An oscilloscope that displays the amplified ECG signal. A high resolution monochrome or colour monitor is used.

Mechanism of action

1. Proper attachment of ECG electrodes involves cleaning the skin, gently abrading the stratum corneum and ensuring adequate contact using conductive gel.
2. The ECG monitor can have two modes:
   a) The **monitoring mode** has a limited frequency response of 0.5–40 Hz. Filters are used to narrow the bandwidth to reduce environmental artifacts. The high-frequency filters reduce distortions from muscle movement, mains current and electromagnetic interference from other equipment. The low-frequency filters help provide a stable baseline by reducing respiratory and body movement artifacts.
   b) The **diagnostic mode** has a wider frequency response of 0.05–100 Hz. The high frequency limit allows the assessment of the ST segment, QRS morphology and tachy-arrhythmias. The low frequency limit allows representation of P and T-wave morphology and ST-segment analysis.
3. There are many ECG electrode configurations. Usually during anaesthesia, three skin electrodes are used (right arm, left arm and indifferent leads). Lead II is ideal for detecting arrythmias. CM5 configuration is able to detect 89% of ST-segment changes due to left ventricular ischaemia. In CM5, the right arm electrode is positioned on the manubrium

(chest lead from **m**anubrium), the left arm electrode is on V5 position (**5th** interspace in the left anterior axillary line) and the indifferent lead is on the left shoulder or any convenient position (Fig. 10.5).
4. The CB5 configuration is useful during thoracic anaesthesia. The right arm electrode is positioned over the centre of the right scapula and the left arm electrode is over V5.
5. A display speed of 25 mm/s and a sensitivity of 1 mV/cm are standard in the UK.

Problems in practice and safety features

1. Incorrect placement of the ECG electrodes in relation to the heart is a common error, leading to false information.
2. Electrical interference can be a 50 Hz (in UK) mains line interference because of capacitance or inductive coupling

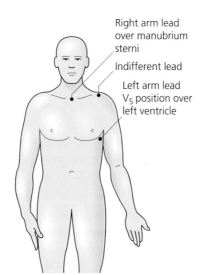

Right arm lead over manubrium sterni

Indifferent lead

Left arm lead V$_5$ position over left ventricle

Fig. 10.5 The CM5 ECG lead configuration (reproduced with permission from Aitkenhead R, Smith G. Textbook of Anaesthesia, 3rd edn. Churchill Livingstone, 1996).

effect. Any electrical device powered by AC can act as one plate of a capacitor and the patient acts as the other plate. Interference can also be because of high frequency current interference from diathermy. Most modern monitors have the facilities to avoid interference. Shielding of cables and leads, differential amplifiers and electronic filters all help to produce an interference-free monitoring system. Differential amplifiers measure the difference between the potential from two different sources. If there is interference common to the two input terminals (e.g. mains frequency), it can be eliminated as only the differences between the two terminals is amplified. This is called *common mode rejection*.

Table 10.1 shows the various types and sources of interference and how to reduce the interference.
3. Muscular activity, such as shivering, can produce artifacts. Positioning the electrodes over bony prominences and the use of low-pass filters can reduce these artifacts.
4. High and low ventricular rate alarms and an audible indicator of ventricular rate are standard on most designs. More advanced monitors have the facility to monitor the ST segment (Fig. 10.6). Continuous monitoring and measurement of the height of the ST segment allows early diagnosis of ischaemic changes.
5. Absence of or improperly positioned patient diathermy plate can cause burns at the site of ECG skin electrodes. This is because of the passage of the diathermy current via the electrodes causing a relatively high current density.

Table 10.1 ECG signal interference

Type of interference	Sources of interference	How to reduce interference
Electromagnetic induction	Any electrical cable or light	Use long ECG and twisted leads (rejecting the induced signal as common mode) Use selective filters in amplifiers
Electrostatic induction and capacitance coupling	Stray capacitances between table, lights, monitors, patients and electrical cables	ECG leads are surrounded by copper screens
Radiofrequency interference (>100 Hz)	Diathermy enters the system by: • mains supply • direct application by probe • radio transmission via probe and wire	High frequency filters clean up signal before entering input Filtering power supply of amplifiers Double screen electronic components of amplifiers and earth outer screen. Newer machines operate at higher frequencies

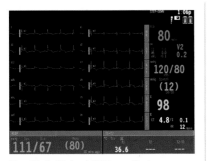

Fig. 10.6 12-lead ECG monitoring.

ECG

- Silver and silver chloride skin electrodes detect the electrical activity of the heart, 0.5–2 mV at the skin surface.
- The signal is boosted by an amplifier and displayed by an oscilloscope.
- The ECG monitor can have two modes, the monitoring mode (frequency range 0.5–40 Hz) and the diagnostic mode (frequency range 0.05–100 Hz).
- CM5 configuration is used to monitor left ventricular ischaemia.
- Electrical interference can be due either to diathermy or mains frequency.
- Differential amplifiers are used to reduce interference (common mode rejection).

Arterial blood pressure

Oscillometry is the commonest method used to measure blood pressure non-invasively during anaesthesia. The systolic, diastolic and mean arterial pressures and pulse rate are measured, calculated and displayed. These devices give reliable trend information about the blood pressure. The term DINAMAP (Device for Indirect Non-invasive Automatic Mean Arterial Pressure) is used for such devices.

Components

1. A cuff with a tube used for inflation and deflation. Some designs have an extra tube for transmitting pressure fluctuations to the pressure transducer.
2. The case where the microprocessor and pressure transducer are housed. It contains the display and a timing mechanism which adjusts the frequency of measurements. Alarm limits can be set for both high and low values.

Mechanism of action

1. The microprocessor is set to control the sequence of inflation and deflation.
2. The cuff is inflated to a pressure above the previous systolic pressure, then it is deflated incrementally. The return of blood flow causes oscillation in cuff pressure (Fig. 10.7).
3. The transducer senses the pressure changes which are interpreted by the microprocessor. This transducer has an accuracy of ± 2%.
4. The mean arterial blood pressure corresponds to the maximum oscillation at the lowest cuff pressure. The systolic pressure

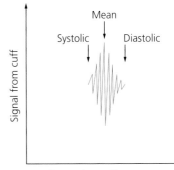

Fig. 10.7 Diagram showing how oscillations in cuff pressure correspond to mean, systolic and diastolic pressures.

corresponds to the onset of rapidly increasing oscillations.
5. The diastolic pressure corresponds to the onset of rapidly decreasing oscillations. In addition, it is mathematically computed from the systolic and mean pressure values (mean blood pressure = diastolic blood pressure + 1/3 pulse pressure).
6. The cuff must be of the correct size (Table 10.2). It should cover at least 2/3 of the upper arm. The width of the cuff's bladder should be 40% of the mid-circumference of the limb. The middle of the cuff's bladder should be positioned over the brachial artery.
7. Some designs have the ability to apply venous stasis to facilitate intravenous cannulation.

Problems in practice and safety features

1. For the device to measure the arterial blood pressure accurately, it should have a fast cuff inflation and a slow cuff deflation (at a rate of 3 mmHg/s or 2 mmHg/beat). The former is to avoid venous congestion and the latter provides enough time to detect the arterial pulsation.
2. If the cuff is too small, the blood pressure is over-read, while it is under-read if the cuff is too large. The error is greater with too small than too large a cuff.
3. The systolic pressure is over-read at low pressures (systolic pressure less than 60 mmHg) and under-read at high systolic pressures.

Table 10.2 A guide to the correct blood pressure cuff size

3 cm	Infant
5 cm	Infant
6 cm	Child
9 cm	Small adult
12 cm	Standard adult
15 cm	Large adult

4. Atrial fibrillation and other arrhythmias affect performance.
5. External pressure on the cuff or its tubing can cause inaccuracies.
6. Frequently repeated cuff inflations can cause ulnar nerve palsy and petechial haemorrhage of the skin under the cuff.

The Finapres uses a combination of oscillometry and a servo control unit. The inflation and deflation of a finger cuff is controlled, producing non-invasive continuous blood pressure measurement.

THE VON RECKLINGHAUSEN OSCILLOTONOMETER

During the pre-microprocessor era, the *Von Recklinghausen Oscillotonometer* was widely used (Fig. 10.8).

Components

1. Two cuffs; the upper, occluding cuff (5 cm wide) overlaps a lower, sensing cuff (10 cm wide). An inflation bulb is attached.
2. The case which contains:
   a) two bellows, one connected to the atmosphere (bellows A), the other connected to the lower sensing cuff (bellows B)
   b) a mechanical amplification system
   c) the oscillating needle and dial
   d) the control lever
   e) the release valve.

Mechanism of action

1. With the control lever at rest, air is pumped into both cuffs and the airtight case of the instrument using the inflation bulb to a pressure exceeding systolic arterial pressure. By operating the control lever, the lower sensing cuff is isolated and the pressure in the upper cuff and instrument case is allowed to decrease slowly through an adjustable leak controlled by the release valve. As systolic pressure is reached, pulsation of the artery under the lower cuff results in pressure oscillations within the cuff and bellows B. The pressure oscillations are transmitted via a mechanical amplification system to the needle. As the pressure in the upper cuff decreases below diastolic pressure, the pulsation ceases (Fig. 10.9).
2. The mean pressure is at the point of maximum oscillation.

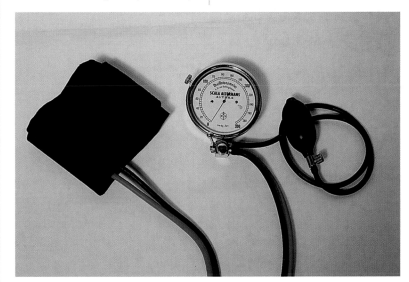

Fig. 10.8 The Von Recklinghausen oscillotonometer.

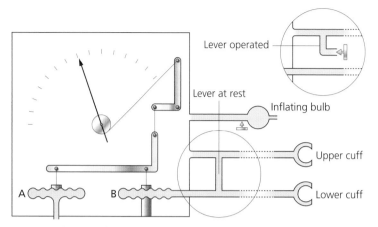

Fig. 10.9 Mechanism of action of the oscillotonometer. See text for details (reproduced with permission from Aitkenhead R, Smith G. Textbook of Anaesthesia, 2nd edn. Churchill Livingstone, 1990).

3. This method is reliable at low pressures. It is useful to measure trends in blood pressure.

Problems in practice and safety features

1. In order for the device to operate accurately, the cuffs must be correctly positioned and attached to their respective tubes.
2. The diastolic pressure is not measured accurately with this device.

Arterial blood pressure

- Oscillometry is the method used.
- Mean arterial pressure corresponds to maximum oscillation.
- A cuff with a tube(s) is connected to a transducer and a microprocessor.
- Accurate within the normal range of blood pressure.
- Arrhythmias and external pressure affect the performance.

Pulse oximetry

This is a non-invasive measurement of the arterial blood oxygen saturation at the level of the arterioles. A continuous display of the oxygenation is achieved by a simple, accurate and rapid method (Fig. 10.10).

Pulse oximetry has proved to be a powerful monitoring tool in the operating theatre, recovery wards, intensive care units, general wards and during the transport of critically ill patients. It is considered to be the greatest technical advance in monitoring of the last decade. It enables the detection of incipient and

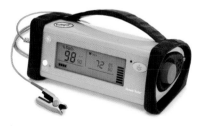

Fig. 10.10 Datex-Ohmeda Trusat oximeter.

unsuspected arterial hypoxaemia, allowing treatment before tissue damage.

Components

1. A probe is positioned on the finger, toe, ear lobe or nose (Fig. 10.11). Two light emitting diodes (LEDs) produce beams at red and infrared frequencies (660 nm and 940 nm respectively) on one side and there is a sensitive photodetector on the other side. The LEDs operate in sequence at a rate of about 30 times per second (Fig. 10.12).
2. The case houses the microprocessor. There is a display of the oxygen saturation, pulse rate and a plethysmographic waveform of the pulse. Alarm limits can be set for a low saturation value and for both high and low pulse rates.

Mechanism of action

1. The oxygen saturation is estimated by measuring the transmission of light, through a pulsatile vascular tissue bed (e.g. finger). This is based on Beer's law (the relation between the light absorbed and the concentration of solute in the solution) and Lambert's law (relation between absorption of light and the thickness of the absorbing layer).
2. The amount of light transmitted depends on many factors. The light absorbed by non-pulsatile tissues (e.g. skin, soft tissues, bone and venous blood) is constant (DC). The non-constant absorption (AC) is the result of arterial blood pulsations (Fig. 10.13). The sensitive photodetector generates a voltage proportional to the transmitted light. The AC component of the wave is about 1–5% of the total signal.

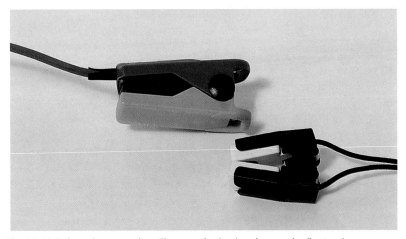

Fig. 10.11 Pulse oximeter probes. Finger probe (top) and ear probe (bottom).

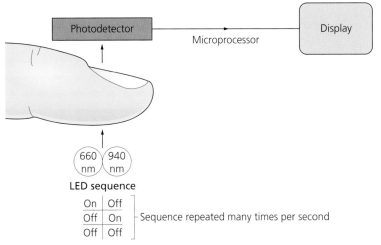

Fig. 10.12 Working principles of the pulse oximeter. The LEDs operate in sequence and when both are off the photodetector measures the background level of ambient light.

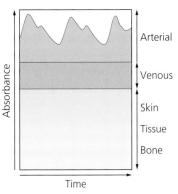

Fig. 10.13 Schematic representation of the contribution of various body components to the absorbance of light (reproduced with permission from Aitkenhead R, Smith G. Textbook of Anaesthesia, 3rd edn. Churchill Livingstone, 1996).

Masimo Rad-57 oximeter uses eight light wavelengths.
6. A variable pitch beep provides an audible signal of changes in saturation.

Problems in practice and safety features

1. It is accurate (± 2%) in the 70–100% range. Below the saturation of 70%, readings are extrapolated.
2. The absolute measurement of oxygen saturation may vary from one probe to another but with accurate trends. This is due to the variability of the centre wavelength of the LEDs.
3. Carbon monoxide poisoning (including smoking), coloured nail varnish, intravenous injections of certain dyes (e.g. methylene blue, indocyanine green), and drugs responsible for the production of methaemoglobinaemia are all sources of error (Table 10.3).
4. Hypoperfusion and severe peripheral vasoconstriction affect the performance of the pulse oximeter. This is because

3. The high frequency of the LEDs allows the absorption to be sampled many times during each pulse beat. This is used to enable running averages of saturation to be calculated many times per second. This decreases the 'noise' (e.g. movement) effect on the signal.
4. The microprocessor is programmed to mathematically analyse both the DC and AC components at 660 and 940 nm. The result is related to the arterial saturation. The absorption of oxyhaemoglobin and deoxyhaemoglobin at these two wavelengths is very different. This allows these two wavelengths to provide good sensitivity. 805 nanometres is one of the isobestic points of oxyhaemoglobin and deoxyhaemoglobin. The OFF part allows a baseline measurement for any changes in ambient light.
5. A more recent design uses multiple wavelengths to eradicate false readings from carboxy haemoglobin and methaemoglobinaemia. The

Table 10.3 Sources of error in pulse oximetry

HbF	No significant clinical change (absorption spectrum is similar to the adult Hb over the range of wavelengths used)
MetHb	False low reading
CoHb	False high reading
SulphHb	Not a clinical problem
Bilirubin	Not a clinical problem
Dark skin	No effect
Methylene blue	False low reading
Indocyanine green	False low reading
Nail varnish	May cause false low reading

the AC signal sensed is about 1–5% of the DC signal when the pulse volume is normal. This makes it less accurate during vasoconstriction when the AC component is reduced.

5. The device monitors the oxygen saturation with no direct information regarding oxygen delivery to the tissues.

6. Pulse oximeters average their readings every 10–20 seconds. They can not detect acute desaturation. The response time to desaturation is longer with the finger probe (more than 60 seconds) whereas the ear probe has a response time of 10–15 seconds.

7. Excessive movement or malposition of the probe is a source of error. Newer designs such as the Masimo oximeter claim more stability despite motion. External fluorescent light can be a source of interference.

8. Inaccurate measurement can be caused by venous pulsation. This can be because of high airway pressures, the Valsalva manoeuvre or other consequences of impaired venous return. Pulse oximeters assume that any pulsatile absorption is caused by arterial blood pulsation only.

9. The site of the application should be checked at regular intervals as the probe can cause pressure sores with continuous use. Some manufacturers recommend changing the site of application every 2 hours especially in patients with impaired microcirculation.

10. Pulse oximetry only gives information about a patient's oxygenation. It does not give any indication of a patient's ability to eliminate carbon dioxide.

Pulse oximetry

- Consists of a probe with two LEDs and a photodetector.
- A microprocessor analyses the signal.
- Accurate within the clinical range.
- Inaccurate readings in carbon monoxide poisoning, the presence of dyes and methaemoglobinaemia.
- Hypoperfusion and severe vasoconstriction affect the reading.

End-tidal carbon dioxide analysers (capnographs)

Gases with molecules that contain at least two dissimilar atoms absorb radiation in the infrared region of the spectrum. Using this property, both inspired and exhaled carbon dioxide concentration can be measured directly and continuously throughout the respiratory cycle (Fig. 10.14).

The end-tidal CO_2 is less than alveolar CO_2 because the end-tidal CO_2 is always diluted with alveolar dead space gas from unperfused alveoli. These alveoli do not take part in gas exchange and so contain no CO_2. Alveolar CO_2 is less than arterial CO_2 as the blood from unventilated alveoli and lung parenchyma (both have higher CO_2 contents) mixes with the blood from ventilated alveoli. In healthy adults with normal lungs, end-tidal CO_2 is 0.3–0.6 kPa less than arterial CO_2. This difference is reduced if the lungs are ventilated with large tidal volumes. The Greek root kapnos, meaning 'smoke', give us the term capnography (CO_2 can be thought as the 'smoke' of cellular metabolism).

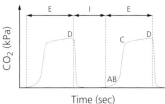

Fig. 10.14 Diagram of an end-tidal carbon dioxide waveform. I – inspiration; E – expiration; A–B represents the emptying of the upper dead space of the airways. As this has not undergone gas exchange the CO_2 concentration is zero. B–C represents the gas mixture from the upper airways and the CO_2-rich alveolar gas. The CO_2 concentration rises continuously. C–D represents the alveolar gas and is described as the 'alveolar plateau'. The curve rises very slowly. D is the end-tidal CO_2 partial pressure where the highest possible concentration of exhaled CO_2 is achieved at the end of expiration. It represents the final portion of gas which was involved in the gas exchange in the alveoli. Under certain conditions (see text) it represents a reliable index of the arterial CO_2 partial pressure. D–A represents inspiration where the fresh gas contains no CO_2.

$$End\text{-}tidal\ CO_2 < Alveolar\ CO_2 < PaCO_2$$

In reality, the devices used cannot determine the different phases of respiration but simply report the minimum and maximum CO_2 concentrations during each respiratory cycle.

Components

1. The sampling chamber can either be positioned within the patient's gas stream (main stream version Fig. 10.15) or connected to the distal end of the breathing system via a sampling tube (side stream version, Fig. 10.16).
2. A photodetector measures light reaching it from a light source at the correct infrared wavelength (using optical filters) after passing through two chambers. One acts as a reference whereas the other one is the sampling chamber (Fig. 10.17).

Mechanism of action

1. Carbon dioxide absorbs the infrared radiation particularly at a wavelength of $4.3\,\mu m$.
2. The amount of infrared radiation absorbed is proportional to the number of carbon dioxide molecules (partial pressure of carbon dioxide) present in the chamber.
3. The remaining infrared radiation falls on the thermopile detector, which in turn produces heat. The heat is measured by a temperature sensor and is proportional to the partial pressure of carbon dioxide gas present in the mixture in the sample chamber. This produces an electrical output. This means that the amount of gas present is inversely proportional to the amount of infrared light present at the detector in the sample chamber (see Fig 10.18).
4. In the same way a beam of light passes through the reference chamber which contains room air. The absorption detected from the sample chamber is compared to that in the reference chamber. This allows the calculation of carbon dioxide values.
5. The inspired and exhaled carbon dioxide forms a square wave, with a zero baseline unless there is rebreathing (Fig. 10.19A).

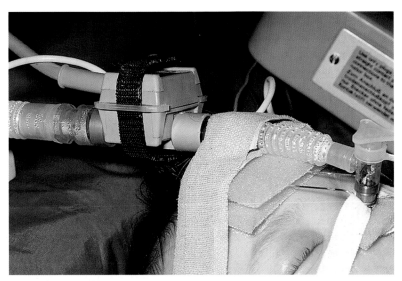

Fig. 10.15 A main stream end-tidal carbon dioxide analyser.

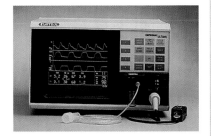

Fig. 10.16 The Datex-Ohmeda Capnomac Ultima which measures end-tidal carbon dioxide, patient oxygenation and inhalational agent concentration via a side stream sampling tube and connection (forefront). A pulse oximeter is also incorporated.

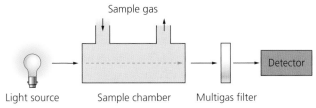

Fig. 10.17 Components of a gas analyser using an infrared light source suitable for end-tidal carbon dioxide measurement. The reference chamber has been omitted for the sake of clarity.

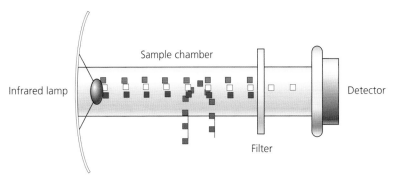

Fig. 10.18 Principles of infrared detector: due to the large amount of infrared absorption in the sample chamber by the carbon dioxide, little infrared finally reaches the detector.

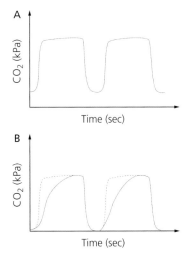

Fig. 10.19 (A) An end-tidal carbon dioxide waveform which does not return to the baseline during inspiration indicating that rebreathing is occurring. (B) An end-tidal carbon dioxide waveform which illustrates the sloping plateau seen in patients with chronic obstructive airways disease. The normal waveform is superimposed (dotted line) reproduced with permission Aitkenhead R and Smith G. Text book of Anaesthesia, 2nd edn. (Churchill Livingstone, 1990.)

6. A microprocessor-controlled infrared lamp is used. This produces a stable infrared source with a constant output. The current is measured with a current-sensing resistor, the voltage across which is proportional to the current

flowing through it. The supply to the light source is controlled by the feedback from the sensing resistor maintaining a constant current of 150 mA.
7. Using the rise and fall of the carbon dioxide during the respiratory cycle, monitors are designed to measure the respiratory rate.
8. Alarm limits can be set for both high and low values.
9. To avoid drift, the monitor should be calibrated regularly with known concentrations of CO_2 to ensure accurate measurement.

Photo-acoustic spectroscopy. In these infrared absorption devices, the sample gas is irradiated with pulsatile infrared radiation, of a suitable wavelength. The periodic expansion and contraction produces a pressure fluctuation of audible frequency that can be detected by a microphone.

The advantages of photo-acoustic spectrometry over conventional infrared absorption spectrometry are:

1. The photo-acoustic technique is extremely stable and its calibration remains constant over much longer periods of time.

2. The very fast rise and fall times give a much more accurate representation of any change in CO_2 concentration.

Carbon dioxide analysers can be either side stream or main stream analysers.

SIDE STREAM ANALYSER

1. This consists of a 1.2 mm internal diameter tube that samples the gases (both inspired and exhaled) at a constant rate (e.g. 150–200 mL/min). The tube is connected to a lightweight adapter near the patient's end of the breathing system (with a pneumo-tachograph for spirometry) with a small increase in the dead space. It delivers the gases to the sample chamber. It is made of Teflon so it is impermeable to carbon dioxide and does not react with anaesthetic agents.
2. As the gases are humid, there is a moisture trap with an exhaust port, allowing gas to be vented to the atmosphere or returned to the breathing system.
3. In order to accurately measure end-tidal carbon dioxide, the sampling tube should be positioned as close as possible to the patient's trachea.
4. A variable time delay before the sample is presented to the sample chamber is expected. The delay depends on the length (which should be as short as possible, e.g. 2 m) and diameter of the sampling tube and the sampling rate. A delay of less than 3.8 s is acceptable.
5. Other gases and vapours can be analysed from the same sample.
6. Portable hand-held side stream analysers are available (Fig. 10.20). They can be used during patient transport and out-of-hospital situations.

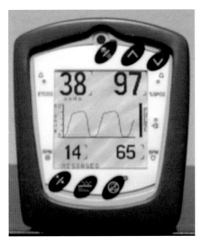

Fig. 10.20 Smith's Medical hand-held side stream end-tidal carbon dioxide analyser.

MAIN STREAM ANALYSER

1. The sample chamber is positioned within the patient's gas stream, increasing the dead space. In order to prevent water vapour condensation on its windows, it is heated to about 41°C.
2. Since there is no need for a sampling tube, there is no transport time delay in gas delivery to the sample chamber.
3. Other gases and vapours are not measured simultaneously.

See Table 10.4 for a comparison of side stream and main stream analysers.

Uses (Table 10.5)

In addition to its use as an indicator for the level of ventilation (hypo-, normo- or hyperventilation), end-tidal carbon dioxide measurement is useful:

1. To diagnose oesophageal intubation (no or very little carbon dioxide is detected). Following manual ventilation or the ingestion of carbonated drinks, some carbon dioxide might be present in the stomach. Characteristically, this may result in up to 5–6 waveforms with an abnormal shape and decreasing in amplitude.
2. As a disconnection alarm for a ventilator or breathing system. There is sudden absence of the end-tidal carbon dioxide.
3. To diagnose lung embolism as a sudden decrease in end-tidal carbon dioxide assuming that the arterial blood pressure remains stable.
4. To diagnose malignant hyperpyrexia as a gradual increase in end-tidal carbon dioxide.

Problems in practice and safety features

1. In patients with chronic obstructive airways disease, the wave form shows a sloping trace and does not accurately reflect the end-tidal carbon dioxide (Fig. 10.19B). An ascending plateau usually indicates impairment of ventilation: perfusion ratio because of uneven emptying of the alveoli.
2. During paediatric anaesthesia, it can be difficult to produce and interpret end-tidal carbon dioxide because of the high respiratory rates and small tidal volumes. The patient's tidal breath can be diluted with fresh gas.
3. During a prolonged expiration or end-expiratory pause, the gas flow exiting the trachea approaches zero. The sampling line may aspirate gas from the trachea and the inspiratory limb, causing ripples on the expired CO_2 trace (cardiogenic oscillations). They appear during the alveolar plateau in synchrony with the heart beat. It is thought to be due to mechanical agitation of deep lung regions that expel CO_2-rich gas. Such fluctuations can be smoothed over by increasing lung volume using PEEP.

Table 10.4 Comparison of various qualities between side stream and main stream analysers

	Side stream	Main stream
Disconnection possible	Yes	Yes
Sampling catheter leak common	Yes	No
Calibration gas required	Yes	No
Sensor damage common	No	Some
Multiple gas analysis possible	Yes	No
Use on non-intubated patients	Yes	No

Table 10.5 Summary of the uses of end-tidal CO_2

Increased end-tidal carbon dioxide	Decreased end-tidal carbon dioxide
Hypoventilation	Hyperventilation
Rebreathing	Pulmonary embolism
Sepsis	Hypoperfusion
Malignant hyperpyrexia	Hypometabolism
Hyperthermia	Hypothermia
Skeletal muscle activity	Hypovolaemia
Hypermetabolism	Hypotension

4. Dilution of the end-tidal carbon dioxide can occur whenever there are loose connections and system leaks.

5. Nitrous oxide (may be present in the sample for analysis) absorbs infrared light with an absorption spectrum partly overlapping that of carbon dioxide (Fig. 10.21). This causes inaccuracy of the detector, nitrous oxide being interpreted as carbon dioxide. By careful choice of the wavelength using special filters, this can be avoided. This is not a problem in most modern analysers.

6. Collision broadening or pressure broadening is a cause of error. The absorption of carbon dioxide is increased because of the presence of nitrous oxide or nitrogen. Calibration with a gas mixture that contains the same background gases as the sample solves this problem.

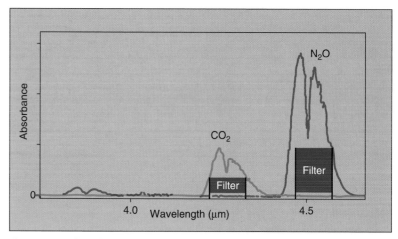

Fig. 10.21 Carbon dioxide and nitrous oxide infrared absorption spectrum.

End-tidal carbon dioxide measurement

- Uses the principle of infrared absorption by carbon dioxide.
- The infrared radiation falls on a temperature sensor producing an electrical output.
- Photo-acoustic spectroscopy with a microphone can also be used.
- Sampling can be either side stream or main stream.
- It reflects accurately the arterial carbon dioxide partial pressure in healthy individuals. End-tidal CO_2 < alveolar CO_2 < arterial CO_2.
- It is used to monitor the level of ventilation, affirm tracheal intubation, as a disconnection alarm, and to diagnose lung embolization and malignant hyperpyrexia.
- Nitrous oxide can distort the analysis in some designs.

Oxygen concentration analysers

It is fundamental to monitor oxygen concentration in the gas mixture delivered to the patient during general anaesthesia. The inspired oxygen concentration (FiO_2) is measured using a galvanic, polarographic or paramagnetic method (Fig. 10.22). The galvanic and polarographic analysers have a slow response time (20–30 sec) because they are dependent on membrane diffusion. The paramagnetic analyser has a rapid response time. The paramagnetic analyser is currently more widely used. These analysers measure the oxygen partial pressure, displayed as a percentage.

PARAMAGNETIC (PAULING) OXYGEN ANALYSERS

Components

1. Two chambers separated by a sensitive pressure transducer. The gas sample containing oxygen is delivered to the measuring chamber. The reference (room air) is delivered to the other chamber. This is accomplished via a sampling tube.

2. An electromagnet is rapidly switched on and off (a frequency of about 100–110 Hz) creating a changing magnetic field to which the gases are subjected. The electromagnet is designed to have its poles in close proximity, forming a narrow gap.

Mechanism of action (Fig. 10.23)

1. Oxygen is attracted to the magnetic field (paramagnetism) because of the fact that it has two electrons in unpaired orbits. Most of the gases used in anaesthesia are repelled by the magnetic field (diamagnetism).

2. The magnetic field causes the oxygen molecules to be attracted and agitated. This leads to changes in pressure on both sides of the transducer. The pressure difference across the transducer is proportional to the oxygen partial pressure difference between the sample and reference gases. The transducer converts this pressure force to an electrical signal that is displayed as oxygen partial

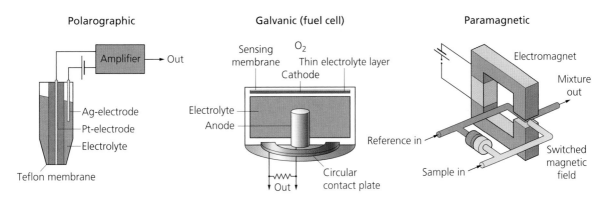

Polarographic

Amplifier → Out

Ag-electrode
Pt-electrode
Electrolyte
Teflon membrane

Galvanic (fuel cell)

Sensing membrane O_2
Thin electrolyte layer
Cathode
Electrolyte
Anode

Reference in
Circular contact plate
Out

Paramagnetic

Electromagnet
Mixture out
Switched magnetic field
Sample in

Fig. 10.22 Different types of oxygen analysers.

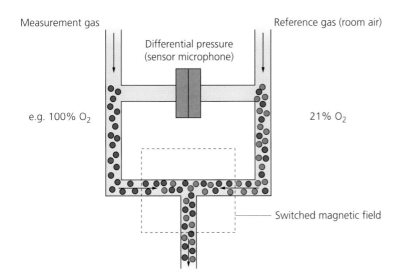

Measurement gas

Differential pressure (sensor microphone)

Reference gas (room air)

e.g. 100% O_2

21% O_2

Switched magnetic field

Fig. 10.23 Paramagnetic oxygen analyser.

mirror attached to the wire and a light deflected from the mirror falls on a calibrated screen for measuring oxygen concentration.

THE GALVANIC OXYGEN ANALYSER (FUEL CELL)

1. It generates a current proportional to the partial pressure of oxygen (so acting as a battery requiring oxygen for the current to flow).
2. It consists of a noble metal cathode and a lead anode in a potassium chloride electrolyte solution. An oxygen-permeable membrane separates the cell from the gases in the breathing system.
3. The oxygen molecules diffuse through the membrane and electrolyte solution to the gold cathode (Fig. 10.22), generating an electrical current proportional to the partial pressure of oxygen:

$$O_2 + 4e^- + 2H_2O \rightarrow 4(OH)^-$$
$$Pb + 2(OH)^- \rightarrow PbO + H_2O + 2e^-$$

4. Calibration is achieved using 100% oxygen and room air (21% oxygen).
5. It reads either the inspiratory or expiratory oxygen concentration.
6. Water vapour does not affect its performance.
7. It is depleted by continuous exposure to oxygen because of

pressure or converted to a reading in volume percentage.
3. They are very accurate and highly sensitive. The analyser should function continuously without any service breaks.
4. The recently designed paramagnetic oxygen analysers have a rapid response making it possible to analyse the inspired and expired oxygen concentration on a breath-to-breath basis. The older designs of oxygen analysers had a slow response time (nearly 1 minute).
5. The audible alarms can be set for low and high concentration

limits (e.g. 28% low and 40% high).

The old version of the paramagnetic analyser consists of a container with two spheres filled with nitrogen (a weak diamagnetic gas). The spheres are suspended by a wire allowing them to rotate in a non-uniform magnetic field.

When the sample enters the container, it is attracted by the magnetic field, causing the spheres to rotate. The degree of rotation depends on the number of oxygen molecules present in the sample. The rotation of the spheres displaces a

exhaustion of the cell, so limiting its life span to about 1 year.
8. The fuel cell has a slow response time of about 20 s with an accuracy of ± 3%.

POLAROGRAPHIC (CLARK ELECTRODE) OXYGEN ANALYSERS

1. They have similar principles to the galvanic analysers (Fig. 10.22). A platinum cathode and a silver anode in an electrolyte solution are used. The electrodes are polarized by a 600–800 mV power source. An oxygen-permeable Teflon membrane separates the cell from the sample.
2. The number of oxygen molecules that traverse the membrane is proportional to its partial pressure in the sample. An electric current is produced when the cathode donates electrons that are accepted by the anode. For every molecule of oxygen, four electrons are supplied making the current produced proportional to the oxygen partial pressure in the sample.
3. They give only one reading, which is the average of inspiratory and expiratory concentrations.
4. Their life expectancy is limited (about 3 years) because of the deterioration of the membrane.
5. The positioning of the oxygen analyser is debatable. It has been recommended that slow responding analysers are positioned on the inspiratory limb of the breathing system and fast responding analysers are positioned as close as possible to the patient.

Problems in practice and safety features

1. Regular calibration of the analysers is vital.

2. Paramagnetic analysers are affected by water vapour therefore a water trap is incorporated in their design.
3. The galvanic and the polarographic cells have limited life spans and need regular service.
4. The fuel cell and the polarographic electrode have slow response times of about 20–30 s with an accuracy of ± 3 %.

Oxygen analysers

- Paramagnetic, galvanic and polarographic cells are used. The former is more widely used.
- The galvanic and polarographic analysers have a slow response time because of membrane diffusion. The paramagnetic analyser has a rapid response time.
- Oxygen is attracted by the magnetic field whereas the gases or vapours are repelled.
- The paramagnetic cell measures the inspired and expired oxygen concentration simultaneously on a breath-by-breath basis.

Nitrous oxide and inhalational agent concentration analysers

Modern vaporizers are capable of delivering accurate concentrations of the anaesthetic agent(s) with different flows. It is important to monitor the inspired and end-tidal concentrations of the agents. This is of vital importance in the circle system as the exhaled inhalational agent is recirculated and added to the fresh gas flow. In addition, because of the low flow, the inhalational agent concentration the patient is receiving is different from the setting of the vaporizer.

Modern analysers can measure the concentration of all the agents available, halothane, enflurane, isoflurane, sevoflurane and desflurane, on a breath-by-breath basis (Fig. 10.24) using infrared.

Components

1. A sampling tube from an adapter within the breathing system which delivers gas to the analyser.
2. A sample chamber to which gas for analysis is delivered.
3. An infrared light source.
4. Optical filters.
5. A photodetector.

Mechanism of action

1. Infrared absorption analysers are used (Fig. 10.25). The sampled gas enters a chamber where it is exposed to infrared light. A photodetector measures the light reaching it across the correct infrared wavelength band. Absorption of the infrared light is proportional to the vapour concentration. The electrical signal is then analysed and processed to give a measurement of the agent concentration.
2. Optical filters are used to select the desired wavelengths. Different analyser designs use different wavelengths for

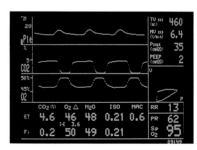

Fig. 10.24 Anaesthetic agent display of the Datex-Ohmeda Capnomac Ultima. Inspired (Fi) and end-tidal (ET) values are displayed for carbon dioxide, oxygen and isoflurane (ISO).

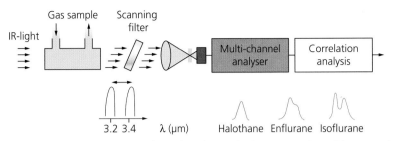

Fig. 10.25 Mechanism of action of an infrared anaesthetic agent monitor with automatic agent identification properties. Agents absorb infrared light differently over a wavelength band of 3.2–3.4 mm. The monitor can therefore identify the agent in use automatically by analysing its unique absorbance pattern.

Optical filters are used to filter the desirable wavelengths. Because of the auto-detection, individual calibration for each agent is not necessary.

5. The sample gas can be returned to the breathing system, making the analysers suitable for use with the circle breathing system.
6. No individual calibration for each agent is necessary.
7. Water vapour has no effect on the performance and accuracy of the analyser.

anaesthetic agent analysis. An infrared light of a wavelength of 4.6 μm is used for N₂O. For the inhalational agents higher wavelengths are used, between 8 and 9 μm. This is to avoid interference from methane and alcohol that happen at the lower 3.3 μm band.

3. Modern sensors can automatically identify and measure concentrations of up to three agents present in a mixture and produce a warning message to the user. Five sensors are used to produce a spectral shape where the five outputs are compared and the shape produced represents the spectral signal of the agent present in the sample. This is compared with the spectral shapes stored in the memory of the sensor and used to identify the agent. Currently, it is possible to detect and measure the concentrations of halothane, enflurane, isoflurane, sevoflurane and desflurane (see Figs 10.26 and 10.27).

4. The amplitude of the spectral shape represents the amount of vapour present in the mixture. The amplitude is inversely proportional to the amount of agent present. The output of the infrared lamp is kept constant with a constant supply of current.

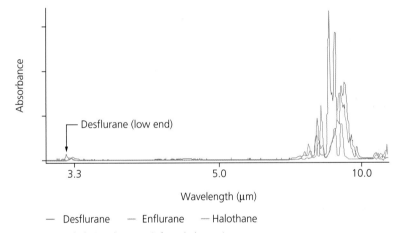

Fig. 10.26 Inhalational agents infrared absorption spectrum.

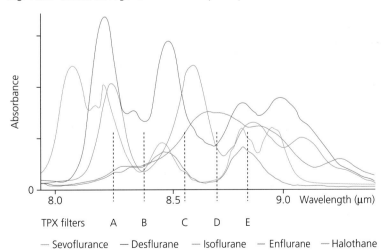

Fig. 10.27 Agent identification and measurement: to measure and identify the agents, all five sensors are used to produce a spectral shape. When the detectors at all five outputs are compared, A, B, C, D and E, a spectral shape is produced, representing the spectral signal of the agent present in the sample.

PIEZOELECTRIC QUARTZ CRYSTAL OSCILLATION

Piezoelectric quartz crystal oscillation can be used to measure the concentration of inhalational agents. A lipophilic-coated piezoelectric quartz crystal undergoes changes in natural resonant frequency when exposed to the lipid-soluble inhalational agents. This change in frequency is directly proportional to the partial pressure of agent. Such a technique lacks agent specificity and sensitivity to water vapour.

Raman spectroscopy and ultraviolet absorption (in the case of halothane) are other methods used for measuring inhalational agent concentration.

Problems in practice and safety features

1. Some designs of infrared light absorption analysers are not agent specific. These must be programmed by the user for the specific agent being administered. Incorrect programming results in erroneous measurements.
2. Alarms can be set for inspired and exhaled inhalational agent concentration.

Inhalational agent concentration analysers

- A sample of gas is used to measure the concentration of inhalational agent using infrared light absorption.
- By selecting light of the correct wavelengths, the inspired and expired concentrations of the agent(s) can be measured.
- An infrared light of a wavelength of 4.6 μm is used for N_2O. For other inhalational agents higher wavelengths are used, between 8 and 9 μm.

- Ultraviolet absorption, mass spectrometry and quartz crystal oscillation are other methods of measuring the inhalational agents' concentration.

MASS SPECTROMETER

This can be used to identify and measure, on a breath-to-breath basis, the concentrations of the gases and vapours used during anaesthesia. The principle of action is to charge the particles of the sample (bombard them with an electron beam) and then separate the components into a spectrum according to their specific mass:charge ratios.

The creation and manipulation of the ions is done in a high vacuum (10^{-5} mmHg) to avoid interference by outside air and to minimize random collisions among the ions and the residual gas. The relative abundance of ions at certain specific mass:charge ratios is determined and is related to the fractional composition of the original gas mixture.

A permanent magnet is used to separate the ion beam into its component ion spectra. Because of the high expense, multiplexed mass spectrometer systems are used with several patient sampling locations on a time-shared basis.

Table 10.6 summarizes the methods used in gas and vapour analysis.

Wright respirometer

This compact and light (weighs less than 150 g) respirometer is used to

---

Table 10.6 The various methods used in gas and vapour analysis

Technology	O_2	CO_2	N_2O	Inhalational agent
Infrared		√	√	√
Paramagnetic	√			
Polarography	√			
Fuel cell	√			
Mass spectrometry	√	√	√	√
Raman spectroscopy	√	√	√	√
Piezoelectric resonance				√

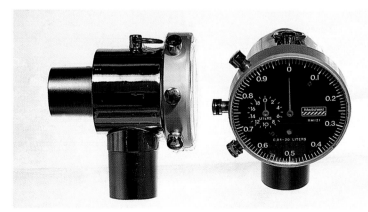

Fig. 10.28 A Wright respirometer. An arrow on the side of the casing indicates the direction of gas flow.

measure the tidal volume and minute volume (Fig. 10.28).

Components

1. The respirometer consists of an inlet and outlet.
2. A rotating vane surrounded by slits (Fig. 10.29). The vane is attached to a pointer.
3. Buttons on the side of the respirometer to turn the device on and off and reset the pointer to the zero position.

Mechanism of action

1. The Wright respirometer is a one-way system. It allows the measurement of the tidal volume if the flow of the gases is in one direction only. The correct direction for gas flow is indicated by an arrow.
2. The slits surrounding the vane are to create a circular flow in order to rotate the vane. The vane does 150 revolutions for each litre of gas passing through. This causes the pointer to rotate round the respirometer display.
3. The outer display is calibrated at 100 mL per division. The small inner display is calibrated at 1 litre per division.

4. It is usually positioned on the expiratory side of the breathing system, which is at a lower pressure than the inspiratory side. This minimizes the loss of gas volume due to leaks and expansion of the tubing.
5. For clinical use, the respirometer reads accurately the tidal volume and minute volume (± 5–10%) within the range of 4–24 L/min. A minimum flow of 2 L/min is required for the respirometer to function accurately.
6. To improve accuracy, the respirometer should be positioned as close to the patient's trachea as possible.
7. The resistance to breathing is very low at about $2\,cmH_2O$ at 100 L/min.
8. A paediatric version exists with a capability of accurate tidal volume measurements between 15 and 200 mL.
9. A more accurate version of the Wright respirometer uses light reflection to measure the tidal volume. The mechanical causes of inaccuracies (friction and inertia) and the accumulation of water vapour are avoided. Other designs use a semi-conductive device that is sensitive to changes in magnetic field. Tidal volume and minute volume can be measured by converting these

changes electronically. An alarm system can also be added.

Problems in practice and safety features

1. The Wright respirometer tends to over-read at high flow rates and under-read at low flows.
2. Water condensation from the expired gases causes the pointer to stick, thus preventing it from rotating freely.

Wright respirometer

- Rotating vane attached to a pointer.
- Fitted on the expiratory limb to measure the tidal and minute volume with an accuracy of ± 5–10%.
- The flow is unidirectional.
- It over-reads at high flows and under-reads at low flows.

Pneumotachograph

This measures gas flow. From this, gas volume can be calculated.

Components

1. A tube with a fixed resistance. The resistance can be a bundle of parallel tubes (Fig. 10.30).
2. Two sensitive pressure transducers on either side of the resistance.

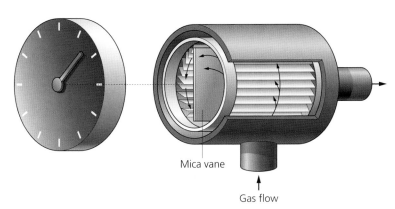

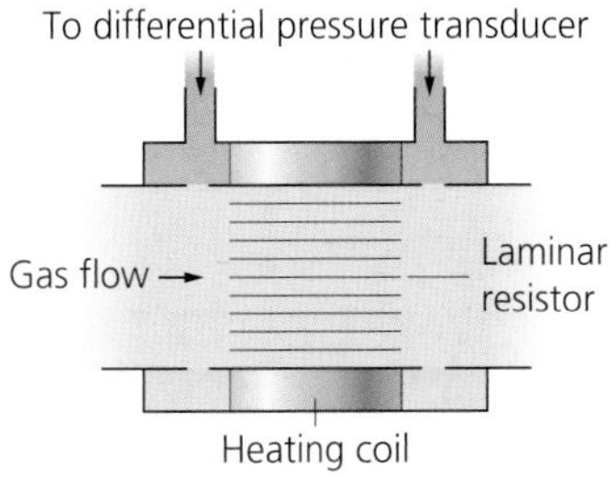

Fig. 10.30 A pneumotachograph. See text for details (reproduced with permission from Aitkenhead R, Smith G. Textbook of Anaesthesia, 3rd edn. Churchill Livingstone, 1996).

Mica vane

Gas flow

Fig. 10.29 Mechanism of action of the Wright respirometer (reproduced with permission from Aitkenhead R, Smith G. Textbook of Anaesthesia, 3rd edn. Churchill Livingstone, 1996).

Mechanism of action

1. The principle of its function is sensing the change in pressure across a fixed resistance through which gas flow is laminar.
2. The pressure change is only a few millimetres of water and is linearly proportional, over a certain range, to the flow rate of gas passing through the resistance.
3. The tidal volumes can be summated over a period of a minute to give the minute volume.
4. It can measure flows in both inspiration and expiration (i.e. bidirectional).

Problems in practice and safety features

Water vapour condensation at the resistance will encourage the formation of turbulent flow affecting the accuracy of the measurement. This can be avoided by heating the parallel tubes.

Combined pneumotachograph and Pitot tube

This combination is designed to improve accuracy and calculate and measure the compliance, airway pressures, gas flow, volume/pressure and flow/volume loops. Modern devices can be used accurately even in neonates and infants.

THE PITOT TUBE

Components

1. Two pressure ports—one facing the direction of gas flow, the other perpendicular to the gas flow. This is used to measure gas flow in one direction only.

2. In order to measure bidirectional flows (inspiration and expiration), two pressure ports face in opposite directions within the gas flow (Fig. 10.31).
3. These pressure ports are connected to pressure transducers.

Mechanism of action

The pressure difference between the ports is proportional to the square of the flow rate.

Problems in practice and safety features

The effects of the density and viscosity of the gas(es) can alter the accuracy. This can be compensated for by continuous gas composition analysis via a sampling tube.

Pneumotachograph

- A bidirectional device to measure the flow rate, tidal and minute volume.
- A laminar flow across a fixed resistance causes changes in pressure which are measured by transducers.
- Condensation at the resistance can cause turbulent flow and inaccuracies.
- Improved accuracy is achieved by adding a Pitot tube(s) and continuous gas composition analysis.

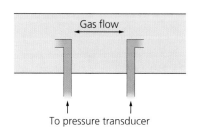

Fig. 10.31 Cross-section of a Pitot tube flowmeter. The two ports are facing in opposite directions within the gas flow.

Ventilator alarms

It is mandatory to use a ventilator alarm during IPPV to guard against patient disconnection, leaks, obstruction or malfunction. These can be pressure and/or volume monitoring alarms. Clinical observation, end-tidal carbon dioxide concentration, airway pressure and pulse oximetry are also ventilator monitors.

PRESSURE MONITORING ALARM

Components

1. The case where the pressure alarm limits are set, an automatic on/off switch. A light flashes with each ventilator cycle (Fig. 10.32).
2. The alarm is pressurized by a sensing tube connecting it to the inspiratory limb of the ventilator system.

Mechanism of action

1. In this alarm, the peak inspiratory pressure is usually measured and monitored during controlled ventilation.
2. A decrease in peak inspiratory pressure activates the alarm. This indicates that the ventilator is unable to achieve the preset threshold pressure in the breathing system. Causes can be disconnection, gas leak or inadequate fresh gas flow.
3. An increase in the peak inspiratory pressure usually indicates an obstruction.
4. The low pressure alarm can be set to $7\,cmH_2O$, $7\,cmH_2O$ plus time delay or $13\,cmH_2O$. The high pressure alarm is set at $60\,cmH_2O$.

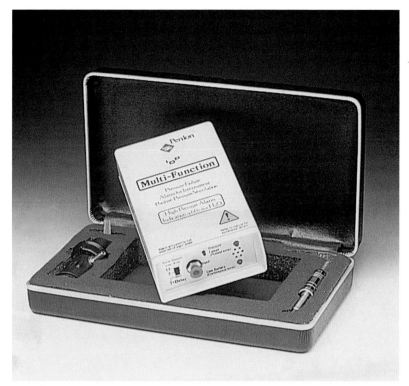

Fig. 10.32 The Penlon pressure monitoring ventilator alarm.

Problems in practice and safety features

Disconnection of the breathing system with partial obstruction of the alarm sensing tube may lead to a condition where the alarm is not activated despite inadequate ventilation.

VOLUME MONITORING ALARM

The expired gas volume can be measured and monitored. Gas volume can be measured either directly using a respirometer or indirectly by integration of the gas flow (pneumotachograph).

These alarms are usually inserted in the expiratory limb with a continuous display of tidal and minute volume. The alarm limits are set for a minimum and maximum tidal and/or minute volume.

Ventilator alarms

- They can be pressure and/or volume monitoring alarms.
- They detect disconnection (low pressure) or obstruction (high pressure) in the ventilator breathing system.
- The pressure alarms are fitted on the inspiratory limb whereas the volume alarms are fitted on the expiratory limb of the breathing system.
- Regular servicing is required.

Peripheral nerve stimulators

These devices are used to monitor transmission across the neuromuscular junction. The depth, adequate reversal and type of neuromuscular blockade can be established (Fig. 10.33).

Components

1. Two surface electrodes (small ECG electrodes) are positioned over the nerve and connected via the leads to the nerve stimulator.
2. Alternatively skin contact can be made via ball electrodes which are mounted on the nerve stimulator casing.
3. The case consists of an on/off switch, facility to deliver a twitch, train-of-four (at 2 Hz) and tetanus (50 Hz). The stimulator is battery operated.

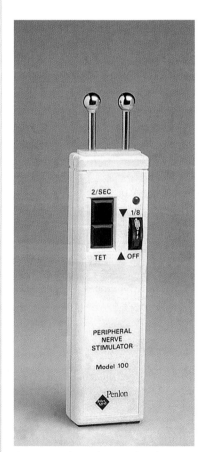

Fig. 10.33 The Penlon peripheral nerve stimulator with detachable ball electrodes.

Mechanism of action

1. A supramaximal stimulus is used to stimulate a peripheral nerve. This ensures that all the motor fibres of the nerve are depolarized. The response of the muscle(s) supplied by the nerve is observed. A current of 15–40 mA is used for the ulnar nerve (a current of 50–60 mA may have to be used in obese patients).
2. This device should be battery powered and capable of delivering a constant current. It is the current magnitude that determines whether the nerve depolarizes or not, so delivering a constant current is more important than delivering a constant voltage as the skin resistance is variable (Ohm's Law).
3. The muscle contraction can be observed visually, palpated, measured using a force transducer, or the electrical activity can be measured (EMG).
4. The duration of the stimulus is less than 0.2–0.3 ms. The stimulus should have a monophasic square wave shape to avoid repetitive nerve firing.
5. Superficial, accessible peripheral nerves are most commonly used for monitoring purposes, e.g. ulnar nerve at the wrist, common peroneal nerve at the neck of the fibula, posterior tibial nerve at the ankle and the facial nerve.
6. The negative electrode is positioned directly over the most superficial part of the nerve. The positive electrode is positioned along the proximal course of nerve to avoid direct muscle stimulation.
7. Consider the ulnar nerve at the wrist. Two electrodes are positioned over the nerve, with the negative electrode placed distally and the positive electrode positioned about 2 cm proximally. Successful ulnar

nerve stimulation causes the contraction of the adductor pollicis brevis muscle.

More advanced devices offer continuous monitoring of the transmission across the neuromuscular junction. A graphical and numerical display of the train-of-four (see below) and the trend provide optimal monitoring. Skin electrodes are used. A reference measurement should be made where the device calculates the supramaximal current needed before the muscle relaxant is given. The device can be used to locate nerves and plexuses with a much lower

current (e.g. a maximum of 5.0 mA) during regional anaesthesia. In this mode, a short stimulus can be used, e.g. 40 ms, to reduce the patient's discomfort.

NEUROMUSCULAR MONITORING

There are various methods for monitoring the neuromuscular transmission using a nerve stimulator (Fig. 10.34).

1. Twitch: a short duration (0.1–0.2 ms) square wave stimulus of a frequency of 0.1–

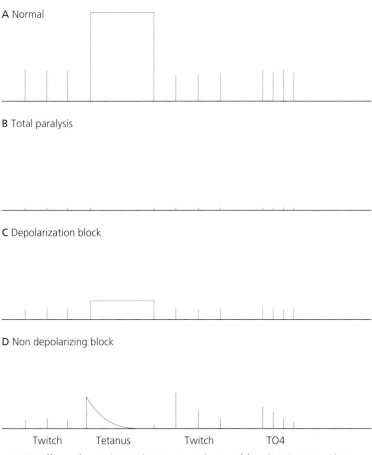

A Normal

B Total paralysis

C Depolarization block

D Non depolarizing block

Twitch   Tetanus   Twitch   TO4

Fig. 10.34 Effects of a single twitch, tetanus and train-of-four (TO4) assessed by a force transducer recording contraction of the adductor pollicis muscle (reproduced with permission from Aitkenhead R, Smith G. Textbook of Anaesthesia, 2nd edn. Churchill Livingstone, 1990).

1 Hz (1 stimulus every 10 seconds to 1 stimulus every 1 second) is applied to a peripheral nerve. When used on its own, it is of limited use. It is the least precise method of assessing partial neuromuscular block.

2. Tetanic stimulation: a tetanus of 50–100 Hz is used to detect any residual neuromuscular block. Fade will be apparent even with normal response to a twitch. Tetanus is usually applied to anaesthetized patients because of the discomfort caused.

3. Train-of-four (TOF): used to monitor the degree of the neuromuscular block clinically. The ratio of the 4th to the 1st twitch is called the **TOF ratio**:
   a) four twitches of 2 Hz each applied over 2 s. A gap of 10 s between each TOF
   b) as the muscle relaxant is administered, fade is noticed first, followed by the disappearance of the 4th twitch. This is followed by the disappearance of the 3rd then the 2nd and last by the 1st twitch
   c) on recovery, the 1st twitch appears first then the 2nd followed by the 3rd and 4th; reversal of the neuromuscular block is easier if the 2nd twitch is visible
   d) for upper abdominal surgery, at least three twitches must be absent to achieve adequate surgical conditions
   e) the TOF ratio can be estimated using visible or tactile means. Electrical recording of the response is more accurate.

4. Post-tetanic facilitation or potentiation: this is used to assess more profound degrees of neuromuscular block.

5. Double burst stimulation (Fig. 10.35): this allows a more accurate visual assessment than TOF for residual neuromuscular

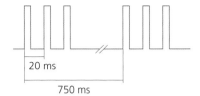

Fig. 10.35 The pattern of double-burst stimulation. Three impulses of 50 Hz tetanus, at 20 ms intervals, every 750 ms is shown (reproduced with permission from Aitkenhead R, Smith G. Textbook of Anaesthesia, 3rd edn. Churchill Livingstone, 1996).

blockade. Two short bursts of 50 Hz tetanus are applied with a 750 ms interval. Each burst compromises of two or three square wave impulses lasting for 0.2 ms.

Problems in practice and safety features

As the muscles of the hand are small in comparison with the diaphragm (the main respiratory muscle), monitoring the neuromuscular block peripherally does not reflect the true picture of the depth of the diaphragmatic block. The smaller the muscle is, the more sensitive it is to a muscle relaxant.

> Peripheral nerve stimulators
> - Used to ensure adequate reversal, and to monitor the depth and the type of the block.
> - Supramaximal stimulus is used to stimulate the nerve.
> - The contraction of the muscle is observed visually, palpated or measured by a pressure transducer.
> - The ulnar, facial, posterior tibial and the common peroneal nerves are often used.

Various methods are used to monitor the neuromuscular transmission: twitch, tetanic stimulation, train-of-four, post-tetanic facilitation and double burst stimulation.

Bispectral index (BIS) analysis (Fig. 10.36)

The Bis monitor is a device to monitor the electrical activity and the level of sedation in the brain and to assess the risk of awareness while under sedation/anaesthesia. In addition it allows titration of hypnotics based on individual requirements to reduce under- and over-dosing. BIS has been shown to correlate with measures of sedation/hypnosis, awareness, and recall end points likely to be reflected in the cortical EEG. It can provide a continuous and consistent measure of sedation/hypnosis induced by most of the widely used sedative-hypnotic agents. Although BIS can measure the hypnotic components, it is less sensitive to the analgesic/opiate components of an anaesthetic.

Components

1. Display
   a) BIS (as a single value or trend)
   b) Facial electromyogram, EMG (in decibels)

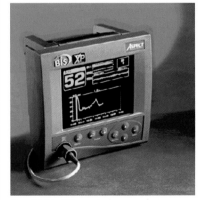

Fig. 10.36 BIS monitor.

c) EEG suppression measured
d) Signal Quality Index (SQI) which indicates the amount of interference from EMG.

2. A forehead sensor with four numbered electrodes (elements) and a smart chip. The sensor uses small tines, which part the outer layers of the skin, and a hydrogel to make electrical contact. It is designed to lower the impedance and to optimize the quality of the signal.

3. A smaller paediatric sensor with three electrodes is available. It has a flexible design to adjust to various head sizes and contours.

Mechanism of action

1. Bispectral analysis is a statistical method that quantifies the level of synchronization of the underlying frequencies in the signal.

2. BIS is a value derived mathematically using information from EEG power and frequency as well as bispectral information. Along with the traditional amplitude and frequency variables, it provides a more complete description of complex EEG patterns.

3. BIS is an empirical, statistically derived measurement. It uses a linear, dimensionless scale from 0 to 100. The lower the value, the greater the hypnotic effect. A value of 100 represents an awake EEG while zero represents complete electrical silence (cortical suppression). BIS values of 65–85 are recommended for sedation, whereas values of 40–60 are recommended for general anaesthesia. At BIS values of less than 40, cortical suppression becomes discernible in raw EEG as a burst suppression pattern (see Fig. 10.37).

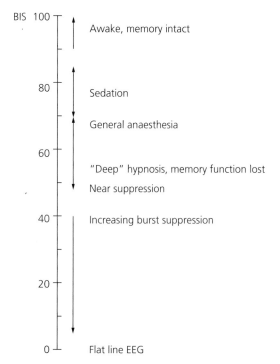

Fig. 10.37 BIS values scale.

4. BIS measures the state of the brain, not the concentration of a particular drug. So a low value for BIS indicates hypnosis irrespective of how it was produced.

5. It has been shown that return of consciousness occurs consistently when the BIS is above 60 and, interestingly, at the same time, changes in blood pressure and heart rate are poor predictors for response.

6. The facial electromyogram (in decibels) is displayed to inform the user of possible interference affecting the BIS value.

7. The sensor is applied on the forehead at an angle. It can be placed on either the right or left side of the head. Element *number 1* is placed at the centre of the forehead, 5 cm above the nose. Element *number 4* is positioned just above and adjacent to the eyebrow. Element *number 2* is positioned between *number 1* and *number 4*. Element *number 3* is positioned on either temple between the corner of the eye and the hairline. The sensor will not function beyond the hairline. Each element should be pressed for 5 seconds with the fingertip.

8. Cerebral ischaemia from any cause can result in a decrease in the BIS value if severe enough to cause a global EEG slowing or outright suppression.

9. BIS is being 'incorporated' as an additional monitoring module that can be added to the existing modular patient monitors such as Datex-Ohmeda S/5, Philips Viridia or GE Marquette Solar 8000M. In addition to its use in the operating theatre, BIS has also been used in the intensive care setting to assess the level of sedation in mechanically ventilated patients.

Problems and safety features

1. Hypothermia of less than 33°C results in a decrease in BIS levels as the brain processes slow. In such situations, e.g. during cardiac bypass procedures, BIS reflects the synergistic effects of hypothermia and hypnotic drugs. A rapid rise in BIS usually occurs during rewarming.

2. Interference from non-EEG electrical signals such as electromyogram. High frequency facial electromyogram activity may be present in sedated, spontaneously breathing patients and during awakening, causing BIS to increase in conjunction with higher electromyogram. Significant electromyogram interference can lead to a faulty high BIS despite the patient being still unresponsive. EEG signals are considered to exist in the 0.5–30 Hz band whereas electromyogram signals exist in the 30–300 Hz band. Separation is not absolute and low-frequency electromyogram signals can occur in the conventional EEG band range. The more recent BIS XP is less affected by electromyogram.

3. BIS cannot be used to monitor hypnosis during ketamine anaesthesia. This is due to ketamine being a dissociative anaesthetic with excitatory effects on the EEG.

4. Sedative concentrations of nitrous oxide (up to 70%) do not appear to affect BIS.

5. There are conflicting data regarding opioid dose–response and interaction of opioids with hypnotics on BIS.

6. Currently there are insufficient data to evaluate the use of BIS in patients with neurological diseases.

7. When the SQI value goes below 50%, the BIS is not stored in the trend memory. The BIS value on the monitor appears in 'reverse video' to indicate this.

8. Interference from surgical diathermy. A recent version, BIS XP, is better protected from the diathermy.

9. As with any other monitor, the use of BIS does not obviate the need for critical clinical judgment.

BIS

- Monitors the electrical activity in the brain.
- Uses a linear dimensionless scale from 0 to 100. The lower the value, the greater the hypnotic effect. General anaesthesia is at 40–60.
- Interference can be from diathermy or EMG.
- Changes in body temperature and cerebral ischaemia can affect the value.

FURTHER READING

Hemmings Jr H, Hopkins P. Foundations of Anesthesia. Basic and Clinical Sciences, 1st edn. London: Mosby, 2000.

McGrath CD, Hunter JM. Monitoring of neuromuscular block. Continuing Education in Anaesthesia, Critical Care and Pain 2006;6(1):7–12.

Walker SD. Anesthetic and respiratory gas measurements by infrared technology. Biomedical Instrumentation and Technology 1989;23(6):466–469.

MCQs

In the following lists, which of the statements (a) to (e) are true?

1. Concerning capnography
   a) Capnography is a more useful indicator of ventilator disconnection and oesophageal intubation than pulse oximetry.
   b) Capnography typically works on the absorption of CO_2 in the ultraviolet region of the spectrum.
   c) In side stream analysers, a delay in measurement of less than 38 seconds is acceptable.
   d) The main stream analyser type can measure other gases simultaneously.
   e) In patients with chronic obstructive airways disease, the wave form can show a sloping trace instead of the square shape wave.

2. Concerning oxygen concentration measurement
   a) An infrared absorption technique is used.
   b) Paramagnetic analysers are commonly used because oxygen is repelled by the magnetic field.
   c) The galvanic (fuel cell) analyser has a slow response time of about 20 seconds and a life span of about 1 year.
   d) The fast responding analysers should be positioned as near the patient as possible.
   e) Paramagnetic analysers can provide breath-to-breath measurement.

3. Pulse oximetry
   a) The probe consists of two emitting diodes producing beams at red and infrared frequencies.
   b) Accurately reflects the ability of the patient to eliminate CO_2.
   c) The measurements are accurate within the clinical range of 70–100%.
   d) Carbon monoxide in the blood causes a false under-reading.
   e) The site of the probe has to be checked frequently.

4. Arterial blood pressure
   a) Mean blood pressure is the systolic pressure plus one third of the pulse pressure.
   b) Too small a cuff causes a false high pressure.
   c) Oscillotonometry is widely used to measure blood pressure.
   d) The Finapres technique uses ultraviolet light absorption to measure the blood pressure.
   e) A slow cuff inflation followed by a fast deflation are needed to improve the accuracy of a non-invasive blood pressure technique.

5. Pneumotachograph
   a) It is a fixed orifice variable pressure flowmeter.
   b) It consists of two sensitive pressure transducers positioned on either side of a resistance.
   c) It is capable of the flow in one direction only.
   d) A Pitot tube can be added to improve accuracy.
   e) Humidity and water vapour condensation have no effect on its accuracy.

6. Polarographic oxygen electrode
   a) It can measure oxygen partial pressure in a blood or gas sample.
   b) The electrode acts as a battery requiring no power source.
   c) Oxygen molecules pass from the sample to the sodium chloride solution across a semi-permeable membrane.
   d) It uses a silver cathode and a platinum anode.
   e) The amount of electrical current generated is proportional to the oxygen partial pressure.

7. Wright respirometer
   a) It is best positioned on the inspiratory limb of the ventilator breathing system.
   b) It is a bidirectional device.
   c) It is accurate for clinical use.
   d) It over-reads at high flow rates and under-reads at low flow rates.
   e) It can measure both tidal volume and minute volume.

8. Paramagnetic gases include
   a) Oxygen
   b) Sevofluorane.
   c) Nitrous oxide.
   d) Carbon dioxide.
   e) Halothane.

9. Oxygen in a gas mixture can be measured by
   a) Fuel cell.
   b) Ultraviolet absorption.
   c) Mass spectrometer.
   d) Clark oxygen (polarographic) electrode.
   e) Infrared absorption.

10. The concentrations of volatile agents can be measured using
    a) Fuel cell.
    b) Piezoelectric crystal.
    c) Ultraviolet spectroscopy.
    d) Infrared spectroscopy.
    e) Clark electrode.

11. A patient with healthy lungs and a $PaCO_2$ of 40 mmHg will have which of the following percentages of CO_2 in the end expiratory mixture?
    a) 4%
    b) 5%
    c) 2%
    d) 1%
    e) 7%

12. BIS monitor
    a) It uses a linear dimensionless scale from 0 to 100 Hz.
    b) Hypothermia can increase the BIS value.
    c) The BIS value is not accurate during ketamine anaesthesia.
    d) Interference can occur due to EMG or diathermy.
    e) BIS can measure the drug concentration of a particular drug.

13. Concerning ECG
    a) The monitoring mode of ECG has a wider frequency response range than the diagnostic mode.
    b) The electrical potentials have a range of 0.5–2 V.
    c) Interference due to electrostatic induction can be reduced by surrounding ECG leads with copper screens.
    d) Silver and silver chloride electrodes are used.
    e) It is standard in the UK to use a display speed of 25 cm/s and a sensitivity of 1 mV/cm.

14. Infrared spectrometry
    a) CO_2 absorbs infrared radiation mainly at a wavelength of 4.3 mm.
    b) Photo-acoustic spectrometry is more stable than the conventional infrared spectrometry.
    c) Sampling catheter leak is a potential problem with the side stream analysers.
    d) A wavelength of 4.6 μm is used for nitrous oxide measurement.
    e) A wavelength of 3.3 μm is used to measure the concentration of inhalational agents.

Answers

1. Concerning capnography
   a) *True. Capnography gives a fast warning in cases of disconnection or oesophageal intubation. The end-tidal CO_2 will decrease sharply and suddenly. The pulse oximeter will be very slow in detecting disconnection or oesophageal intubation as the arterial oxygen saturation will remain normal for longer periods especially if the patient was pre-oxygenated.*
   b) *False. CO_2 is absorbed in the infrared region.*
   c) *False. In side stream analysers, a delay of less than 3.8 seconds is acceptable. The length of the sampling tubing should be as short as possible, e.g. 2 m, with an internal diameter of 1.2 mm and a sampling rate of about 150 mL/min.*
   d) *False. Only CO_2 can be measured by the main stream analyser. CO_2, N_2O and inhalational agents can be measured simultaneously with a side stream analyser.*
   e) *True. In patients with chronic obstructive airways disease, the alveoli empty at different rates because of the differing time constants in different regions of the lung with various degrees of altered compliance and airway resistance.*

2. Concerning oxygen concentration measurement
   a) *False. Oxygen does not absorb infrared radiation. Only molecules with two differing atoms can absorb infrared radiation.*
   b) *False. Oxygen is attracted by the magnetic field because it has two electrons in unpaired orbits.*
   c) *True. The fuel cell is depleted by continuous exposure to oxygen due to the exhaustion of the cell giving it a life span of about 1 year.*
   d) *True. Although the positioning of the oxygen analyser is still debatable, it has been recommended that the fast responding ones are positioned as close to the patient as possible. The slow responding analysers are positioned on the inspiratory limb of the breathing system.*
   e) *True. Modern paramagnetic analysers have a rapid response allowing them to provide breath-to-breath measurement. Older versions have a 1 minute response time.*

3. Pulse oximetry
   a) *True. The probe uses light emitting diodes (LEDs) that emit light at red (660 nm) and infrared (940 nm) frequencies. The LEDs operate in sequence with an 'off' period when the photodetector measures the background level of ambient light. This sequence happens at a rate of about 30 times per second.*
   b) *False. Pulse oximetry is a measurement of the arterial oxygen saturation.*
   c) *True. Readings below 70% are extrapolated by the manufacturers.*
   d) *False. Using a pulse oximeter, carbon monoxide causes a false high reading of the arterial oxygen saturation.*
   e) *True. The probe can cause pressure sores with continuous use so its site should be checked at regular intervals. Some recommend changing the site every 2 hours.*

4. Arterial blood pressure
   a) *False.* The mean blood pressure is the diastolic pressure plus one third of the pulse pressure (systolic pressure – diastolic pressure).
   b) *True.* The opposite is correct also.
   c) *True.* Most of the non-invasive blood pressure measuring devices use oscillometry as the basis for measuring blood pressure. Return of the blood flow during deflation causes pressure changes in the cuff. The transducer senses the pressure changes which are interpreted by the microprocessor.
   d) *False.* The Finapres uses oscillometry and a servo control unit is used.
   e) *False.* Slow cuff inflation leads to venous congestion and inaccuracy. A fast cuff deflation might miss the oscillations caused by the return of blood flow (i.e. systolic pressure). A fast inflation and slow deflation of the cuff is needed. A deflation rate of 3 mmHg/s or 2 mmHg/beat is adequate.

5. Pneumotachograph
   a) *True.* The pneumotachograph consists of a tube with a fixed resistance, usually as a bundle of parallel tubes, and is therefore a 'fixed orifice' device. As the fluid (gas or liquid) passes across the resistance, the pressure across the resistance changes, therefore it is a 'variable pressure' flowmeter.
   b) *True.* The two pressure transducers measure the pressures on either side of the resistance. The pressure changes are proportional to the flow rate across the resistance.
   c) *False.* It can measure flows in both directions; i.e. it is bidirectional.
   d) *True.* The combined design improves accuracy and allows the measurement and calculation of other parameters: compliance, airway pressure, gas flow, volume/pressure and flow/volume loops.
   e) *False.* A laminar flow is required for the pneumotachograph to measure accurately. Water vapour condensation at the site of the resistance leads to the formation of turbulent flow thus reducing the accuracy of the measurement.

6. Polarographic oxygen electrode
   a) *True.* The polarographic (Clark) electrode analysers can be used to measure oxygen partial pressure in a gas sample (e.g. on an anaesthetic machine giving an average inspiratory and expiratory concentration) or in blood in a blood gas analyser.
   b) *False.* A power source of about 700 mV is needed in a polarographic analyser. The galvanic analyser (fuel cell) acts as a battery requiring no power source.
   c) *True.* The oxygen molecules pass across a Teflon semi-permeable membrane at a rate proportional to their partial pressure in the sample into the sodium chloride solution. The performance of the electrode is affected as the membrane deteriorates or perforates.
   d) *False.* The opposite is correct: the anode is made of silver and the cathode is made of platinum.
   e) *True.* When the oxygen molecules pass across the membrane, very small electrical currents are generated as electrons move from the cathode to the anode.

7. Wright respirometer
   a) *False. The wright respirometer is best positioned on the expiratory limb of the ventilator breathing system. This minimizes the loss of gas volume due to leaks and expansion of the tubing on the inspiratory limb.*
   b) *False. It is a unidirectional device allowing the measurement of the tidal volume if the flow of gases is in one direction only. An arrow on the device indicates the correct direction of the gas flow.*
   c) *True. It is suitable for routine clinical use with an accuracy of ± 5–10% within a range of flows of 4–24 L/min.*
   d) *True. Over-reading at high flows and under-reading at low flows is due to the effect of inertia on the rotating vane. Using a Wright respirometer based on light reflection or the use of a semi-conductive device sensitive to changes in magnetic field, instead of the mechanical components, improves the accuracy.*
   e) *True. The wright respirometer can measure the volume per breath and if the measurement is continued for one minute, the minute volume can be measured as well.*

8. Paramagnetic gases include
   a) *True. Oxygen is attracted by the magnetic field because it has two electrons in unpaired orbits causing it to possess paramagnetic properties.*
   b) *False.*
   c) *False.*
   d) *False.*
   e) *False.*

9. Oxygen in a gas mixture can be measured by
   a) *True. The oxygen molecules diffuse through a membrane and electrolyte solution to reach the cathode. This generates a current proportional to the partial pressure of oxygen in the mixture.*
   b) *False. Oxygen does not absorb ultraviolet radiation. Halothane absorbs ultraviolet radiation.*
   c) *True. Mass spectrometry can be used for the measurement of any gas. It separates the gases according to their molecular weight. The sample is ionized and then the ions are separated. Mass spectrometry allows rapid simultaneous breath-to-breath measurement of oxygen concentration.*
   d) *True. Although polarographic analysers are used mainly to measure oxygen partial pressure in a blood sample in blood gas analysers, they can also be used to measure the partial pressure in a gas sample. See Question 6 above.*
   e) *False. Gases that absorb infrared radiation have molecules with two different atoms (e.g. carbon and oxygen in CO_2). An oxygen molecule has two similar atoms.*

10. The concentrations of volatile agents can be measured using
   a) *False. The fuel cell is used to measure the oxygen concentration.*
   b) *True. A piezoelectric quartz crystal with a lipophilic coat undergoes changes in natural frequency when exposed to a lipid soluble inhalational agent. It lacks agent specificity. It is not widely used in current anaesthetic practice.*
   c) *True. Halothane can absorb ultraviolet radiation. It is not used in current anaesthetic practice.*
   d) *True. Infrared radiation is absorbed by all the gases with dissimilar atoms in the molecule. Infrared analysers can be either side stream or main stream.*
   e) *False. The clark polarographic electrode is used to measure oxygen concentration.*

11. A patient with healthy lungs and a $PaCO_2$ of 40 mmHg will have which of the following percentages of CO_2 in the end expiratory mixture?
   a) *False.*
   b) *True. In a patient with healthy lungs, the end-tidal CO_2 concentration is a true reflection of the arterial CO_2. A $PaCO_2$ of 40 mmHg (5.3 kPa) is therefore equivalent to an end-tidal CO_2 of about 5 kPa. One atmospheric pressure is 760 mmHg or 101.33 kPa. That makes the end-tidal CO_2 percentage about 5%.*
   c) *False.*
   d) *False.*
   e) *False.*

12. BIS monitor
   a) *False. BIS uses a linear dimensionless scale of 0–100 without any units. The lower the BIS value, the greater the hypnotic effect. General anaesthesia is between 40 and 60.*
   b) *False. Hypothermia below 33°C decreases the BIS value as the electrical activity in brain is decreased by the low temperature.*
   c) *True. The BIS value is not accurate during ketamine anaesthesia. Ketamine is a dissociative anaesthetic with excitatory effects on the EEG.*
   d) *True. Newer versions have better protection from diathermy and EMG.*
   e) *False. BIS monitors the electrical activity in the brain and not the concentration of a particular drug.*

13. Concerning ECG
   a) *False. The monitoring mode has a limited frequency response of 0.5–40 Hz whereas the diagnostic mode has a much wider range of 0.05–100 Hz.*
   b) *False. The electrical activity of the heart has an electrical potentials range of 0.5–2 mV.*
   c) *True. Surrounding the ECG leads with copper screens reduces interference due to electrostatic induction and capacitance coupling.*
   d) *True. Silver and silver chloride form a stable electrode combination. They are held in a cup and separated from the skin by a foam pad soaked in conducting gel.*
   e) *False. The standard in the UK is to use a display speed of 25 mm/s and a sensitivity of 1 mV/cm.*

14. Infrared spectrometry
   a) *False. CO_2 absorbs infrared radiation mainly at a wavelength of 4.3 μm.*
   b) *True. Photo-acoustic spectrometry is more stable than the conventional infrared spectrometry. Its calibration remains constant over much longer periods of time.*
   c) *True. This is not the case with the main stream analysers.*
   d) *True. Optical filters are used to select the desired wavelengths to avoid interference from other vapours or gases.*
   e) *False. For the inhalational agents, higher wavelengths are used, such as 8–9 μm, to avoid interference from methane and alcohol (at 3.3 μm).*

Chapter 11

Invasive monitoring

Invasive arterial pressure monitoring

Invasive arterial pressure monitoring provides beat-to-beat real-time information with sustained accuracy.

Components

1. An indwelling Teflon arterial cannula (20 or 22 G) is used. The cannula has parallel walls to minimize the effect on blood flow to the distal parts of the limb. Cannulation can be achieved by directly threading the cannula (either by direct insertion method or a transfixation technique) or by using a modified Seldinger technique with a guidewire to assist in the insertion as in some designs (Fig. 11.1).
2. A column of bubble-free heparinized saline at a pressure of 300 mmHg, incorporating a flushing device.
3. Via the fluid column, the cannula is connected to a transducer (Figs 11.2, 11.3, 11.4). This in

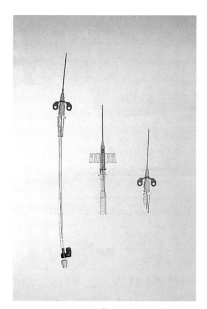

Fig. 11.1 A range of arterial cannulae.

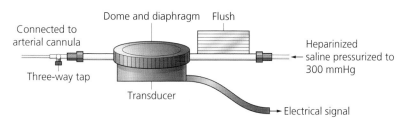

Fig. 11.2 Components of a pressure measuring system.

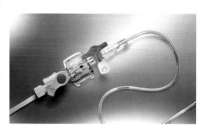

Fig. 11.3 Smith's Medex single use disposable integrated pressure transducer.

turn is connected to an amplifier and oscilloscope. A strain gauge variable resistor transducer is used.
4. The diaphragm (a very thin membrane) acts as an interface between the transducer and the fluid column.
5. The pressure transducer is a device that changes either electrical resistance or capacitance in response to changes in pressure on a solid-state device. The moving part of the transducer is very small and has little mass.

Mechanism of action

1. The saline column moves back and forth with the arterial pulsation causing the diaphragm to move. This causes changes in the resistance and current flow through the wires of the transducer.
2. The transducer is connected to a Wheatstone bridge circuit (Fig. 11.5). This is an electrical circuit for the precise comparison of

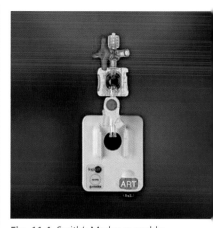

Fig. 11.4 Smith's Medex re-usable pressure transducer.

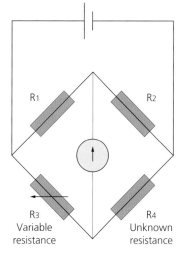

Fig. 11.5 The Wheatstone bridge circuit where null deflection of the galvanometer implies R1/R2 = R3/R4.

resistors. It uses a null-deflection system consisting of a very sensitive galvanometer and four resistors in two parallel branches: two constant resistors, a variable resistor, and the unknown resistor. Changes in resistance and current are measured, electronically converted and displayed as systolic, diastolic and mean arterial pressures. The Wheatstone bridge circuit is ideal for measuring the small changes in resistance found in strain gauges. Most pressure transducers contain four strain gauges that form the four resistors of the Wheatstone bridge.

3. The flushing device allows 3–4 mL per hour of heparinized saline to flush the cannula. This is to prevent clotting and backflow through the catheter. Manual flushing of the system is also possible when indicated.

4. The radial artery is the most commonly used artery because the ulnar artery is the dominant artery in the hand. The ulnar artery is connected to the radial artery through the palmar arch in 95% of patients. The brachial, femoral, ulnar or dorsalis pedis arteries are used occasionally.

5. The information gained from invasive arterial pressure monitoring includes heart rate, pulse pressure, the presence of a respiratory swing, left ventricular contractility, vascular tone (SVR) and stroke volume.

The arterial pressure waveform

1. This can be characterized as a complex sine wave that is the summation of a series of simple sine waves of different amplitudes and frequencies.

2. The fundamental frequency (or 1st harmonic) is equal to the heart rate, so a heart rate of 60 beats per minute = 1 beat/sec or 1 cycle/sec or 1 Hz. The first ten harmonics of the fundamental frequency contribute to the waveform.

3. The system used to measure arterial blood pressure should be capable of responding to a frequency range of 0.5–40 Hz in order to display the arterial waveform correctly.

4. The dicrotic notch in the arterial pressure waveform represents changes in pressure because of vibrations caused by the closure of the aortic valve.

5. The rate of rise of the upstroke part of the wave (dP/dt) reflects the myocardial contractility. A slow rise upstroke might indicate a need for inotropic support. A positive response to the inotropic support will show a steeper upstroke. The maximum upward slope of the arterial waveform during systole is related to the speed of ventricular ejection.

6. The position of the dicrotic notch on the downstroke of the wave reflects the peripheral vascular resistance. In vasodilated patients, e.g. following an epidural block or in septic patients, the dicrotic notch is positioned lower on the curve. The notch is higher in vasoconstricted patients.

7. The downstroke slope indicates resistance to outflow. A slow fall is seen in vasoconstriction.

8. The stroke volume can be estimated by measuring the area from the beginning of the upstroke to the dicrotic notch. Multiply that by the heart rate and the cardiac output can be estimated.

9. Mean blood pressure is the average pressure throughout the cardiac cycle. As systole is shorter than diastole, the mean arterial pressure (MAP) is slightly less than the value half way between systolic and diastolic pressures. An estimate of MAP can be obtained by adding a third of the pulse pressure (systolic − diastolic pressure) to the diastolic pressure.

MAP can also be determined by integrating a pressure signal over the duration of one cycle, divided by time.

The natural frequency

This is the frequency at which the monitoring system itself resonates and amplifies the signal by up to 20–40%. This determines the frequency response of the monitoring system. The natural frequency should be at least ten times the fundamental frequency. The natural frequency of the measuring system is much higher than the primary frequency of the arterial waveform which is 1–2 Hz, corresponding to a heart rate of 60–120 beats/min. Stiffer (low compliance) tubing or a shorter length of tubing (less mass) produce higher natural frequencies. This results in the system requiring a much higher pulse rate before amplification.

The natural frequency of the monitoring system is:

1. directly related to the catheter diameter
2. inversely related to the square root of the system compliance
3. inversely related to the square root of the length of the tubing
4. inversely related to the square root of the density of the fluid in the system.

Problems in practice and safety features

1. The arterial pressure waveform should be displayed (Fig. 11.6) in order to detect damping or resonance. The monitoring system should be able to apply an optimal damping value of 0.64.
   a) **Damping** is caused by dissipation of stored energy. Anything that takes energy out of the system results in a progressive diminution of amplitude of oscillations.

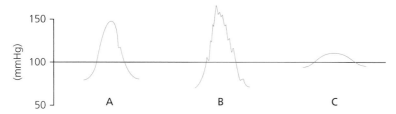

Fig. 11.6 Arterial pressure waveform. (A) Correct, optimally damped waveform. (B) Underdamped waveform. (C) Overdamped waveform (reproduced with permission from Aitkenhead R, Smith G. Textbook of Anaesthesia, 3rd edn. Churchill Livingstone, 1996).

Increased damping lowers the systolic and elevates the diastolic pressures with loss of detail in the waveform. Damping can be caused by an air bubble (air is more compressible in comparison to the saline column), clot or a highly compliant, soft transducer diaphragm and tube.

b) **Resonance** occurs when the frequency of the driving force coincides with the resonant frequency of the system. If the natural frequency is less than 40 Hz, it falls within the range of the blood pressure and a sine wave will be superimposed on the blood pressure wave. Increased resonance elevates the systolic and lowers the diastolic pressures. The mean pressure should stay unchanged. Resonance can be due to a stiff, non-compliant diaphragm and tube. It is worse with tachycardia.

2. The transducer should be positioned at the level of the right atrium as a reference point that is at the level of the midaxillary line. Raising or lowering the transducer above or below the level of the right atrium gives error readings equivalent to 7.5 mmHg for each 10 cm.

3. Ischaemia distal to the cannula is rare but should be monitored for. Multiple attempts at insertion and haematoma formation increase the risk of ischaemia.

4. Arterial thrombosis occurs in 20–25% of cases with very rare adverse effects such as ischaemia or necrosis of the hand. Cannulae in place for less than 24 hours very rarely cause thrombosis.

5. The arterial pressure wave narrows and increases in amplitude in peripheral vessels. This makes the systolic pressure higher in the dorsalis pedis than in the radial artery.

6. There is risk of bleeding due to disconnection.

7. Inadvertent drug injection causes distal vascular occlusion and gangrene. An arterial cannula should be clearly labelled.

8. Local infection is thought to be less than 20%. Systemic infection is thought to be less than 5%. This is more common in patients with an arterial cannula for more than 4 days with a traumatic insertion.

9. Arterial cannulae should not be inserted in sites with evidence of infection and trauma or through a vascular prosthesis.

10. Periodic checks and re-zeroing are carried out to prevent baseline drift of the transducer electrical circuits.

Invasive arterial blood pressure

- Consists of an arterial cannula, a heparinized saline column, a flushing device, a transducer, an amplifier and an oscilloscope.
- In addition to blood pressure, other parameters can be measured and estimated such as myocardial contractility, vascular tone and stroke volume.
- The waveform should be displayed to detect any resonance or damping.
- The measuring system should be able to cover a frequency range of 0.5–40 Hz.
- The monitoring system should be able to apply an optimal damping value of 0.64.

Central venous catheterization and pressure (CVP)

The CVP is the filling pressure of the right atrium. It can be measured directly using a central venous catheter. The catheter can also be used to administer fluids, blood, drugs, parenteral nutrition and sample blood. Specialized catheters can be used for haemofiltration, haemodialysis (see Chapter 13, Haemofiltration), and transvenous pacemaker placement.

The tip of the catheter is usually positioned in the superior vena cava at the entrance to the right atrium. The internal jugular, subclavian and basilic veins are possible routes for central venous catheterization. The subclavian route is associated with the highest rate of complications but

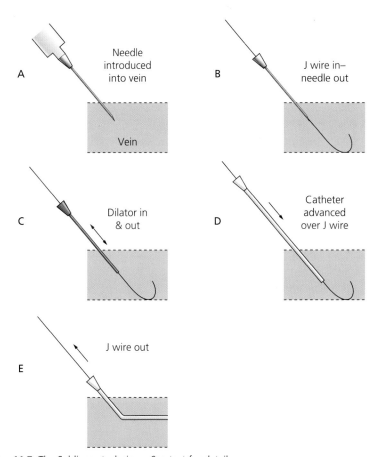

A — Needle introduced into vein / Vein

B — J wire in– needle out

C — Dilator in & out

D — Catheter advanced over J wire

E — J wire out

Fig. 11.7 The Seldinger technique. See text for details.

is convenient for the patient and for the nursing care.

The Seldinger technique is the common and standard method used for central venous catheterization (Fig. 11.7) regardless of catheter type. The procedure should be done under sterile conditions:

1. Introduce the needle into the vein using the appropriate landmarks or an ultrasound-locating device.
2. A J-shaped soft tip guidewire is introduced through the needle (and syringe in some designs) into the vein. The needle can then be removed. The J-shaped tip is designed to minimize trauma to the vessels' endothelium.

3. After a small incision in the skin, has been made, a dilator is introduced over the guidewire to make a track through the skin and subcutaneous tissues and is then withdrawn.
4. The catheter is then railroaded over the guidewire into its final position before the guidewire is withdrawn.
5. Blood should be aspirated easily from all ports which should then be flushed with saline or heparin solution. All the port sites that are not intended for immediate use are sealed. A port should never be left open to air during insertion because of the risk of air embolism.

6. The catheter is secured onto the skin and covered with a sterile dressing.
7. A chest X-ray is performed to ensure correct positioning of the catheter and to detect pneumo- and/or haemothorax.

The CVP is read using either a pressure transducer or a water manometer.

PRESSURE TRANSDUCER

1. A similar measuring system to that used for invasive arterial pressure monitoring (catheter, heparinized saline column, transducer, diaphragm, flushing device and oscilloscope system). The transducer is positioned at the level of the right atrium.
2. A measuring system of limited frequency range is adequate because of the shape of the waveform and the values of the central venous pressure.

FLUID MANOMETER (FIG. 11.8)

1. A giving set with either normal saline or 5% dextrose is connected to the vertical manometer via a three-way tap. The latter is also connected to the central venous catheter.
2. The manometer has a spirit level side arm positioned at the level of the right atrium (zero reference point). The upper end of the column is open to air via a filter. This filter must stay dry to maintain direct connection with the atmosphere.
3. The vertical manometer is filled to about the 20 cm mark. By opening the three-way tap to the patient, a swing of the column should be seen with respiration. The CVP is read in cmH_2O when the fluid level stabilizes.

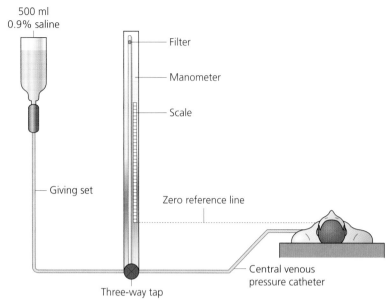

500 ml
0.9% saline

Filter

Manometer

Scale

Giving set

Zero reference line

Central venous
pressure catheter

Three-way tap

Fig. 11.8 Measurement of CVP using a water manometer. The manometer's fluid level falls until the height of the fluid column above the zero reference point is equal to the CVP (reproduced with permission from Aitkenhead R, Smith G. Textbook of Anaesthesia, 3rd edn. Churchill Livingstone, 1996).

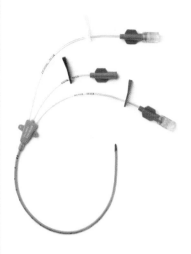

Fig. 11.9 Smith's Medex silver impregnated triple lumen central venous catheter. Both the inside and outside surfaces are impregnated with silver.

4. The manometer uses a balance of forces: downward pressure of the fluid (determined by density and height) against pressure of the central venous system (caused by hydrostatic and recoil forces).

In both techniques the monitoring system has to be zeroed at the level of the right atrium (usually at the midaxillary line). This eliminates the effect of hydrostatic pressure on the CVP value.

CATHETERS

There are different types of catheters used for central venous cannulation and CVP measurement. They differ in their lumen size, length, number of lumens, the presence or absence of a subcutaneous cuff and the material they are made of. The vast majority of catheters are designed to be inserted using the Seldinger technique although some are designed as 'long' intravenous

cannulae (cannula over a needle, see Fig. 11.12).

Antimicrobial-coated catheters have been designed to reduce the incidence of catheter-related blood stream infection. These can be either antiseptic coated (e.g. chlorhexidine/silver sulfadiazine, benzalkonium chloride, platinum/silver) or antibiotic coated (e.g. minocycline/rifampin) on either the internal or external surface or both. The antibiotic coated central lines are thought to be more effective in reducing the incidence of infection (Fig. 11.9).

Multi-lumen catheter

1. The catheter has two or more lumens of different sizes, e.g. 16 G and 18 G (Fig. 11.10). Paediatric sizes also exist (Fig. 11.11).
2. The different lumens should be flushed with heparinized saline before insertion.

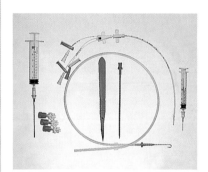

Fig. 11.10 A triple lumen catheter and insertion set.

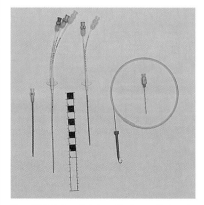

Fig. 11.11 Paediatric catheters, dilator, J wire and introducing needle. 12 cm triple lumen (left), 8 cm double lumen (right).

3. Single and double lumen versions exist.
4. Simultaneous administration of drugs and CVP monitoring is possible. It does not allow the insertion of a pulmonary artery catheter.
5. These catheters are made of polyurethane. This provides good tensile strength, allowing larger lumens for smaller internal diameter.

Long central catheters/peripherally inserted central catheters (PICC)

1. These catheters, 60 cm in length, are designed to be inserted through an introducing cannula via an antecubital fossa vein, usually the basilic vein (Fig. 11.12).
2. They are used when a central catheter is required in situations when it is undesirable to gain access via the internal jugular or the subclavian veins, for example during head and neck surgery or prolonged antibiotic therapy. They are made of soft flexible polyurethane or silicone

Hickman catheters

1. These central catheters are made of polyurethane or silicone and are usually inserted into the subclavian vein. The catheter can have one, two or three lumens (Fig. 11.13).
2. The proximal end is tunnelled under the skin for a distance of about 10 cm.
3. A Dacron cuff is positioned 3–4 cm from the site of entry into the vein under the skin. It induces a fibroblastic reaction to anchor the catheter in place (Fig. 11.14). The cuff also reduces the risk of infection as it stops the spread of infection from the site of entry to the skin. Some catheters also have a silver impregnated cuff that acts as an antimicrobial barrier.
4. They are used for long-term chemotherapy, parenteral nutrition, blood sampling or as a readily available venous access especially in children requiring frequent anaesthetics during cancer treatment.
5. These lines are designed to remain in situ for several months

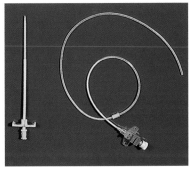

Fig. 11.13 A single lumen Dacron cuffed Hickman catheter (right). Dilator/introducer (left).

unless they become infected but require some degree of daily maintenance.

Dialysis catheters

These are large calibre catheters designed to allow high flow rates of at least 300 mL/min. They are made of silicone or polyurethane. Most of them are dual lumen with staggered end and side holes to prevent admixture of blood at the inflow and outflow portions reducing recirculation

Problems in practice and safety features

1. Inaccurate readings can be due to catheter blockage, catheter inserted too far or using the wrong zero level.
2. Pneumo-haemothorax (with an incidence of 2–10 with subclavian vein catheterization and 1–2 with internal jugular catheterization), trauma to the arteries (carotid, subclavian and brachial), air embolism, haematoma and tracheal puncture are complications of insertion.
3. Sepsis and infection are common complications with an incidence of 2.8–20%. *Staphylococcus aureus* and *Enterococcus* are the most common organisms.

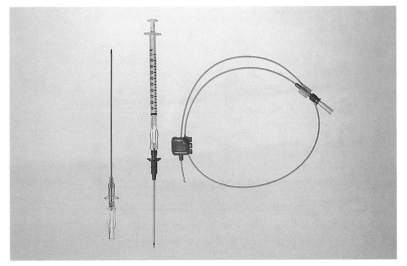

Fig. 11.12 A cannula over a needle CVP line (left). A long central venous catheter (right) with introducing cannula (centre).

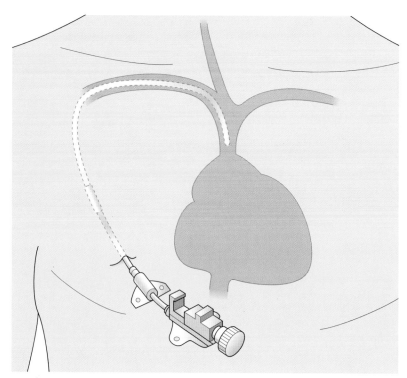

Fig. 11.14 Final position of a tunnelled Hickman catheter (reproduced with permission from Viggo-Spectramed, a division of BOC Health Care).

serious but unusual complication such as venous or cardiac perforation can be lethal.

6. Catheter-related venous thrombosis is thought to be up to 40% depending on the site, the duration of placement, the technique and the condition of the patient.

7. Microshock. A central venous catheter presents a direct pathway to the heart muscle. Faulty electrical equipment can produce minute electrical currents (less than 1 ampere) which can travel via this route to the myocardium. This can produce ventricular fibrillation (VF) if the tip of the catheter is in direct contact with the myocardium (see Chapter 14). This very small current does not cause any adverse effects if applied to the body surface but if passed directly to the heart, the current density will be high enough to cause VF, hence the name microshock.

Guidelines for reduction in sepsis and infection rates with the use of central venous catheters (Centers for Disease Control and Prevention. Guidelines for the prevention of intravascular catheter-related infections, 2002)

- Education and training of staff who insert and maintain the catheters.
- Use the maximum sterile barrier precautions during central venous catheter insertion.
- Use of 2% chlorhexidine preparations for skin antisepsis.
- Avoidance of routine replacement of central venous catheters as a strategy to prevent infection.
- Use of antimicrobial coated short-term central venous catheters if

rate of infection is high despite adherence to other strategies.
- Antimicrobial coated catheters are recommended when catheter is expected to remain in place for more than 5 days.

4. A false passage may be created if the guidewire or dilator are advanced against resistance. The insertion should be smooth.

5. There may be cardiace complications such as self-limiting arrhythmias due to the irritation caused by the guidewire or catheter. Gradual withdrawal of the device is usually adequate to restore normal rhythm. More

Central venous catheterization and pressure

- There are different routes of insertion, e.g. the internal jugular, subclavian and basilic veins.
- The Seldinger technique is the most commonly used.
- The catheters differ in size, length, number of lumens and material.
- A pressure transducer or water manometer is used to measure CVP.
- Sepsis and infection are common.
- Antibiotic and/or antiseptic coated catheters can reduce the incidence of infections.

Balloon-tipped flow-guided pulmonary artery catheter

Pulmonary artery (PA) catheters are usually inserted via the internal jugular or subclavian veins via an introducer. They are floated through the right atrium and ventricle into the pulmonary artery.

Indications for using a PA catheter include

- Ischaemic heart disease, cardiogenic shock and right ventricle failure.
- Sepsis and septic shock.
- Adult respiratory distress syndrome.
- Oliguria and unexplained hypotension.
- Perioperative monitoring, e.g. CABG, vascular surgery.

Components

PA catheters are available in sizes 5–8 G and are usually 110 cm in length (Fig. 11.15). They have up to five lumens and are marked at 10 cm intervals.

1. The distal lumen ends in the pulmonary artery. It is used to measure PA and pulmonary capillary wedge (PCW) pressures and to sample mixed venous blood.
2. The proximal lumen should ideally open in the right atrium, being positioned about 30 cm from the tip of the catheter. It can be used to continuously monitor the CVP, to administer the injectate to measure the cardiac output (by thermodilution) or to infuse fluids. Depending on the design, a second proximal lumen may be present which is usually dedicated to infusions of drugs.
3. Another lumen contains two insulated wires leading to a thermistor that is about 3.7 cm from the catheter tip. Proximally

it is connected to a cardiac output computer.
4. The balloon inflation lumen is used to inflate the balloon which is situated at the catheter tip.

Up to 1.5 mL of air is needed. When the balloon is inflated, the catheter floats with the blood flow into a pulmonary artery branch (Fig. 11.16).

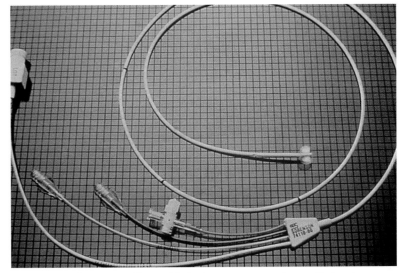

Fig. 11.15 A balloon-tipped flow-guided pulmonary artery catheter with four lumens (proximal, distal, thermistor and balloon inflation).

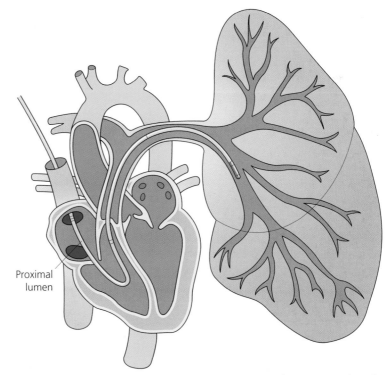

Proximal lumen

Fig. 11.16 Position of the pulmonary artery catheter tip in a pulmonary artery branch. The desired position of the proximal lumen in the right atrium is indicated by an arrow.

Mechanism of action

1. Before insertion, flush all the lines and test the balloon with 1–1.5 mL of air.
2. The distal lumen of the catheter is connected to a transducer pressure measuring system for continuous monitoring as the catheter is advanced. As the catheter passes via the superior vena cava to the right atrium, low pressure waves (mean of 3–8 mmHg normally) are displayed (Fig. 11.17). The distance from the internal jugular or the subclavian vein to the right atrium is about 15–20 cm.
3. The balloon is partly inflated, enabling the blood flow to carry the catheter tip through the tricuspid valve into the right ventricle. Tall pressure waves (15–25 mmHg systolic, and 0–10 mmHg diastolic) are displayed.
4. As the balloon tip floats through the pulmonary valve into the PA, the pressure waveform changes with higher diastolic pressure (10–20 mmHg), but similar systolic pressures. The dicrotic notch, caused by the closure of the pulmonary valve, can be noted. The distance from the right ventricle to the pulmonary artery should be less than 10 cm, unless there is cardiomegaly.

5. The balloon is fully inflated enabling the blood flow to carry the tip of the catheter into a pulmonary artery branch, where it wedges. This is shown as a damped pressure waveform (PCWP, mean pressure of 4–12 mmHg). This reflects the left atrial filling pressure. The balloon should then be deflated so the catheter floats back into the PA. The balloon should be kept deflated until another PCWP reading is required.
6. The cardiac output can be measured using thermodilution. 10 mL of cold injectate is administered upstream via the proximal lumen. The thermistor (in the pulmonary artery) measures the change in temperature of the blood downstream. A temperature–time curve is displayed from which the computer can calculate the cardiac output (Fig. 11.18). The volume of injectate should be known accurately and the whole volume injected quickly. Usually the mean of three readings is taken. Because of the relatively high incidence of complications, less invasive techniques are being developed to measure the cardiac output. Thermodilution remains the standard method for measuring the cardiac output.

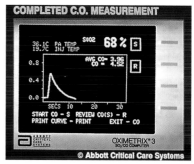

Fig. 11.18 The Abbott cardiac output computer. Cardiac output is measured using a thermodilution technique which produces a temperature–time curve. Cardiac output is computed from this information. When connected to the appropriate catheter, mixed venous oxygen saturation (SvO$_2$) can also be monitored.

7. Some designs have the facility to continuously monitor the mixed venous oxygen saturation using fibreoptic technology (Figs 11.19 and 11.20). Cardiac pacing capability is present in some designs.

Information gained from PA catheter

The responses to fluid challenges and therapeutic regimens are monitored in preference to isolated individual readings. The following can be measured:

CVP, right ventricular (RV) pressure, PA pressure, PCWP, cardiac output, cardiac index, stroke volume, stoke volume index, left and right ventricular stroke work index, systemic vascular resistance, pulmonary vascular resistance, mixed venous oximetry (SvO$_2$), blood temperature and degree of shunt.

Problems in practice and safety features

The overall morbidity of such catheters is 0.4%.

1. Complications due to central venous cannulation (as above).

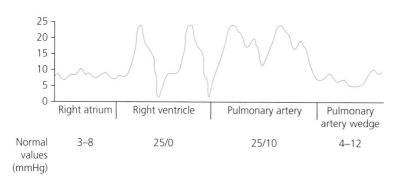

	Right atrium	Right ventricle	Pulmonary artery	Pulmonary artery wedge
Normal values (mmHg)	3–8	25/0	25/10	4–12

Fig. 11.17 Diagrammatic representation of the pressure waveforms seen as a pulmonary artery flotation catheter is advanced until it wedges in a branch of the pulmonary artery (reproduced with permission from Aitkenhead R, Smith G. Textbook of Anaesthesia, 3rd edn. Churchill Livingstone, 1996).

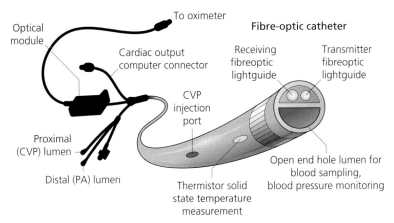

Fig. 11.19 Mechanism of action of the Abbott Oximetrix pulmonary artery catheter. This uses fibreoptic technology to measure mixed venous oxygen saturation (SvO$_2$).

Balloon-tipped flow-guided pulmonary artery catheter

- Inserted via a large central vein into the right atrium, right ventricle, pulmonary artery and branch with contiguous pressure monitoring.
- Used to measure left ventricular filling pressure in addition to other parameters.
- Complications are due to central venous cannulation, the passage of the catheter through different structures and the presence of the catheter in the circulation.
- PCWP does not accurately reflect left ventricular (LV) filling pressure in certain conditions.

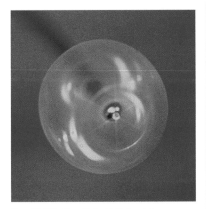

Fig. 11.20 The Abbott Oximetrix pulmonary artery catheter tip.

2. Complications due to catheter passage and advancement. These include arrhythmias (ventricular ectopics, ventricular tachycardia and others), heart block, knotting/ kinking (common in low-flow states and patients with large hearts; a 'rule of thumb' is that the catheter should not be advanced more than 10–15 cm without a change in the pressure waveform), valvular damage and perforation of PA vessel.

3. Complications due to the presence in the PA. These include thrombosis (can be reduced by the use of heparin-bonded catheters), PA rupture (more common in the elderly, may present as haemoptysis and is often fatal), infection, balloon rupture, pulmonary infarction, valve damage and arrhythmias.

4. In certain conditions, the PCWP does not accurately reflect left ventricular filling pressure. Such conditions include mitral stenosis and regurgitation, left atrial myxoma, ball valve thrombus, pulmonary veno-occlusive disease, total anomalous pulmonary venous drainage, cardiac tamponade and acute right ventricular dilatation resulting from right ventricular infarction, massive pulmonary embolism and acute severe tricuspid regurgitation.

5. **Catheter whip** can occur because of the coursing of the pulmonary catheter through the right heart. Cardiac contractions can produce 'shock transients' or 'whip' artifacts. Negative deflections due to a whip artifact may lead to an underestimation of pulmonary artery pressures.

Oesophageal Doppler haemodynamic measurement

An estimate of cardiac output can be quickly obtained using the minimally invasive oesophageal Doppler. Patient response to therapeutic manoeuvres (e.g. fluid challenge) can also be rapidly assessed. The technique has the advantage of the smooth muscle tone of the oesophagus acting as a natural means of maintaining the probe in position for repeated measurements. In addition, the oesophagus is in close anatomical proximity to the aorta so that signal interference from bone, soft tissue and lung is minimized. Over the past three decades the oesophageal Doppler has evolved from an experimental technique to a relatively simple bedside procedure with the latest models incorporating both Doppler and echo-ultrasound in a single probe.

The measurement of cardiac output using the oesophageal

Doppler method correlates well with that obtained from a pulmonary artery catheter. Oesophageal Doppler ultrasonography has been used for intravascular volume optimization in both the perioperative period and in the critical care setting. Its use in cardiac, general and orthopaedic surgery has been associated with a reduction in morbidity and hospital stay. Because of the mild discomfort associated with placing the probe and maintaining it in a fixed position, patients require adequate sedation.

Components

1. A monitor housing:
   a) a screen for visual verification of correct signal measurement (Fig. 11.21)
   b) technology that enables beat-to-beat calculation of the stroke volume and cardiac output.
2. An insulated thin latex-free silicone oesophageal probe containing a Doppler transducer angled at 45° (Fig. 11.21). The probe has a diameter of 6 mm with an internal spring coil to ensure flexibility and rigidity.

Mechanism of action

1. The device relies on the Doppler principle. There is an increase in observed frequency of a signal when the signal source approaches the observer and a decrease when the source moves away.
2. The changes in the frequency of the transmitted ultrasound result from the encounter of the wavefront with moving red blood cells. If the transmitted sound waves encounter a group of red cells moving towards the source, they are reflected back at a frequency higher than that at which they were sent, producing a **positive Doppler shift**. The opposite effect occurs when a given frequency sent into tissues encounters red cells moving away. The result is the return of a frequency lower than that transmitted, resulting in a **negative Doppler shift**. Analysis of the reflected frequencies allows determination of velocity of flow.
3. The lubricated probe is inserted via the mouth with the bevel of the tip facing up at the back of the patient's throat into the distal oesophagus to a depth of about 35–40 cm from the teeth.
4. The probe is rotated and slowly pulled back while listening to the audible signal. The ideal probe tip location is at the level between the fifth and sixth thoracic vertebrae because at that level the descending aorta is adjacent and parallel to the distal oesophagus.

This location is achieved by superficially landmarking the distance to the third sternocostal junction anteriorly. A correctly positioned probe can measure the blood flow in this major vessel using a high ultrasound frequency of 4 MHz.

5. The Doppler signal waveform is analysed and the stroke volume and total cardiac output is computed using the Doppler equation and a normogram which corrects for variations found with differing patient age, sex and body surface area.

The Doppler equation

$$v = \frac{cf_d}{2\,f_T\cos\theta}$$

where

v is flow velocity
c is speed of sound in body tissue (1540 m/s)
f_d Doppler frequency shift
$\cos\theta$ is cosine of angle between sound beam and blood flow (45°)
f_T is frequency of transmitted ultrasound (Hz)

6. The parameters obtained from analysis of the Doppler signal waveform allow the operator to gain an assessment of cardiac

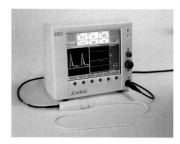

Fig. 11.21 The CardioQ oesophageal Doppler machine and attached probe (foreground).

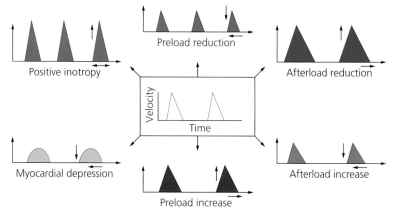

Fig. 11.22 Changes in oesophageal Doppler waveform associated with a variety of clinical situations (reproduced with permission from Dr M. Singer).

output, stroke volume, volaemic status, systemic vascular resistance and myocardial function (Fig. 11.22).

Problems in practice and safety features

1. The probe is fully insulated and safe when diathermy is being used.
2. The probe cannot easily be held in the correct position for long periods. Frequent repositioning may be necessary if continuous monitoring is required.
3. Oesophageal Doppler measurement can only be used in an adequately sedated, intubated patient. Its use in awake patients has been described using local anaesthesia. A suprasternal probe is also available and can be used in awake patients.
4. Insertion of the probe is not recommended in patients with pharyngo-oesophageal pathology (e.g. oesophageal varices).
5. The role of the oesophageal Doppler in children is still being evaluated.

Oesophageal Doppler

- Minimally invasive and rapid estimate of cardiac output using the Doppler principle.
- Insulated Doppler probe lies in the distal oesophagus emitting a high ultrasound frequency of 4 MHz.
- Continuous monitoring is possible, although frequent probe repositioning is a problem.

Temperature probes

Monitoring a patient's temperature during surgery is a common and

routine procedure. Different types of thermometers are available.

THERMISTOR

Components

1. A small bead of a temperature-dependent semiconductor.
2. Wheatstone bridge circuit.

Mechanism of action

1. The thermistor has electrical resistance which changes non-linearly with temperature. The response is made linear electronically.
2. It can be made in very small sizes.
3. It is mounted in a plastic or stainless steel probe making it mechanically robust, and it can be chemically sterilized.
4. It is used in PA catheters to measure cardiac output.
5. In the negative thermal conductivity thermistors, such as cobalt oxide, copper oxide and manganese oxide, the electrical resistance decreases as the temperature increases. In the positive thermal conductivity thermistors, such as barium titanate, the electrical resistance increases with the temperature.

Problems in practice and safety features

Thermistors need to be stabilized as they age.

INFRARED TYMPANIC THERMOMETER

Components

1. A small probe with a disposable and transparent cover is inserted into the external auditory meatus.
2. The detector (which consists of a series of thermocouples called a thermopile).

Mechanism of action

1. The detector receives infrared radiation from the tympanic membrane.
2. The infrared signal detected is converted into an electrical signal that is processed to measure accurately the core temperature within 3 seconds.

Problems in practice and safety features

1. Non-continuous intermittent readings.
2. The probe has to be accurately aimed at the tympanic membrane. False low readings from the sides of the ear canal can be a problem.
3. Wax in the ear can affect the accuracy.

THERMOCOUPLES

Components

1. Two strips of dissimilar metals of different specific heats and in contact from both ends. Usually copper-constantan (copper with 40% nickel) junctions are used.
2. A galvanometer.

Mechanism of action

1. One junction is used as the measuring junction whereas the other one is the reference. The latter is kept at a constant temperature.
2. The metals expand and contract to different degrees with change in temperature producing an electrical potential that is compared to a reference junction. The current produced is directly proportional to the temperature difference between the two junctions.
3. The voltage produced is called the Seebeck effect.

4. The measuring junction produces a potential of 40 μv per °C. This potential is measured by an amplifier.
5. They are stable and accurate to 0.1°C.

Body core temperature can be measured using different sites.

1. **Rectal** temperature does not accurately reflect the core temperature in anaesthetized patients. During an operation, changes in temperature are relatively rapid and the rectal temperature lags behind.
2. **Oesophageal** temperature accurately reflects the core temperature with the probe positioned in the lower oesophagus (at the level of the left atrium). Here the probe is not affected by the cooler tracheal temperature (Fig. 11.23).
3. **Tympanic membrane** temperature is closely associated with brain temperature. It accurately reflects core temperature, compared with lower oesophageal temperature. Thermocouple and thermistor probes as well as the infrared probe can be used (Fig. 11.24).

4. **Bladder** temperature correlates well with the core temperature when there is a normal urine output (Fig. 11.25).
5. **Skin** temperature, when measured with the core temperature, can be useful in determining the volaemic status of the patient (Fig. 11.26).

The axilla is the best location for monitoring muscle temperature, making it most suitable for detecting malignant hyperthermia.

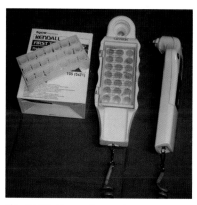

Fig. 11.24 Tympanic membrane thermometer.

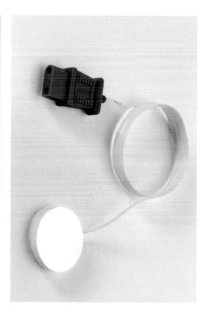

Fig. 11.26 Skin temperature probe.

Temperature probes

- They can be thermistors, thermocouples or infrared thermometers.
- Core and skin temperatures can be measured.
- Core temperature can be measured from the rectum, oesophagus, tympanic membrane or the bladder.

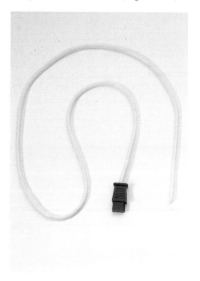

Fig. 11.23 Oesophageal/rectal temperature probe.

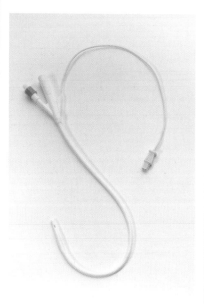

Fig. 11.25 Smith's Medical bladder catheter with a temperature probe.

FURTHER READING

O'Grady NP, Alexander M, Dellinger JL et al. Centers for Disease Control and Prevention. Guidelines for the prevention of intravascular catheter-related infections. MMWR 2002;51: RR-10;1–34.

Hemmings Jr H, Hopkins P. Foundations of Anesthesia. Basic and Clinical Sciences, 1st edn. London: Mosby, 2000.

Shoemaker WC, Velmahos GC, Demetriades D. Procedures and Monitoring for the Critically Ill, 1st edn. Philadelphia: WB Saunders, 2002.

Nanavai N. The oesophageal Doppler. CPD Anaesthesia 2004;6(1):25–30.

MCQs

In the following lists, which of the statements (a) to (e) are true?

1. Thermometers
   a) The electrical resistance of a thermistor changes non-linearly with temperature.
   b) Thermocouples are used in measuring cardiac output using the thermodilution method.
   c) The Seebeck effect is used to measure the temperature with thermocouples.
   d) Thermometers can be used to measure core and peripheral temperatures at the same time.
   e) A galvanometer is used to measure the potential in a thermocouple.

2. Concerning direct arterial blood pressure measurement
   a) A 16 G radial artery cannula is suitable.
   b) The position of the dicrotic notch in the wave form can reflect the vascular tone.
   c) The monitoring system should be capable of responding to a frequency range of up to 40 Hz.
   d) Increased damping of the wave form causes an increase in systolic pressure and a decrease in diastolic pressure.
   e) Air bubbles produce an overdamped waveform.

3. Balloon-tipped flow-guided pulmonary artery catheter
   a) They can have up to five separate lumens.
   b) They measure the cardiac output using the Doppler technique.
   c) The balloon should be left wedged and inflated in order to get a continuous reading of the left ventricular filling pressure.
   d) Mixed venous blood oxygen saturation can be measured.
   e) They use a thermocouple at the tip to measure the temperature of the blood.

4. If the mean arterial blood pressure is 100 mmHg, pulmonary capillary wedge pressure is 10 mmHg, mean pulmonary artery pressure is 15 mmHg, cardiac output is 5 L/min, and CVP is 5 mmHg, which of the following statements are correct?
   a) The unit for vascular resistance is dyne sec^{-1} cm^5.
   b) The pulmonary vascular resistance is about 800.
   c) The peripheral vascular resistance is about 1500.
   d) The patient has pulmonary hypertension.
   e) The patient has normal peripheral vascular resistance.

5. Concerning central venous pressure and cannulation
   a) 10 mmHg is equivalent to 7.5 cmH$_2$O.
   b) During cannulation, the left internal jugular vein is the approach of choice since the heart lies mainly in the left side of the chest.
   c) Subclavian vein cannulation has a higher incidence of pneumothorax than the internal jugular vein.
   d) The 'J' shaped end of the guidewire is inserted first.
   e) The Dacron cuff used in a Hickman's line is to anchor the catheter only.

6. In an invasive pressure measurement system, the following is correct
   a) A clot causes high systolic and low diastolic pressures.
   b) A transducer diaphragm with very low compliance causes low systolic and high diastolic pressures.
   c) A soft wide lumen catheter causes low systolic and high diastolic pressures.
   d) An air bubble causes low systolic and diastolic pressures.
   e) A short and narrow lumen catheter is ideal.

7. Concerning the oesophageal Doppler
   a) The ideal probe location is at the level between the 5th and 6th thoracic vertebrae.
   b) It emits a pulsed ultrasound wave of 4 Hz.
   c) Red cells moving towards the ultrasound source reflect the sound back at a frequency lower than that at which it was sent, producing a positive Doppler shift.
   d) The oesophageal probe tip is located at a depth of about 40 cm.
   e) The angle between the ultrasound beam and blood flow is 75°.

Answers

1. Thermometers
   a) *True. The response is non-linear but can be made linear electronically.*
   b) *False. Thermistors are used in measuring the cardiac output by thermodilution. Thermocouples are not used in measuring the cardiac output by thermodilution.*
   c) *True. The Seebeck effect is when the electrical potential produced at the junction of two dissimilar metals is dependent on the temperature of the junction. This is the principle used in thermocouples.*
   d) *True. The gradient between the core and peripheral temperatures is useful in assessing the degree of skin perfusion and the circulatory volume. For example, hypovolaemia causes a decrease in skin perfusion which reduces the peripheral temperature and thus increases the gradient. The normal gradient is about 2–4°C.*
   e) *True. The galvanometer is placed between the junctions of the thermocouple, the reference and the measuring junctions. This allows the current to be measured. Changes in current are calibrated to measure the temperature difference between the two junctions.*

2. Concerning direct arterial blood pressure measurement
   a) *False. A 16 G cannula is far too big to be inserted in an artery. 20 G or 22 G cannulae are usually used allowing adequate blood flow to pass by the cannula distally.*
   b) *True. The position of the dicrotic notch (which represents the closure of the aortic valve) is on the down stroke curve. A high dicrotic notch can be seen in vasoconstricted patients with high peripheral vascular resistance. A low dicrotic notch can be seen in vasodilated patients (e.g. patients with epidurals or sepsis).*
   c) *True. The addition of the shape of the dicrotic notch to an already simple wave form makes a maximum frequency of 40 Hz adequate for such a monitoring system. Because of the complicated waveform of the ECG, the monitoring system requires a much wider range of frequencies (maximum of 100 Hz).*
   d) *False. Increased damping leads to a decrease in systolic pressure and an increase in diastolic pressure. Decreased damping causes the opposite. The mean pressure remains the same.*
   e) *True. This is due to the difference in the compressibility of the two media, air and saline. Air is more compressible in contrast to the saline column.*

3. Balloon-tipped flow-guided pulmonary artery catheter
   a) *True. The most distal lumen is in the pulmonary artery, there are one or two proximal lumens in the right atrium, one lumen carries the insulated wires leading to the thermistor proximal to the tip of the catheter and another lumen is used to inflate the balloon at the tip of the catheter.*
   b) *False. The cardiac output is measured by thermodilution. A 'cold' injectate (e.g. saline) is injected via the proximal lumen. The changes in blood temperature are measured by the thermistor in the pulmonary artery. A temperature–time curve is displayed from which the cardiac output can be calculated.*
   c) *False. Leaving the balloon wedged and inflated is dangerous and should not be done. This is due to the risk of ischaemia to the distal parts of the lungs supplied by the pulmonary artery or its branches.*
   d) *True. Using fibreoptics, the mixed venous oxygen saturation can be measured on some designs. This allows the calculation of oxygen extraction by the tissues.*
   e) *False. A thermistor is used to measure the temperature of the blood. Thermistors are made to very small sizes.*

4. If the mean arterial blood pressure is 100 mmHg, pulmonary capillary wedge pressure is 10 mmHg, mean pulmonary artery pressure is 15 mmHg, cardiac output is 5 L/min, and CVP is 5 mmHg, which of the following statements are correct?

a) *False. The unit for vascular resistance is dyne sec cm^{-5}.*

b) *False. The pulmonary vascular resistance = mean pulmonary artery pressure-left atrial pressure × 80/cardiac output (15 – 10 × 80/5 = 80 dyne sec cm^{-5}).*

c) *True. The peripheral vascular resistance = mean arterial pressure–right atrial pressure × 80/cardiac output (100 – 5 × 80/5 = 1520 dyne sec cm^{-5}.*

d) *False. The normal mean pulmonary artery pressure is about 15 mmHg (systolic pressure of about 25 and a diastolic pressure of about 10 mmHg) and pulmonary vascular resistance is 80–120 dyne sec cm^{-5}.*

e) *True. The normal peripheral vascular resistance is 1000–1500 dyne sec cm^{-5}.*

5. Concerning central venous pressure and cannulation

a) *False. 10 cmH$_2$O is equivalent to 7.5 mmHg or 1 kPa.*

b) *False. The right internal jugular is usually preferred first as the internal jugular, the brachiocephalic veins and the superior vena cava are nearly in a straight line.*

c) *True. The higher incidence of pneumothorax with the subclavian approach makes the internal jugular the preferred vein.*

d) *True. The 'J' shaped end of the guidewire is inserted first because it is atraumatic and soft.*

e) *False. In addition to anchoring the catheter, the cuff also reduces the risk of infection by stopping the spread of infection from the site of skin entry. Some catheters have a silver impregnated cuff that acts as an antimicrobial barrier.*

6. In an invasive pressure measurement system, the following is correct

a) *False. A clot will cause damping of the system as pressure changes are not accurately transmitted. The systolic pressure is decreased and the diastolic pressure is increased.*

b) *False. A too rigid diaphragm will cause the system to resonate. This leads to high systolic and low diastolic pressures.*

c) *True. A soft wide lumen catheter will increase the damping of the system (see 'a').*

d) *False. An air bubble will increase the damping of the system (see 'a').*

e) *True. A catheter that is short and narrow allows transmission of pressure changes accurately. For clinical use, a maximum length of 2 m is acceptable.*

7. Concerning the oesophageal Doppler

a) *True. The ideal probe tip location is at the level between the 5th and 6th thoracic vertebrae. At that level the descending aorta is adjacent and parallel to the distal oesophagus. This location is achieved by superficially landmarking the distance to the third sternocostal junction anteriorly.*

b) *False. The frequency used is 4 MHz.*

c) *False. Red cells moving towards the ultrasound source reflect the sound back at a frequency higher than that at which they were sent, producing a positive Doppler shift. The opposite produces a negative Doppler shift.*

d) *True. The tip of the probe is positioned in the distal oesophagus at about 40 cm depth.*

e) *False. The angle between the ultrasound beam and blood flow is 45°.*

Chapter 12

Pain management and regional anaesthesia

Patient controlled analgesia (PCA)

PCA represents one of the most significant advances in the treatment of post-operative pain. Improved technology enables pumps to accurately deliver boluses of opioid when a demand button is activated by the patient.

It is the patient who determines the plasma concentration of the opioid, this being a balance between the dose required to control the pain and that which causes side-effects. The plasma concentration of the opioid is maintained at a relatively constant level with the dose requirements being generally smaller.

Components

1. A pump with an accuracy of at least ± 5% of the programmed dose (Fig. 12.1).
2. The remote demand button connected to the pump and activated by the patient.
3. An antisiphon and backflow valve.

Mechanism of action

1. Different modes of analgesic administration can be employed
   a) patient controlled on-demand bolus administration (PCA)

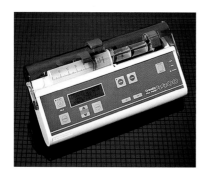

Fig. 12.1 The Graseby Omnifus PCA pump.

b) continuous background infusion and patient controlled bolus administration.
2. The initial programming of the pump must be tailored for the individual patient. The mode of administration, the amount of analgesic administered per bolus, the 'lock-out' time (i.e. the time period during which the patient is prevented from receiving another bolus despite activating the demand button), the duration of the administration of the bolus and the maximum amount of analgesic permitted per unit time are all variable settings on a PCA device.
3. Some designs have the capability to be used as a PCA pump for a particular variable duration then switching automatically to a continuous infusion as programmed.
4. The history of the drug administration including the total dose of the analgesic, the number of boluses and the number of successful and failed attempts can be displayed.
5. The devices have memory capabilities so they retain their programming during syringe changing.
6. Tamper-resistant features are included.
7. Some designs have a safety measure where an accidental triggering of the device is usually prevented by the need for the patient to make two successive presses on the hand control within 1 second.
8. PCA devices operate on mains or battery.
9. Different routes of administration can be used for PCA, e.g. intravenous, intramuscular, subcutaneous or epidural routes.
10. Alarms are included for malfunction, occlusion and disconnection.

Problems in practice and safety features

1. The ability of the patient to cooperate and understand is essential.
2. Availability of trained staff to programme the device and monitor the patient is vital.
3. In the PCA mode, the patient may awaken in severe pain because no boluses were administered during sleep.
4. Some PCA devices require special giving sets and syringes.
5. Technical errors can be fatal.

DISPOSABLE AND PORTABLE PATIENT CONTROLLED ANALGESIA

This is a wrist-mounted lightweight PCA device (Fig. 12.2).

Components

1. A 65 mL balloon sheath where the opioid is stored.
2. A kink-resistant tubing connecting the sheath to the patient control module. This has a built-in filter.
3. A 0.5 mL reservoir housed in the patient control module.

Mechanism of action

1. The balloon sheath is under pressure delivering the opioid through the filter.
2. The bolus dose is preset at 0.5 mL with a lockout time of 6 minutes.
3. Depression of the demand button empties the reservoir. Upon release of the button, the reservoir again begins to fill with the opioid. The outlet is connected to a venous cannula.
4. The design eliminates programming errors and electrical malfunction.
5. The device features a tamper-resistant design.

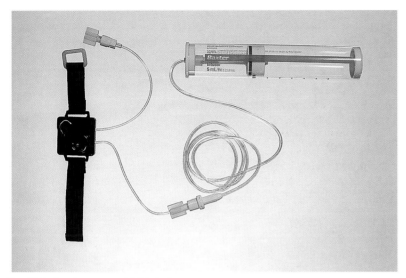

Fig. 12.2 A wrist-mounted PCA device.

6. The maximum weartime is 5 days but drug stability has to be taken into consideration.

Patient controlled analgesia (PCA)

● The patient has the ability to administer the opioid as required.
● The device is programmed by the anaesthetist.
● Different modes of administration.
● Tamper-resistant designs are featured.
● Portable versions exist.
● Technical errors can be fatal.

SYRINGE PUMPS

These are programmable pumps that can be adjusted to give variable rates of infusion and also bolus administration (Fig. 12.3). They are used to maintain continuous infusions of analgesics (or other drugs). The type of flow is pulsatile continuous delivery and their accuracy is within ± 2–5%. Some designs can accept a variety of

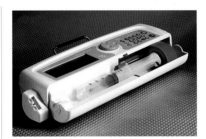

Fig. 12.3 The Graseby syringe pump.

different size syringes. The power source can be battery and/or mains.

It is important to prevent free flow from the syringe pump. Anti-siphon valves are usually used to achieve that. Inadvertent free flow can occur if the syringe barrel or plunger is not engaged firmly in the pump mechanism. The syringe should be securely clamped to the pump. Syringe drivers should not be positioned above the level of the patient. If the pump is more than 100 cm above the patient, a gravitational pressure can be generated that overcomes the friction between a non-secured plunger and barrel. Siphoning can also occur if there is a crack in the syringe allowing air to enter.

Some pumps have a 'back-off' function that prevents the pump from administering a bolus following an obstruction due to increased pressure in the system. An anti-reflux valve should be inserted in any other line that is connected to the infusion line. Anti-reflux valves prevent back-flow up the secondary and often lower pressure line should a distal occlusion occur and they avoid a subsequent inadvertent bolus.

VOLUMETRIC PUMPS

These are programmable pumps designed to be used with specific giving set tubing (Fig. 12.4). They are more suitable for infusions where accuracy of total volume is more important than precise flow rate. Their accuracy is generally within ± 5–10%. Volumetric pump accuracy is sensitive to the internal diameter of the giving set tubing. Various mechanisms of action exist. Peristaltic, cassette and reservoir systems are commonly used.

The power source can be battery and/or mains.

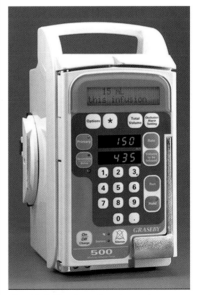

Fig. 12.4 The Graseby volumetric pump

TARGET CONTROLLED INFUSION PUMPS

These pumps have advanced software technology where the age and the weight of the patient are entered in addition to the drug's desired plasma concentration. They are mainly used with a propofol infusion technique. The software is capable of estimating the plasma and effect (brain) concentrations allowing the anaesthetist to adjust the infusion rate accordingly.

Epidural needles

Epidural needles are used to identify and cannulate the epidural space. The Tuohy needle is widely used in the UK (Fig. 12.5).

Components

1. The needle is 10 cm in length with a shaft of 8 cm (with 1 cm markings). A 15 cm version exists for obese patients.
2. The needle wall is thin in order to allow a catheter to be inserted through it.
3. The needle is provided with a stylet introducer to prevent occlusion of the lumen by a core of tissue as the needle is inserted.
4. The bevel (called a Huber point) is designed to be slightly oblique at 20° to the shaft, with a rather blunt leading edge.
5. Some designs allow the wings at the hub to be added or removed.
6. The commonly used gauges are either 16 G or 18 G.

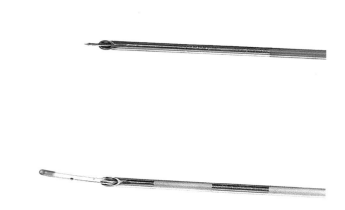

Fig. 12.6 Detail of a spinal needle introduced through a Tuohy needle (top); an epidural catheter passing through a Tuohy needle (bottom).

Mechanism of action

1. The markings on the needle enable the anaesthetist to determine the distance between the skin and the epidural space. Hence the length of the catheter left inside the epidural space can be estimated.
2. The shape and design of the bevel (Figs 12.6 and 12.9) enable the anaesthetist to direct the catheter within the epidural space (either in a cephalic or caudal direction).
3. The bluntness of the bevel also minimizes the risk of accidental dural puncture.
4. Some anaesthetists prefer winged epidural needles for better control and handling of the needle during insertion.
5. A paediatric 19 G 5 cm long Tuohy needle (with 0.5 cm markings), allowing the passage of a 21 G nylon catheter, is available.
6. A combined spinal–epidural technique is possible using a 26 G spinal needle of about 12 cm length with a standard 16 G Tuohy needle. The Tuohy needle is first positioned in the epidural space then the spinal needle is introduced through it into the subarachnoid space (Fig. 12.6). A relatively high pressure is required to inject through the spinal needle because of its small bore. This might lead to accidental displacement of the tip of the needle from the subarachnoid space leading to a failed or partial block. To prevent this happening, in some designs, the spinal needle is 'anchored' to the epidural needle to prevent displacement (Fig. 12.7).

Problems in practice and safety features

1. During insertion of the catheter through the needle, if it is necessary to withdraw the

Fig. 12.5 16 G Tuohy needle. Note the eight 1 cm markings along its shaft (reproduced with permission from Aitkenhead R, Smith G. Textbook of Anaesthesia, 3rd edn. Churchill Livingstone, 1996).

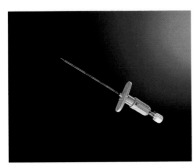

Fig. 12.7 The Portex 'Secure' combined spinal–epidural device.

catheter, the needle must be withdrawn simultaneously. This is because of the risk of the catheter being transected by the oblique bevel.

2. In accidental dural puncture, there is a high incidence of post-dural headache due to the epidural needle's large bore (e.g. 16 G or 18 G).

Epidural needle

● 10 cm Tuohy needle with the oblique bevel (Huber point) is most popular. 5 and 15 cm lengths exist.
● It has 1 cm markings to measure the depth of the epidural space.
● A stylet introducer is provided with the needle.
● A combined epidural–spinal technique is becoming more popular.

Epidural catheter, filter and syringe

THE CATHETER

Components

1. 90 cm transparent, malleable tube made of either nylon or Teflon and biologically inert. The 16 G

version has an external diameter of about 1 mm and an internal diameter of 0.55 mm.
2. The distal end has two or three side ports with a closed and rounded tip in order to reduce the risk of vascular or dural puncture (Fig. 12.6). Paediatric designs, 18 G or 19 G, have closer distal side ports.
3. Some designs have an open end.
4. The distal end of the catheter is marked clearly at 5 cm intervals,

with additional 1 cm markings between 5 and 15 cm.
5. The proximal end of the catheter is connected to a Luer lock and a filter (Fig. 12.8).
6. In order to prevent kinking, some designs incorporate a coil-reinforced catheter.
7. Some designs are radio-opaque. These catheters tend to be more rigid than the normal design. They can be used in patients with chronic pain to ensure correct placement of the catheter.

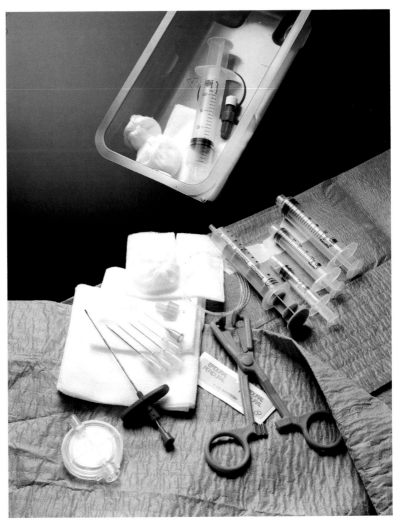

Fig. 12.8 The Portex epidural set containing Tuohy needle, loss of resistance syringe and a range of other syringes and needles, epidural catheter and filter, drape, swabs and epidural catheter label.

Mechanism of action

1. The catheters are designed to pass easily through their matched gauge epidural needles.
2. The markings enable the anaesthetist to place the desired length of catheter within the epidural space (usually 3–5 cm).
3. There are catheters with a single port at the distal tip. These offer a rather sharp point and increase the incidence of catheter-induced vascular or dural puncture.
4. An epidural fixing device can be used to prevent the catheter falling out. The device clips on the catheter. It has an adhesive flange that secures it to the skin. The device does not occlude the catheter and does not increase the resistance to injection (Fig. 12.9).

Problems in practice and safety features

1. The patency of the catheter should be tested prior to insertion.
2. The catheter can puncture an epidural vessel or the dura at the time of insertion or even days later.
3. The catheter should not be withdrawn through the Tuohy needle once it has been threaded beyond the bevel as that can transect the catheter. Both needle and catheter should be removed in unison.

4. It is almost impossible to predict in which direction the epidural catheter is heading when it is advanced.
5. Once the catheter has been removed from the patient, it should be inspected for any signs of breakage. The side ports are points of catheter weakness where it is possible for the catheter to break. Usually, if a portion of the catheter were to remain in the patient after removal, conservative management would be recommended.

THE FILTER

The hydrophilic filter is a 0.22 micron mesh which acts as a bacterial, viral and foreign body (e.g. glass) filter with a priming volume of about 0.7 mL. It is recommended that the filter should be changed every 24 hours if the catheter is going to stay in situ for long periods.

THE SYRINGE (LOSS OF RESISTANCE DEVICE)

The syringe has a special low resistance plunger used to identify the epidural space by loss of resistance to either air or saline. Plastic and glass versions are available.

> Epidural catheter, filter and syringe
> - Marked 90 cm catheter with distal side or end ports.
> - It should not be advanced for more than 5 cm inside the epidural space.
> - The proximal end is connected to a 0.22 micron mesh bacterial, viral and foreign body filter.
> - A low resistance plunger syringe is used to identify the epidural space.

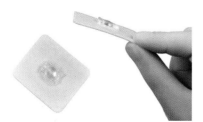

Fig. 12.9 Smith's Portex LockIt Plus epidural catheter fixing device.

Spinal needles

These needles are used to inject local anaesthetic(s) and/or opiates into the subarachnoid space. In addition, they are used to sample cerebrospinal fluid (CSF) or for intrathecal injections of antibiotics and cytotoxics (Fig. 12.10).

Components

1. The needle's length varies from 5 to 15 cm; the 10 cm version is most commonly used. They have a transparent hub in order to identify quickly the flow of CSF.
2. A stylet is used to prevent a core of tissue occluding the lumen of the needle during insertion. It also acts to strengthen the shaft. The stylet is withdrawn once the tip of the needle is (or is suspected to be) in the subarachnoid space.
3. Spinal needles are made in different sizes, from 18 G to 29 G in diameter. 32 G spinal needles have been described but are not widely used.

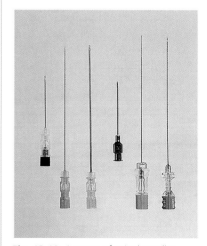

Fig. 12.10 A range of spinal needles and introducers. From left to right: 5 cm paediatric 22 G Yale; 25 G Yale; 18 G Quincke; 20 G introducer; 25 G Whitacre; 24 G Sprotte.

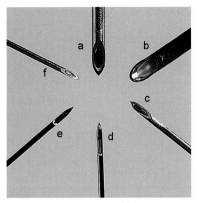

Fig. 12.11 Bevel design of (a) 18 G Quincke; (b) 16 G Tuohy; (c) 22 G Yale; (d) 24 G Sprotte; (e) 25 G Whitacre; (f) 25 G Yale.

4. The 25 G and smaller needles are used with an introducer which is usually an 18 G or 19 G needle.
5. There are two designs for the bevel. The cutting, traumatic bevel is seen in the Yale and Quincke needles. The non-cutting, atraumatic pencil point, with a side hole just proximal to the tip is seen in the Whitacer and Sprotte needles (Fig. 12.11).
6. A 28 G nylon, open-ended microcatheter can be inserted through a Crawford spinal needle (23 G). A stylet inside the catheter is removed during the insertion. This allows top-ups to be administered. The priming volume is 0.03 ml with a length of 910 mm. A 0.2 micron filter is attached to the catheter (Fig 12.12).

Mechanism of action

1. The large 22 G needle is more rigid and easier to direct. It gives a better feedback feel as it passes through the different tissue layers.
2. The CSF is slower to emerge from the smaller sized needles. Aspirating gently with a syringe can speed up the tracking back of CSF.

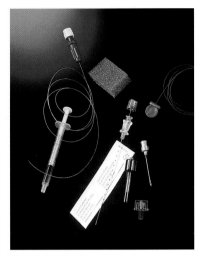

Fig. 12.12 The Portex spinal microcatheter set.

3. Continuous spinal anaesthesia can be achieved by inserting 3–4 cm of the 28 G spinal micro-catheter into the subarachnoid space.

Problems in practice and safety features

Dural headache

1. The incidence of dural headache is directly proportional to the gauge of the needle and the number of punctures made through the dura and indirectly proportional to the age of the patient. There is a 30% incidence of dural headache using a 20 G spinal needle, whereas the incidence is reduced to about 1% when a 26 G needle is used. For this reason smaller gauge spinal needles are preferred.
2. The Whitacer and Sprotte atraumatic needles separate rather than cut the longitudinal fibres of the dura. The defect in the dura has a higher chance of sealing after the removal of the needles. This reduces the incidence of dural headache.
3. Traumatic bevel needles cut the dural fibres, producing a ragged

tear which allows leakage of CSF. Dural headache is thought to be caused by the leakage of CSF.
4. The risk of dural headache is higher during pregnancy and labour, day surgery patients and those who have experienced a dural headache in the past.

Spinal micro-catheters

1. They are difficult to advance.
2. There is a risk of trauma to nerves.
3. Cauda equina syndrome is thought to be due to the potential neurotoxicity from the anaesthetic solutions rather than the microcatheter.

Spinal needles

- They have a stylet and a transparent hub.
- Different gauges from 18 G to 32 G.
- The bevel can be cutting (Yale and Quincke) or pencil-like (Whitacer and Sprotte).
- Can cause dural headache.
- Continuous spinal block using a 28 G microcatheter is possible.

Nerve block needles

These needles are used in regional anaesthesia to identify a nerve plexus or peripheral nerve (Fig. 12.13).

Components

1. They are made of steel with a Luer-lock attachment.
2. They have short, rather blunt bevels in order to cause minimal trauma to the nervous tissue. The bluntness makes skin insertion more difficult. This can be overcome by a small incision.
3. The needles have transparent hubs which allow earlier

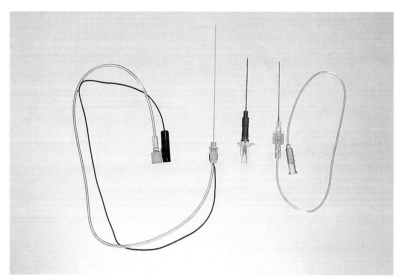

Fig. 12.13 A range of Braun nerve block needles. Insulated 100 mm needle (left); 45 mm catheter over needle design (centre); 50 mm non-insulated needle (right).

recognition of intravascular placement whilst performing blocks.

4. A side port for injecting the local anaesthetic solution is found in some designs.

5. The needles are connected to a nerve stimulator to aid in localizing the nerve using an insulated cable to prevent leakage of current (see Chapter 14).

6. 22 G size needles are optimal for the vast majority of blocks. There are different lengths such as 50, 100 and 150 mm depending on the depth of the nerve or plexus.

7. A pencil-shaped needle tip with a distal side hole for injecting local anaesthetic drugs is available.

Mechanism of action

1. The needle should first be introduced through the skin and subcutaneous tissues and then attached to the lead of the nerve stimulator.

2. An initial high output (e.g. 3–5 mA) from the nerve stimulator is selected. The needle is advanced slowly towards the nerve until nerve stimulation is noticed. The output is then reduced until a maximal stimulation is obtained with the minimal output. This current should be 0.2–0.4 mA. Contractions with such a low current mean that the tip of the needle is touching or very close to the nerve. Higher currents suggest that the needle is unlikely to be near the nerve. Contractions at a current less than 0.2 mA may indicate possible intraneural needle placement.

3. The blunt nerve block needle pushes the nerve ahead of itself as it is advanced, whereas a sharp needle is more likely to pierce the nerve. Blunt needles give a better feedback feel as resistance changes as they pass through the different layers of tissues.

4. As the local anaesthetic solution is injected, the stimulation is markedly reduced after only a small volume (about 2 mL) is injected. This is due to displacement of the nerve by the needle tip. Failure of the twitching to disappear (or pain experienced by the awake patient) after injection may indicate intraneural needle placement.

5. If a nerve stimulator is not used, paresthesia is elicited when the needle tip is in contact with the nerve.

6. Catheters can be inserted and left in situ after localizing the nerve or plexus (Fig. 12.14). Repeat bolus or continuous infusion of local anaesthetic solution can then be administered.

7. The immobile needle technique is used for major nerve and plexus blocks when a large volume of local anaesthetic solution is used. One operator maintains the needle in position, whilst the second operator, after aspiration, injects the local anaesthetic solution through the side port. This technique reduces the possibility of accidental misplacement and intravascular injection.

8. Catheter techniques can be used to enhance the spread (such as in the axillary block) or to prolong the duration of the block.

Nerve block needles can either be insulated with an exposed tip or non-insulated.

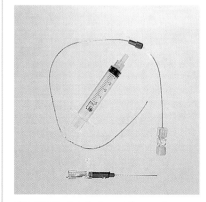

Fig. 12.14 A catheter set for continuous plexus anaesthesia.

INSULATED NEEDLES

These needles are Teflon coated with exposed tips. The current passes through the tip only. The insulated needles have a slightly greater diameter than similar non-insulated needles, which may result in a higher risk of nerve injury. The plexus or nerve can be identified with a smaller current than that required using the non-insulated needles.

NON-INSULATED NEEDLES

These needles allow current to pass through the tip as well the shaft. They are effective in regional anaesthesia because the maximum density of the current is being localized to the tip because of its lower resistance. However, a nerve may be stimulated via the shaft. In this situation, the local anaesthetic solution injected will be placed away from the nerve resulting in an unsuccessful block.

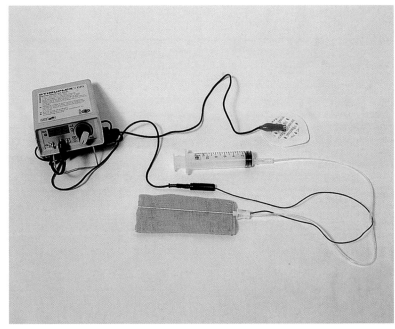

Fig. 12.15 The Braun Stimuplex nerve stimulator connected to a nerve block needle and skin electrode.

Nerve block needles

- Made of steel with short blunt bevel to reduce trauma to nerves and improve feedback feel.
- 22 G is optimal with lengths of 50–150 mm available.
- Can be insulated or non-insulated.
- Immobile needle technique is commonly used.

Nerve stimulator for nerve blocks

This device is designed to produce visible muscular contractions at a predetermined current and voltage once a nerve plexus or peripheral nerve(s) has been located, without actually touching it, thereby providing a greater accuracy for local anaesthetic deposition (Fig. 12.15).

The ideal peripheral nerve stimulator should have

1. Constant current output despite changes in resistance of the external circuit (tissues, needles, connectors, etc.)
2. Clear meter reading (digital) to 0.1 mA.
3. Variable output control.
4. Linear output.
5. Clearly marked polarity.
6. Short pulse width.
7. Pulse of 1–2 Hz.
8. Battery indicator.
9. High quality clips of low resistance.

Components

1. The nerve stimulator case with an on/off switch and a dial selecting the amplitude of the current.
2. Two leads to complete the circuit. One is connected to an ECG skin electrode and the other to the locating needle. The polarity of the leads should be clearly indicated and colour-coded with the negative lead being attached to the needle.

Mechanism of action

1. A small constant current (0.25–0.5 mA) is used to stimulate the nerve fibres causing the motor fibres to contract. Less current is needed if the needle is connected to the negative lead than to the positive lead. When the negative (cathode) lead is used to locate the nerve, the current causes changes in the resting membrane potential of the cells, producing an area of depolarization and so causing an action potential. If the stimulating electrode is positive (anode), the current causes an area of hyper-polarization near the needle tip and a ring of depolarization distal to the tip.

This requires a much higher current.

2. The frequency is set at 1–2 Hz. Tetanic stimuli are not used because of the discomfort caused. Using 2 Hz frequency allows more frequent feedback.

3. The duration of the stimulus should be short (50–100 ms) to generate painless motor contraction.

4. The nerve stimulator is battery operated to improve patient safety.

5. Nerve location can be very accurately defined, especially when low currents are used. The success rate of technically difficult nerve blocks can be increased by using a nerve stimulator. A sciatic nerve block with a success rate of over 90% can be achieved in experienced hands, compared to about 50% without using a nerve stimulator.

6. Nerve blocks can be performed while the patient is anaesthetized or heavily sedated as the response is visibly monitored with no need to elicit paresthesia. However, the use of neuromuscular blocking agents will abolish any muscular contractions.

Problems in practice and safety features

1. Higher currents will stimulate nerve fibres even if the tip of the needle is not adjacent to the nerve. The muscle fibres themselves can also be directly stimulated when a high current is used. In both situations the outcome will be an unsuccessful block once the local anaesthetic solution has been injected.

2. The positive ground electrode should have good contact with clear dry skin. As the current flows between the two electrodes (needle and ground), it is preferable not to position the ground over a superficial nerve. The passage of the current through the myocardium should also be avoided.

3. Most stimulators have a connection/disconnection indicator to ensure that the operator is aware of the delivery or not of stimulus current.

4. It is not recommended to use nerve stimulators designed to monitor the extent of neuromuscular blockade for regional nerve blocks. These are high output devices which can damage the nervous tissue.

5. It should be remembered that using the nerve stimulator is no excuse for not having the sound knowledge of surface and neuroanatomy required to perform regional anaesthesia.

Peripheral nerve stimulator

- It has two leads, the positive one to the skin and the negative to the needle.
- A small current of 0.5 mA or less is used with a frequency of 1–2 Hz.
- The stimulus is of short duration (1–2 msec).

Ultrasound guidance in regional anaesthesia

This relatively new technique uses ultrasound control to locate the nerves/plexuses. It is claimed that a higher success rate can be achieved when it is used, with lower complication rates.

Most nerve blocks need ultrasound frequencies in the range of 10–14 MHz. Many broadband ultrasound transducers with a bandwidth of 5–12 or 8–14 MHz can offer excellent resolution of superficial structures in the upper frequency range and good penetration depth in the lower frequency range.

The true echogenicity of a nerve is only captured if the sound beam is oriented perpendicularly to the nerve axis. This can be achieved best with **linear array transducers** with parallel sound beam emission rather than with **sector transducers**. The latter are characterized by diverging sound waves, such that the echotexture of the nerves will only be displayed in the centre of the image.

Portable ultrasound units are available.

FURTHER READING

Dalrymple P, Chelliah S. Electrical nerve locators. Continuing Education in Anaesthesia, Critical Care and Pain 2006;6(1):32–36.

Keay S, Callander C. The safe use of infusion devices. Continuing Education in Anaesthesia, Critical Care and Pain 2004;4(3):81–85.

Marhofer P, Greher M, Kapral S. Ultrasound guidance in regional anaesthesia. British Journal of Anaesthesia 2005;94(1):7–17.

The Royal College of Anaesthetists. Good practice in the management of continuous epidural analgesia in the hospital setting. November 2004. www.rcoa.ac.uk/docs/Epid.Analg.pdf.

MCQs

In the following lists, which of the statements (a) to (e) are true?

1. Epidural catheters and filters
   a) A minimum of 10 cm of the catheter should be inserted into the epidural space.
   b) The catheter should not be withdrawn through the Tuohy needle once it has been threaded beyond the bevel.
   c) Catheters with a single port at the distal tip reduce the incidence of vascular or dural puncture.
   d) The filter should be changed every 8 hours.
   e) Catheters can be radio-opaque.

2. Regional anaesthesia using a nerve stimulator
   a) The needles used have sharp tips to aid in localizing the nerves/plexuses.
   b) AC current is used to locate the nerve.
   c) A current of 1 A is usually used to locate a nerve.
   d) Paresthesia is not required for successful blocks.
   e) 50 Hz frequency stimuli are used.

3. Nerve stimulators in regional anaesthesia
   a) They enable the block to be performed even without full knowledge of the anatomy.
   b) In the insulated nerve block needle, the current passes through the tip only.
   c) In the non-insulated nerve block needle, the current passes through the tip and the shaft.
   d) A catheter can be used for continuous nerve/plexus blockade.
   e) The immobile needle technique improves the success rate of the block.

4. Incidence of spinal headache
   a) Yale and Quincke needle design have lower incidence of spinal headache.
   b) It is inversely proportional to the size of the needle used.
   c) It is similar in young and elderly patients.
   d) It is proportional to the number of dural punctures.
   e) It is reduced using a pencil-shaped needle tip.

5. The following is true
   a) Using ultrasound guidance in regional anaesthesia, a frequency range of 10–14 kHz is adequate.
   b) It is important to prevent free flow from the syringe pump.
   c) There is no need to use anti-reflux valves in other infusion lines.
   d) Sector transducers can achieve better images when in regional anaesthesia.
   e) Syringe pumps should be positioned at the same level as the patient.

Answers

1. Epidural catheters and filters
   a) *False*. 3–5 cm of the catheter is left in the epidural space. This reduces the incidence of vascular or dural puncture, segmental or unilateral block (as the catheter can pass through an inter-vertebral foramina) and knotting.
   b) *True*. The withdrawal of the catheter through the Tuohy needle after it has been threaded beyond the bevel can lead to the transection of the catheter. This usually happens when the catheter punctures a vessel during insertion. The needle and the catheter should be removed together and another attempt should be made to reinsert the needle and catheter.
   c) *False*. Catheters with a single port at the distal tip increase the incidence of vascular or dural puncture. This is due to the 'sharp' point at the end of the catheter. In contrast, catheters with side ports have a closed and rounded end thus reducing the incidence of vascular or dural puncture.
   d) *False*. The filter can be used for up to 24 hours.
   e) *True*. Some catheters are designed to be radio-opaque. They are more rigid than the standard design. They are mainly used in patients with chronic pain to ensure the correct placement of the catheter.

2. Regional anaesthesia using a nerve stimulator
   a) *False*. There is a need for feedback from the needle as it goes through the different layers of tissue. A sharp needle will pass the different layers of tissues easily with minimal feedback. A blunt needle will provide much better feedback.
   b) *False*. DC current from a battery is used to operate nerve stimulators. By avoiding AC current, patient safety is improved.
   c) *False*. This is a very high current. A current range of up to 5 mA is needed in locating the nerve. A current of 0.25–0.5 mA is used to stimulate the nerve fibres. Using a very high current, the tip of the needle might be far away from the nerve but might still lead to stimulation of the nerve fibres or the muscle fibres directly leading to the failure of the block.
   d) *True*. There is no need for paresthesia in order to achieve a successful block using a nerve stimulator. Paresthesia implies that the needle is touching the nerve. With a nerve stimulator, the nerve can be stimulated electrically without being touched.
   e) *False*. Stimuli with a frequency of 1–2 Hz are used. Tetanic stimuli (e.g. 50 Hz frequency) are not used because of the discomfort caused.

3. Nerve stimulators in regional anaesthesia
   a) *False*. Full knowledge of the anatomical structure is essential for a successful block.
   b) *True*. As the tip is the only non-insulated part of the needle, the current passes only through it. Using a small current, the tip of the needle has to be very close to the nerve before stimulation is visible.
   c) *True*. In a non-insulated needle, the current passes through both the tip and shaft. This might lead to nerve stimulation by current from the shaft even when the tip is far away from the nerve. This obviously leads to a failed block.
   d) *True*. After successful nerve stimulation, a catheter can be inserted. This allows a prolonged and continuous block using an infusion or boluses.
   e) *True*. The immobile needle technique allows one operator to maintain the needle in the correct position whilst the second operator injects the local anaesthetic. This also reduces the risk of accidental intravascular injection.

4. Incidence of spinal headache
   a) *False. Yale and Quincke have a higher incidence of spinal headache. This is due to the traumatic bevel cutting the dural fibres producing a ragged tear which allows CSF leakage.*
   b) *False. The incidence is directly proportional to the size of the needle used. Using a 20 G spinal needle causes a 30% incidence of spinal headache whereas a 26 G needle has a 1% incidence of headache.*
   c) *False. The incidence of spinal headache is much higher in the young than in elderly patients.*
   d) *True. The incidence of spinal headache is increased with multiple dural punctures.*
   e) *True. The pencil-shaped needle tip separates rather than cuts the longitudinal dural fibres. After removal of the needle, the dura has a higher chance of sealing, reducing the incidence of spinal headache.*

5. The following is true
   a) *False. The frequencies needed for nerve blocks are in the range of 10–14 MHz. Most modern ultrasound devices can generate these frequencies.*
   b) *True. Anti-siphon valves are used to prevent free flow from the syringe pump. In addition, the syringe should be securely clamped to the pump. Siphoning can also occur if there is a crack in the syringe allowing air entry.*
   c) *False. An anti-reflux valve should be inserted in any other line that is connected to the infusion line. Anti-reflux valves prevent back-flow up the secondary (usually with lower pressure) should a distal occlusion occur and avoid a subsequent inadvertent bolus.*
   d) *False. Sector transducers emit diverging sound waves, such that the echotexture of the nerves will only be displayed in the centre of the image. The true echogenicity of a nerve is only captured if the sound beam is oriented perpendicularly to the nerve axis. This can be achieved best with linear array transducers with parallel sound beam emission.*
   e) *True. Gravitational pressure can be generated to overcome the friction between a non-secured plunger and barrel especially if the pump is positioned more than 100 cm above the patient.*

Chapter 13

Additional equipment used in anaesthesia and intensive care

Continuous positive airway pressure (CPAP)

CPAP is a spontaneous breathing mode used in the intensive care unit, during anaesthesia and for patients requiring respiratory support at home. It increases the functional residual capacity (FRC) and improves oxygenation. CPAP prevents alveolar collapse and possibly recruits already collapsed alveoli.

Components

1. A flow generator producing high flows of gas (Fig. 13.1), or a large reservoir bag may be needed.
2. Connecting tubing from the flow generator to the inspiratory port of the mask. An oxygen analyser is fitted along the tubing to determine the inspired oxygen concentration.
3. A tight fitting mask with a harness. The mask has both inspiratory and expiratory ports. A CPAP valve is fitted to the expiratory port.
4. If the patient is intubated and spontaneously breathing, a T-piece with a CPAP valve fitted to the expiratory limb can be used.

Mechanism of action

1. Positive pressure within the lungs (and breathing system) is maintained throughout the whole of the breathing cycle.
2. The patient's peak inspiratory flow rate can be met.
3. The level of CPAP varies depending on the patient's requirements. It is usually 5–15 cmH$_2$O.
4. CPAP is useful in weaning patients off ventilators especially when PEEP was used.

Problems in practice and safety features

1. CPAP has cardiovascular effects similar to PEEP but to a lesser extent. Although the arterial oxygenation may be improved, the cardiac output can be reduced. This may reduce the oxygen delivery to the tissues.
2. Barotrauma can occur.
3. A loose-fitting mask allows leakage of gas and loss of pressure.
4. A nasogastric tube is inserted in patients with depressed consciousness level to prevent gastric distension.
5. Skin erosion caused by the tight fitting mask. This is minimized by the use of soft silicone masks or protective dressings. Rhinorrhoea and nasal dryness can also occur.
6. Nasal masks are better tolerated but mouth breathing reduces the effects of CPAP.

Continuous positive airway pressure (CPAP)

- A tight fitting mask, CPAP valve and flow generator are used.
- Barotruma, decrease in cardiac output and gastric distension are some of the complications.

Haemofiltration

Haemofiltration is a process of acute renal support used for critically ill patients. It is the ultrafiltration of blood.

Ultrafiltration is the passage of fluid under pressure across a semipermeable membrane where low molecular weight solutes (up to 20 000 daltons) are carried along with the fluid by solvent drag (convection).

The widespread use of haemofiltration has revolutionized the management of critically ill patients with acute renal failure within the intensive therapy environment. Haemofiltration is popular because of its relative ease of use and higher tolerability in the cardiovascularly unstable patient.

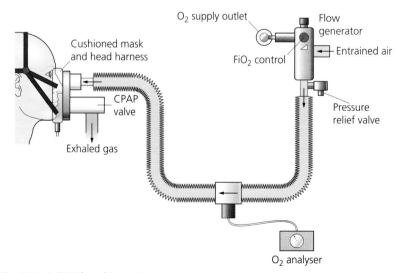

Fig. 13.1 A CPAP breathing system set-up.

Components

1. Intravascular access lines. These can either be arteriovenous lines (such as femoral artery and vein or brachial artery and femoral vein) or venovenous lines (such as the femoral vein or the subclavian vein using a single double lumen catheter). The extracorporeal circuit is connected to the intravascular lines. The lines should be as short as possible to minimize resistance.
2. Filter or membrane (Fig. 13.2). Synthetic membranes are ideal for this process. They are made of polyacrylonitrile (PAN), polysulphone or polymethyl methacrylate. They have a large pore size to allow efficient diffusion (in contrast to the smaller size of dialysis filters).
3. Two roller pumps one on each side of the circuit. Each pump peristaltically propels about 10 mL of blood per revolution and is positioned slightly below the level of the patient's heart.
4. The collection vessel for the ultrafiltrate is positioned below the level of the pump.

Mechanism of action

1. At its most basic form, the haemofiltration system consists of a circuit linking an artery to a vein with a filter positioned between the two.
2. The patient's blood pressure provides the hydrostatic pressure necessary for ultrafiltration of the plasma. This technique is suitable for fluid overloaded patients who have a stable, normal blood pressure.
3. Blood pressure of less than a mean of 60 or 70 mmHg reduces the flow and the volume of filtrate and leads to clotting despite heparin.
4. In the venovenous system, a pump is added making the cannulation of a large artery unnecessary (Fig. 13.3). The speed of the blood pump controls the maintenance of the transmembrane pressure. The risk of clotting is also reduced. This is the most common method used. Blood flows of 30–750 mL/min can be achieved, although flow rates of 150–300 mL/min are generally used. This gives an ultrafiltration rate of 25–40 mL/min.
5. The fluid balance is maintained by the simultaneous reinfusion of a sterile crystalloid fluid. The fluid contains most of the plasma electrolytes present in their normal values (sodium, potassium, calcium, magnesium, chloride, lactate and glucose) with an osmolality of 285–335 mosmol/kg. Large amounts of fluid are needed such as 2–3 L/h.
6. Pressure transducers monitor the blood pressure in access and return lines. Air bubble detection facilities are also incorporated. Low inflow pressures can happen during line occlusion. High and low post-pump pressures can happen in line occlusion or disconnection respectively.

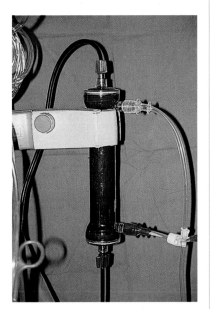

Fig. 13.2 A synthetic haemofilter.

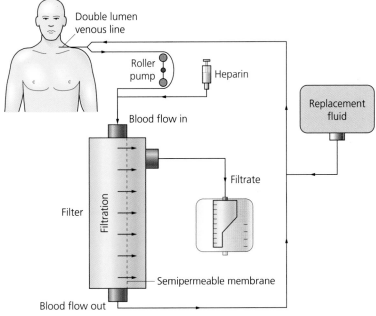

Fig. 13.3 Diagrammatic representation of venovenous haemofiltration.

7. Some designs have the facility to weigh the filtrate and automatically supply the appropriate amount of reinfusion fluid.
8. Heparin is added as the anticoagulant with a typical loading dose of 3000 IU followed by an infusion of 10 IU per kg body weight. Heparin activity is monitored by activated partial thromboplastin time or activated clotting time. Prostacyclin or low molecular weight heparin can be used as alternatives to heparin.
9. The filters are supplied either in a cylinder or flat box casing. The packing of the filter material ensures a high surface area to volume ratio.
   a) They are highly biocompatible causing minimal complement or leucocyte activation.
   b) They are also highly wettable achieving high ultrafiltration rates.
   c) They have large pore size allowing efficient diffusion.
   d) The optimal surface area of the membrane is 0.5–1.5 m².
   e) Both small molecules (e.g. urea, creatinine and potassium) and large molecules (e.g. myoglobin and some antibiotics) are cleared efficiently. Proteins do not pass through the membrane because of their larger molecular size.

Problems in practice and safety features

1. The extracorporeal circuit must be primed with 2 litres of normal saline prior to use. This removes all the toxic ethylene oxide gas still present in the filter. (Ethylene oxide is used to sterilize the equipment after manufacture).
2. Haemolysis of blood components by the roller pump.

3. The risk of cracks to the tubing after long-term use
4. The risk of bleeding must be controlled by optimizing the dose of anticoagulant.

Haemofiltration

- An effective method of renal support in critically ill patients using ultrafiltration of the blood.
- Arteriovenous or venovenous lines are connected to the extracorporeal circuit (filter and a pump).
- Synthetic filters with a surface area of 0.5–1.5 m² are used.

Arterial blood gases analyser (Fig. 13.4)

In order to measure arterial blood gases, a sample of heparinized, anaerobic and fresh arterial blood is needed.

1. Heparin should be added to the sample to prevent clotting during the analysis. The heparin should only fill the dead space of the syringe and form a thin film on its interior. Excess heparin, which is acidic, lowers the pH of the sample.
2. The presence of air bubbles in the sample increases the oxygen

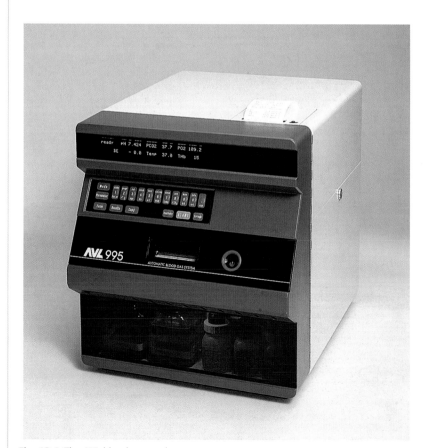

Fig. 13.4 The AVL blood gas analyser.

partial pressure and decreases carbon dioxide partial pressure.
3. An old blood sample has a lower pH and oxygen partial pressure and a higher carbon dioxide partial pressure. If there is a need to delay the analysis (e.g. machine self-calibration), the sample should be kept on ice.

The measured parameters are

1. Arterial blood oxygen partial pressure.
2. Arterial carbon dioxide partial pressure.
3. The pH of the arterial blood.

From these measurements, other parameters can be calculated, e.g. actual bicarbonate, standard bicarbonate, base excess and oxygen saturation.

Polarographic (Clark) oxygen electrode

This measures the oxygen partial pressure in a blood (or gas) sample (Fig. 13.5).

Components

1. A platinum cathode sealed in a glass body.
2. A silver/silver chloride anode.
3. A sodium chloride electrolyte solution.
4. An oxygen-permeable Teflon membrane separating the solution from the sample.
5. Power source of 700 mV.

Mechanism of action

1. Oxygen molecules cross the membrane into the electrolyte solution at a rate proportional to their partial pressure in the sample.
2. A very small electric current flows when the polarization potential is applied across the electrode in the presence of oxygen molecules in the electrolyte solution. Electrons are donated by the **anode** and accepted by the **cathode**, producing an electric current within the solution. The circuit is completed by the input terminal of the amplifier.

Cathode reaction
$$O_2 + 2H_2O + 4e^- = 4OH^-$$
Electrolyte reaction
$$NaCl + OH^- = NaOH + Cl^-$$
Anode reaction
$$Ag + Cl^- = AgCl + e^-$$

3. The oxygen partial pressure in the sample can be measured since the amount of current is linearly proportional to the oxygen partial pressure in the sample.
4. The electrode is kept at a constant temperature of 37°C.

Problems in practice and safety features

1. The membrane can deteriorate and perforate, affecting the performance of the electrode. Regular maintenance is essential.
2. Protein particles can precipitate on the membrane affecting the performance.

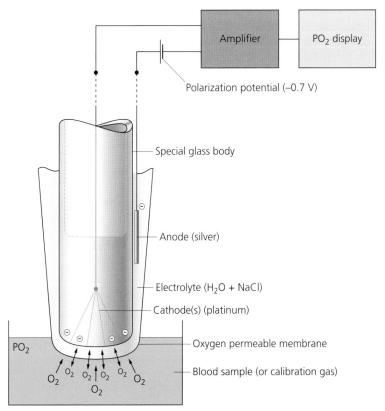

Fig. 13.5 Mechanism of action of the oxygen electrode. (Reproduced with permission from AVL Medical Instruments UK Ltd.)

Polarographic oxygen electrode

● Consists of a platinum cathode, silver/silver chloride anode, electrolyte solution, membrane and polarization potential of 700 mV.
● The flow of the electrical current is proportional to the oxygen partial pressure in the sample.
● Requires regular maintenance.

pH electrode

This measures the activity of the hydrogen ions in a sample. Described mathematically it is

$$pH = -\log [H^+]$$

It is a versatile electrode which can measure samples of blood, urine or CSF (Fig. 13.6).

Components

1. A glass electrode (silver/silver chloride) incorporating a bulb made of pH-sensitive glass holding a buffer solution.
2. A calomel reference electrode (mercury/mercury chloride) which is in contact with a potassium chloride solution via a cotton plug. The arterial blood sample is in contact with the potassium chloride solution via a membrane.
3. A meter to display the potential difference across the two electrodes.

Mechanism of action

1. The reference electrode maintains a constant potential.
2. The pH within the glass remains constant due to the action of the buffer solution. However, a pH gradient exists between the sample and the buffer solution. This gradient results in an electrical potential.
3. Using the two electrodes to create an electrical circuit, the potential can be measured. One electrode is in contact with the buffer and the other is in contact with the blood sample.
4. A linear electrical output of about 60 mV per unit pH is produced.
5. The two electrodes are kept at a constant temperature of 37°C.

Problems in practice and safety features

1. It should be calibrated before use with two buffer solutions.
2. The electrodes must be kept clean.

> pH electrode
>
> - Two half cells linked via the sample.
> - The electrical potential produced is proportional to the pH of the sample.

Carbon dioxide electrode (Severinghaus electrode)

A modified pH electrode is used to measure carbon dioxide partial pressure, as a result of change in the pH of an electrolyte solution (Fig. 13.7).

Components

1. A pH-sensitive glass electrode with a silver/silver chloride reference electrode forming its outer part.

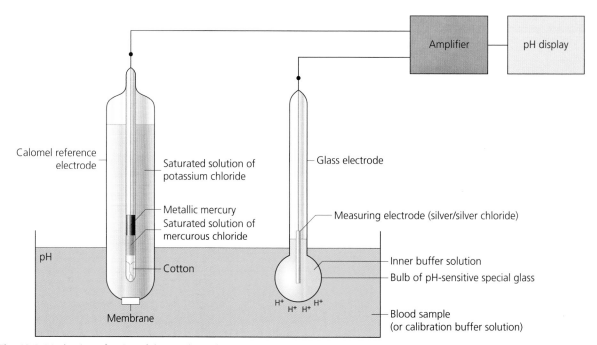

Fig. 13.6 Mechanism of action of the pH electrode.

Amplifier — pH display

Calomel reference electrode
Saturated solution of potassium chloride
Glass electrode
Metallic mercury
Saturated solution of mercurous chloride
Measuring electrode (silver/silver chloride)
pH
Inner buffer solution
Bulb of pH-sensitive special glass
Cotton
H^+ H^+ H^+ H^+
Membrane
Blood sample (or calibration buffer solution)

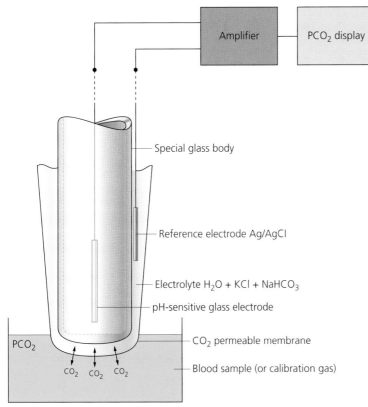

Fig. 13.7 Mechanism of action of the carbon dioxide electrode.

2. The electrodes are surrounded by a thin film of an electrolyte solution (sodium bicarbonate).
3. A carbon dioxide permeable rubber or Teflon membrane.

Mechanism of action

1. Carbon dioxide (not hydrogen ions) diffuses in both directions until equilibrium exists across the membrane between the sample and the electrolyte solution.
2. Carbon dioxide reacts with the water present in the electrolyte solution producing hydrogen ions resulting in a change in pH.

$$CO_2 + H_2O \rightarrow H^+ + HCO_3^-$$

3. The change in pH is measured by the glass electrode.

4. The electrode should be maintained at a temperature of 37°C. Regular calibration is required.

Problems in practice and safety features

1. The integrity of the membrane is vital for accuracy.
2. Slow response time because diffusion of carbon dioxide takes up to 2–3 minutes.

Carbon dioxide electrode

- A modified pH electrode measures changes in pH due to carbon dioxide diffusion across a membrane.
- Maintained at 37°C.
- Slow response time.

Intra-aortic balloon pump (IABP)

This is a catheter incorporating a balloon which is inserted into the aorta to support patients with severe cardiac failure. It is usually inserted using a percutaneous femoral approach, over a guidewire, under fluoroscopic guidance. The correct position of the pump is in the descending aorta, 2–3 cm distal to the left subclavian artery (Fig 13.8).

Components

1. An 8 FG catheter with a balloon.
2. The catheter has two lumens, a central lumen for continuous arterial pressure monitoring and an outer lumen for helium gas exchange to and from the balloon.
3. The usual volume of the balloon is 40 mL. A 34 mL balloon is available for small individuals. The size of the balloon should be 80–90% of the diameter of the aorta.

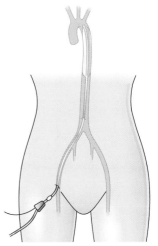

Fig. 13.8 The intra-aortic balloon pump in situ.

The pump is attached to a console (Fig. 13.9) which controls the flow of helium in and out of the balloon and monitors the patient's blood pressure and ECG. The console allows the adjustment of the various parameters in order to optimize counterpulsation.

Mechanism of action

1. The balloon is inflated in early diastole, immediately after the closure of the aortic valve. This leads to an increase in peak diastolic blood pressure (diastolic augmentation) and an increase in coronary artery perfusion pressure. This increases myocardial oxygen supply. Inflation should be at the dicrotic notch on the arterial pressure waveform (Fig. 13.10).

2. The balloon is deflated at the end of diastole just before the aortic valve opens. This leads to a decrease in aortic end-diastolic pressure causing a decrease in left ventricular afterload and

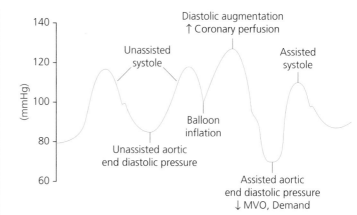

Fig. 13.10 The changes that intra-aortic balloon pump therapy causes to the arterial waveform and their consequences.

decreased myocardial oxygen demand. This will lead to an increase in left ventricular performance, stroke work and ejection fraction. Deflation should be at the lowest point of the arterial diastolic pressure.

3. During myocardial ischaemia, the main benefits of the IABP are the reduction of myocardial oxygen demand (by lowering of the left ventricular pressure) and the increase in myocardial oxygen supply (by increasing the coronary artery perfusion).

4. The effectiveness of the balloon depends on the ratio of the balloon to aorta size, heart rate and rhythm, compliance of the aorta and peripheral vessels and the precise timing of the counterpulsation.

Indications for use of IABP

1. Refractory ventricular failure.
2. Acute myocardial infarction complicated with cardiogenic shock, mitral regurgitation, ventricular septal defect.
3. Impending myocardial infarction.
4. Unstable angina refractory to medical treatment.
5. High risk angioplasty.

6. Ischaemia-related ventricular arrythmias.
7. Pre- and post-coronary bypass surgery, including weaning from cardiopulmonary bypass.

Contraindications for use of IABP

1. Severe aortic regurgitation.
2. Aortic dissection.
3. Major coagulopathy.
4. Severe bilateral peripheral arterial disease.
5. Bilateral femoral-popliteal bypass graft.
6. Sepsis.

Problems in practice and safety features

1. If the balloon is too large, it may damage the aorta. If it is too small, counterpulsation will be ineffective.
2. Limb ischaemia.
3. Thrombosis and embolism. Low dose heparinization is often used to counteract this.
4. Arterial dissection or perforation.
5. Bleeding.
6. Infection.

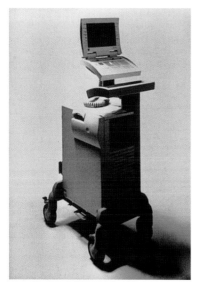

Fig. 13.9 The intra-aortic balloon pump console.

Intra-aortic balloon pump

- 8 FG catheter with a balloon positioned in the descending aorta.
- Two lumens, a central one to monitor blood pressure and an outer one for inflation and deflation of the balloon with helium.
- Balloon inflation occurs at the dicrotic notch of the arterial pressure waveform.
- Balloon deflation occurs at the lowest point of the arterial diastolic pressure.

Intravenous giving sets

These are designed to administer intravenous fluids, blood and blood products (Fig. 13.11).

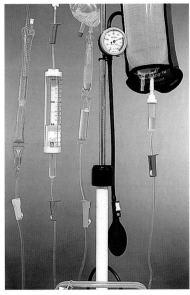

Fig. 13.11 Giving sets (from left to right): paediatric blood giving set; paediatric giving set with burette; adult blood giving set; pressure bag at 300 mmHg containing heparinized saline suitable for use with invasive arterial pressure monitoring systems.

Components

Adult giving set
1. A clear plastic tube of about 175 cm in length and 4 mm in internal diameter. One end is designed for insertion into the fluid bag whereas the other end is attached to an intravascular cannula with a Luer-lock connection.
2. Blood giving sets have a filter with a mesh of about 150 μm and a fluid chamber with a ball float. Giving sets unsuitable for blood administration have no filter and no float and a narrower diameter.
3. A rubber injection site is found at the patient's end. The maximum size needle used for injection should be 23 G.
4. A flow controller determines the drip rate (20 drops of clear fluid is 1 mL and 15 drops of blood is 1 mL).

Paediatric set
1. In order to attain accuracy, a burette (30–200 mL) in 1 mL divisions is used to measure the volume of fluid to be infused. The burette has a filter, air inlet and an injection site on its top. At the bottom, there is a flap/ball valve to prevent air entry when the burette is empty.
2. There are two flow controllers: one is between the fluid bag and the burette and is used to fill the burette; the second is between the burette and the patient and controls the drip rate. An injection site should be close to the patient to reduce the dead space.
3. Drop size is 60 drops per 1 mL of clear fluid. A burette with a drop size similar to the adult's version (15 drops per mL) is used for blood transfusion.
4. 0.2 micron filters can be added in line to filter out air and foreign bodies, e.g. glass or plastic particles. Infusion-related thrombophlebitis can be reduced by the use of these filters.

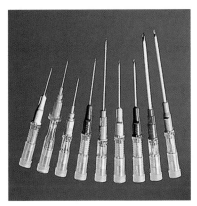

Fig. 13.12 A range of intravenous cannulae.

Intravenous cannulae

Intravenous cannulae are made of plastic. They are made by different manufacturers with different characteristics (Fig. 13.12).

Using distilled water at a temperature of 22°C and under a pressure of 10 kPa, the flow through a 110 cm tubing with an internal diameter of 4 mm is as follows:

20 G: 40–80 mL/min
18 G: 75–120 mL/min
16 G: 130–220 mL/min
14 G: 250–360 mL/min

Recent designs offer protection against the risk of needle stick injuries (Fig. 13.13), covering the sharp needle tip with a blunt end.

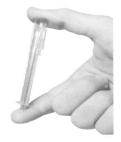

Fig. 13.13 Smith's Medical Protective Acuvance cannula designed to reduce the risk of needle stick injury.

Blood warmers

These are used to warm blood (and other fluids) before administering them to the patient. The aim is to deliver blood/fluids to the patient at 37°C. At this temperature there is no significant haemolysis or increase in osmotic fragility of the red blood cells (Fig. 13.14).

DRY HEAT WARMER

Consists of two plates between which a thin-walled channelled PVC bag can be inserted and sandwiched (Figs 13.15 and 13.16). The bag is heated on both sides with warming elements. The door should not be opened once the bag is primed as the bag swells preventing the closure of the door.

These devices increase the resistance to flow and cause a significant increase in giving set dead space.

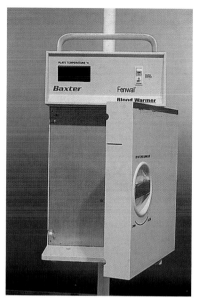

Fig. 13.15 An opened dry heat warmer.

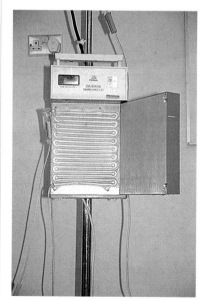

Fig. 13.16 A dry heat warmer fitted with a PVC bag.

COAXIAL FLUID HEATING SYSTEM (FIG. 13.17)

A coaxial tubing is used to heat and deliver the fluids to the patient. The outside tubing carries heated sterile water. The inside tubing carries the intravenous fluid. The sterile water is heated to 40°C and stored by the

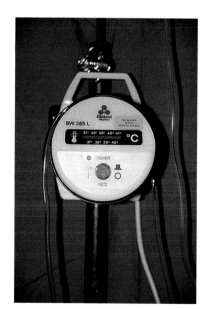

Fig. 13.14 A dry heat warmer around which a giving set extension is coiled.

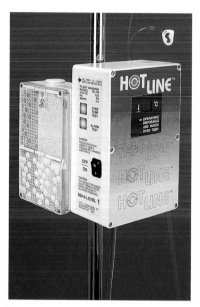

Fig. 13.17 A coaxial fluid heating system.

heating case. The water is circulated through the outside tubing. The intravenous fluid does not come in contact with the circulating water. The coaxial tubing extends to the intravenous cannula reducing the loss of heat as fluid is exposed to room temperature.

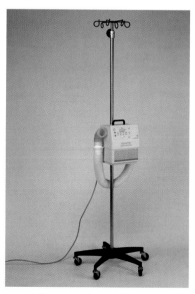

Fig. 13.18 Level 1 forced-air warmer.

Forced-air warmers (Fig. 13.18)

These devices are used to maintain the temperature of patients during surgery. They have been found to be effective even when applied to a limited surface body area. They consist of a case where warm ambient air is pumped at variable temperatures between 32 and 37°C. The warm air is delivered via a hose to a thin-walled channelled bag positioned on the patient' body. There are different bags available depending on which part of the body is covered (e.g. upper or lower body). A thermostat to prevent overheating controls the temperature of the warm air. Cooling versions also exist for surgery where body temperature >37°C is desirable, e.g. neurosurgery.

Defibrillator

This is a device that delivers electrical energy to the heart causing simultaneous depolarization of an adequate number of myocardial cells to allow a stable rhythm to be established (Fig. 13.19).

Components

1. The device has an on/off switch, joules setting control, charge and discharge buttons.
2. Paddles can be either external (applied to the chest wall) or internal (applied directly to the heart). The external paddles are usually 8–8.5 cm in size.

Mechanism of action

1. DC energy rather than AC energy is used. DC energy is more effective causing less myocardial damage and being less arrhythmogenic than AC energy. The lower the energy used, the less the damage to the heart.
2. Transformers are used to step up mains voltage from 240 V AC to 5000 V AC. A rectifier converts it to 5000 V DC. A variable voltage step-up transformer is used so that different amounts of charge may be selected. Most defibrillators have internal rechargeable batteries that supply DC in the absence of mains supply. This is then converted to AC by means of an inverter, and then amplified to 5000 V DC by a step-up transformer and rectifier.
3. The DC shock is of brief duration and produced by discharge from a capacitor. The capacitor stores energy in the form of an electrical charge, and then releases it over a short period of time. The current delivered is maintained for several milliseconds in order to achieve successful defibrillation. As the current and charge delivered by a discharging capacitor decay rapidly and exponentially, inductors are used to prolong the duration of current flow.
4. The external paddles are positioned on the sternum and on the left midaxillary line (5–6th rib). An alternative placement is one paddle positioned anteriorly over the left precordium and the other positioned posteriorly behind the heart. Firm pressure on the paddles is required in order to reduce the transthoracic impedance and achieve a higher peak current flow. Using conductive gel pads helps in reducing the transthoracic impedance. Disposable adhesive defibrillator electrode pads can be used instead of paddles, offering hands-free defibrillation.
5. Most of the current is dissipated through the resistance of the skin and the rest of the tissues and only a small part of the total current (about 35 A) flows through the heart. The impedance to the flow of current is about 50–150 ohms; however, repeated administration of shocks

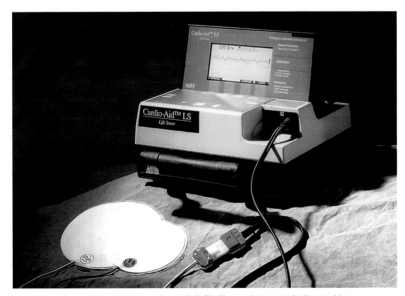

Fig. 13.19 The S & W Vickers Cardio-Aid defibrillator shown with disposable defibrillation electrode pads.

in quick succession reduces impedance.

6. For internal defibrillation, the shock delivered to the heart depends on the size of the heart and the paddles.

7. Some designs have an ECG oscilloscope and paper recording facilities. DC defibrillation can be synchronized with the top of the R-wave in the treatment of certain arrhythmias such as atrial fibrillation.

8. The implantable automatic internal defibrillator is a relatively recent development where a self-contained diagnostic and therapeutic device is placed next to the heart. It consists of a battery and electrical circuitry (pulse generator) connected to one or more insulated wires. The pulse generator and batteries are sealed together and implanted under the skin, usually near the shoulder. The wires are threaded through blood vessels from the implantable cardiac defibrillator (ICD) to the heart muscle. It continuously monitors the rhythm and when malignant tachyarrhythmias are detected, a defibrillation shock is automatically delivered. ICDs are subject to malfunction due to internal short circuit when attempting to deliver an electrical shock to the heart or due to a memory error. Newer devices also provide overdrive pacing to electrically convert a sustained ventricular tachycardia, and 'backup' pacing if bradycardia occurs. They also offer a host of other sophisticated functions (such as storage of detected arrhythmic events and the ability to do 'non-invasive' electrophysiologic testing).

Problems in practice and safety features

1. Skin burns.
2. Further arrythmias.

Defibrillators

- External and internal paddles are available.
- DC energy is discharged from a capacitor.
- Implanted automatic internal defibrillators are becoming more popular.
- Newer versions have pacemaker capabilities.

Chest drain

Used for the drainage of air, blood and fluids from the pleural space.

Components

1. A drainage tubing with distal ports.
2. An underwater seal and a collection chamber of approximately 20 cm diameter.

Mechanism of action

1. An airtight system is required to maintain a subatmospheric intrapleural pressure. This allows re-expansion of the lung and restores haemodynamic stability by minimizing mediastinal shift. The underwater seal acts as a one-way valve through which air is expelled from the pleural space and prevented from re-entering during the next inspiration.
2. Under asepsis, skin and sub-cutaneous tissues are infiltrated with local anaesthetic at the level of the 4–5th intercostal space in the midaxillary line. The chest wall is incised and blunt dissection using artery forceps through to the pleural cavity is performed. Using the tip of finger adherent lung is swept away from the insertion site.

3. The drain is inserted into the pleural cavity and slid into position (usually towards the apex). The drain is then connected to an underwater seal device.
4. Some designs have a flexible trocar to reduce the risk of trauma.
5. The drainage tube is submerged to a depth of 1–2 cm in the collection chamber. This ensures minimum resistance to drainage of air and maintains the underwater seal even in the face of a large inspiratory effort
6. The collection chamber should be about 100 cm below the chest as subatmospheric pressures up to $-80\,cmH_2O$ may be produced during obstructed inspiration.
7. A Heimlich flutter one-way valve can be used instead of an underwater seal, allowing better patient mobility.
8. Drainage can be allowed to occur under gravity or suction of about $-15–20\,mmHg$ may be applied.

Problems in practice and safety features

1. Retrograde flow of fluid may occur if the collection chamber is raised above the level of the patient. The collection chamber should be kept below the level of the patient at all times to prevent fluid being siphoned into the pleural space.
2. Absence of oscillations may indicate obstruction of the drainage system by clots or kinks, loss of sub-atmospheric pressure or complete re-expansion of the lung.
3. Persistent bubbling indicates a continuing bronchopleural air leak.
4. Clamping a pleural drain in the presence of a continuing air leak may result in a tension pneumothorax.

	Vein	Artery
Appearance	Black	Black
Movement	None	Pulsatile
Compressible	Yes	No
Colour flow	Constant flow	Pulsatile

Chest drain

- An airtight system to drain the pleural cavity usually inserted at the 4–5th intercostal space in the midaxillary line.
- The underwater seal chamber should be about 100 cm below the level of the patient.
- Absence of oscillation is seen with complete lung expansion, obstruction of the system or loss of negative pressure.
- Persistent bubbling is seen with a continuing bronchopleural air leak.

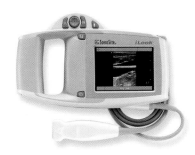

Fig. 13.20 The portable ultrasound Sonosite machine with probe attached.

FURTHER READING

Shoemaker WC, Velmahos GC, Demetriades D. Procedures and monitoring for the critically ill. Philadelphia: WB Saunders, 2002.

Mackay JH, Arrowsmith JE. Core topics in cardiac anaesthesia. Cambridge: Cambridge University Press, 2004.

Bellomo R, Ronco C. Continuous haemofiltration in the intensive care unit. Critical Care 2000;4:339–345.

The Sonosite ultrasound machine (Fig. 13.20)

Components

An ultrasound probe which is connected to a control unit that displays the ultrasound image.

Mechanism of action

1. The probe transmits and receives the ultrasound beam once placed in contact with the skin via 'acoustic coupling' jelly.
2. 2D images of structures are displayed. Procedures requiring precise needle placement such as venous cannulation or nerve blocks can be performed under direct ultrasound control. This helps to minimize the possible risks of the procedure.
3. Structures can then be identified via their ultrasound characteristics and anatomical relationships.
4. Increasing the depth allows visualization of deeper structures. The depth of the image should be optimized so that the target is centered in the display image.

Problems in practice and safety features

1. One of the commonest mistakes in ultrasound imaging is the use of incorrect gain settings. Insufficient gain can result in missed structures of low reflectivity, such as thrombus. Excessive gain can result in artifacts.
2. The characteristics differentiating vein from artery are listed below.

MCQs

In the following lists which of the statements (a) to (e) are true?

1. Concerning defibrillators
   a) Alternating current is commonly used instead of direct current.
   b) The electric current released is measured in watts.
   c) Consists of an inductor which releases the electric current.
   d) Can cause skin burns.
   e) The same amount of electrical energy is used for external and internal defibrillation.

2. Concerning arterial blood gases analysis
   a) Excess heparin in the sample increases the hydrogen ion concentration.
   b) Blood samples with air bubbles have a lower oxygen partial pressure.
   c) If there is delay in the analysis, the blood sample can be kept at room temperature.
   d) Normal H^+ ion concentration is 40 mmol/L.
   e) CO_2 partial pressure can be measured by measuring the pH.

3. Concerning the CO_2 electrode
   a) KCl and $NaHCO_3$ are used as electrolyte solutions.
   b) A carbon dioxide-sensitive glass electrode is used.
   c) The electrical signal generated is directly proportional to the log of CO_2 tension in the sample.
   d) It has a response time of 10 seconds.
   e) It should be kept at room temperature.

4. CPAP
   a) CPAP is a controlled ventilation mode.
   b) It can improve oxygenation by increasing the FRC.
   c) Pressures of up to 15 kPa are commonly used.
   d) It has no effect on the cardiovascular system.
   e) A nasogastric tube can be used during CPAP.

5. Haemofiltration
   a) Solutes of molecular weight up to 20 000 daltons can pass through the filter.
   b) It should not be used in the cardiovascularly unstable patient.
   c) Blood flows of 150–300 mL/min are generally used.
   d) Warfarin is routinely used to prevent the filter clotting.
   e) The optimal membrane surface area is 0.5–1.5 cm^2.

6. Intra-aortic balloon
   a) The usual volume of the balloon is 40 mL.
   b) The inflation of the balloon occurs at the upstroke of the arterial waveform.
   c) The deflation of the balloon occurs at the end of diastole just before the aortic valve opens.
   d) It is safe to use in aortic dissection.
   e) Helium is used to inflate the balloon.

7. Chest drains
   a) The underwater seal chamber can be positioned at any level convenient to the patient.
   b) Persistent air bubbling may be a sign of a continuing bronchopleural air leak.
   c) They function by expelling intra-pleural fluids during deep inspiration.
   d) Negative pressure of about −15–20 mmHg may be applied to help in the drainage.
   e) Clamping a pleural drain in the presence of a continuing air leak may result in a tension pneumothorax.

Answers

1. Concerning defibrillators
   a) *False. DC current is used as the energy generated is more effective and causes less myocardial damage. Also DC energy is less arrhythmogenic than AC energy.*
   b) *False. Joules, not watts, are used to measure the electric energy released.*
   c) *False. The defibrillator consists of a capacitor that stores then discharges the electric energy in a controlled manner. Step-up transformers are used to change mains voltage to a much higher AC voltage. A rectifier converts that to a DC voltage. Inductors are used to prolong the duration of current flow as the current and charge delivered by a discharging capacitor decay rapidly and exponentially.*
   d) *True. Because of the high energy release, skin burns can be caused by defibrillators especially if gel pads are not used.*
   e) *False. The amount of electrical energy used in internal defibrillation is a very small fraction of that used in external defibrillation. In internal defibrillation, the energy is delivered directly to the heart. In external defibrillation, a large proportion of the energy is lost in the tissues before reaching the heart.*

2. Concerning arterial blood gases analysis
   a) *True. Heparin is added to the blood sample to prevent clotting during the analysis. Heparin should only fill the dead space of the syringe and form a thin layer on its interior. Heparin is acidic and in excess will increase the hydrogen ion concentration (lowering the pH) of the sample.*
   b) *False. As air consists of about 21% oxygen in nitrogen, the addition of an air bubble(s) to the blood sample will increase the oxygen partial pressure in the sample.*
   c) *False. At room temperature, the metabolism of the cells in the blood sample will continue. This leads to a low oxygen partial pressure and a high H^+ concentration and CO_2 partial pressure. If there is a delay in the analysis, the sample should be kept on ice.*
   d) *False. The normal H^+ concentration is 40 nanomol/L, which is equivalent to a pH of 7.4.*
   e) *True. CO_2 partial pressure in a sample can be measured by measuring the changes in pH of an electrolyte solution using a modified pH electrode. The CO_2 diffuses across a membrane separating the sample and the electrolyte solution. The CO_2 reacts with the water present producing H^+ ions resulting in changes in pH.*

3. Concerning the carbon dioxide electrode
   a) *True. KCl, $NaHCO_3$ and water are the electrolyte solutions used. The CO_2 reacts with the water producing hydrogen ions.*
   b) *False. A pH-sensitive glass electrode is used to measure the changes in pH caused by the formation of H^+ ions resulting from the reaction between water and CO_2.*
   c) *True. The electrical signal generated at the electrode is directly proportional to the pH of the sample or the –log of H^+ concentration. The latter is related to the CO_2 tension in the sample.*
   d) *False. The CO_2 electrode has a slow response time as the CO_2 takes 2–3 minutes to diffuse across the membrane.*
   e) *False. The CO_2 electrode, like the pH electrode, should be kept at 37°C. Dissociation of acids or bases changes when temperature changes.*

4. CPAP
   a) *False*. CPAP is continuous positive airway pressure used in spontaneously breathing patients via a face mask or a tracheal tube.
   b) *True*. Oxygenation can be improved by CPAP as the alveoli are held open throughout the ventilatory cycle preventing airway closure thus increasing the FRC.
   c) *False*. Pressures of up to $15\,cmH_2O$ are commonly used during CPAP.
   d) *False*. CPAP reduces the cardiac output (similar to PEEP, although to a lesser extent). The arterial oxygenation might improve with the application of CPAP, but oxygen delivery might be reduced because of the reduced cardiac output.
   e) *True*. A nasogastric tube is inserted in patients with depressed consciousness level to prevent gastric distension.

5. Haemofiltration
   a) *True*. Solutes of up to 20 000 daltons molecular weight are carried along the semipermeable membrane with the fluid by solvent drag (convection).
   b) *False*. One of the reasons for the popularity of haemofiltration in the ITU setup is that it has a higher tolerability in cardiovascularly unstable patients.
   c) *True*. Although blood flows of 30–750 mL/min can be achieved during haemofiltration, blood flows of 150–300 mL/min are commonly used. This gives a filtration rate of 25–40 mL/min.
   d) *False*. Heparin is the anticoagulant of choice during haemofiltration. If there is a contraindication for its use, prostacyclin can be used instead.
   e) *False*. The filters have a large surface area with large pore size and are packed in such a way as to ensure a high surface area to volume ratio. The optimal surface area is $0.5–1.5\,m^2$.

6. Intra-aortic balloon
   a) *True*. The usual volume of the balloon is 40 mL. A smaller version, 34 mL, can be used in small patients. The size of the balloon should be 80–90% of the diameter of the aorta.
   b) *False*. The balloon should be inflated in early diastole immediately after the closure of the aortic valve at the dicrotic notch of the arterial waveform. This leads to an increase in coronary artery perfusion pressure.
   c) *True*. This leads to a decrease in aortic end-diastolic pressure so reducing the left ventricular afterload and myocardial oxygen demand.
   d) *False*. Aortic dissection is one of the absolute contraindications to intra-aortic balloon pump.
   e) *True*. Helium is used to inflate the balloon. Because of its physical properties (low density) it allows rapid and complete balloon inflation and deflation.

7. Chest drains
   a) *False*. The collection chamber should be about 100 cm below the chest as subatmospheric pressures up to $-80\,cmH_2O$ may be produced during obstructed inspiration. Retrograde flow of fluid may occur if the collection chamber is raised above the level of the patient.
   b) *True*.
   c) *False*. Deep inspiration helps in expanding the lung whereas deep expiration helps in the drainage of fluids from the pleural space.
   d) *True*. Drainage can be allowed to occur under gravity, or suction of about −15 −20 mmHg may be applied.
   e) *True*.

Chapter 14

Electrical safety

The electrical equipment used in the operating theatre and intensive care unit is designed to improve patient care and safety. At the same time, however, there is the potential of exposing both the patient and staff to an increased risk of electric shock. It is essential for the anaesthetist to have a thorough understanding of the basic principles of electricity, eventhough these devices include specific safety features.

In the UK, mains electricity is supplied as an alternating current with a frequency of 50 Hz. The current travels from the power station to the substation where it is converted to mains voltage by a transformer. From the substation, the current travels in two conductors, the live and neutral wires. The live wire is at a potential of 240 V (or more accurately 240 RMS, root mean square). The neutral is connected to the earth at the substation so keeping its potential approximately the same as earth. The live wire carries the potential to the equipment whereas the neutral wire returns the current back to the source, so completing the circuit.

Principles of electricity

Electric current

An electric current is the flow of electrons through a conductor past a given point per unit of time, propelled by the driving force, i.e. the voltage (potential difference). The current is measured in amperes (A). 1 Ampere represents a flow of 6.24×10^{18} electrons (1 coulomb of charge) past a specific point in 1 second.

- **Direct current (DC)** – the current flows in one direction (e.g. flow from a battery).

- **Alternating current (AC)** – the flow of electrons reverses direction at regular intervals (e.g. mains supply); in the UK the frequency of AC is 50 cycles per second (Hz).

Potential difference

When a current of 1 A is carried along a conductor, such that 1 watt (W) of power is dissipated between two points, the potential difference between those points is 1 volt (V).

Electrical resistance

Electrical resistance is the resistance along a conductor to the flow of electrical current. It is not dependent on the frequency of the current. Electrical resistance is measured in ohms (Ω).

Impedance

Impedance is the sum of the forces that oppose the movement of electrons in an AC circuit. The unit for impedance is the ohm (Ω). The term impedance covers resistors, capacitors and inductors and is dependent on the frequency of the current. Substances with high impedance are known as insulators. Substances with low impedance are known as conductors. The impedance through capacitors and inductors is related to the frequency (hertz, Hz) at which AC reverses direction.

- Capacitor: impedance $\propto$ 1/frequency
- Inductor: impedance $\propto$ frequency.

Ohm's law

Electric potential (volts) = current (amperes) × resistance (ohms)
[$E = I \times R$]

Capacitance

Capacitance is a measure of the ability of a conductor or system to store an electrical charge. A capacitor consists of two parallel conducting plates separated by an insulator (dielectric). The unit for capacitance is the farad.

With AC, the plates change polarity at the same current frequency (e.g. 50/sec). This will cause the electrons to move back and forth between the plates so allowing the current to flow.

The impedance of a capacitor = distance between the plates/current frequency × plate area.

Inductance

Inductance occurs when electrons flow in a wire resulting in a magnetic field being induced around the wire. If the wire is coiled repeatedly around an iron core,] as in a transformer, the magnetic field can be very powerful.

Identification of medical electrical equipment

A **single fault condition** is a condition when a single means for protection against hazard in equipment is defective or a single external abnormal condition is present, e.g. short circuit between the live parts and the applied part.

The following classes of equipment describe the method used to protect against electrocution according to an international standard (IEC 60601).

Class I Equipment

This type of equipment offers basic protection whereby the live, neutral and earth wires do not come into contact with each other. There is a secondary protection whereby parts that can be touched by the user, such as the metal case, are insulated from the live electricity and connected to an earth wire via the plug to the mains supply. There are fuses positioned on the live and neutral supply in the equipment. In addition, in the UK, a third fuse is positioned on the live wire in the mains plug. This fuse melts and disconnects the electrical circuit in the event of a fault, protecting the user from electrical shock. The fault can be due to deteriorating insulation, or a short circuit, making the metal case 'live'. Current will pass to earth causing the fuse to blow (this current is called 'leakage current'). Some tiny non-fault leakage currents are always present as insulation is never 100% perfect. A faultless earth connection is required for this protection to function.

Class II Equipment

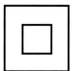

This type of equipment, also called double-insulated equipment, has double or reinforced insulation protecting the accessible parts. There is no need to earth this type of equipment. The power cable has only 'live' and 'neutral' conductors with only one fuse.

Class III Equipment

This type of equipment does not need electrical supply exceeding 24 volts AC or 50 volts DC. The voltage used is called **safety extra low voltage** (**SELV**). Although this does not cause an electrical shock, there is still a risk of a microshock. This equipment may contain an internal power source or be connected to the mains supply by an adaptor or a SELV transformer. The power input port is designed to prevent accidental connection with another cable.

The following types of equipment define the degree of protection according to the maximum permissible leakage current.

Type B Equipment

This may be Class I, II or III mains-powered equipment or equipment with an internal power source. This equipment is designed to have low leakage currents, even in fault conditions, such as 0.5 mA for Class I and 0.1 mA for Class II. It may be connected to the patient externally or internally but is not considered safe for direct connection to the heart.

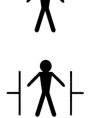

The equipment may be provided with defibrillator protection.

Type BF Equipment

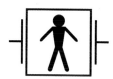

This is similar to Type B equipment, but the part applied to the patient is isolated from all other parts of the equipment using an isolated (or floating) circuit. This isolation means that allowable leakage current under single fault conditions is not exceeded even when 1.1 times the rated mains voltage is applied between the attachment to the patient and the earth. The maximum AC leakage current is 0.1 mA under normal conditions and under a single fault condition is 0.5 mA. It is safer than Type B but still not safe enough for direct connection to the heart.

The equipment may be provided with defibrillator protection.

Type CF equipment

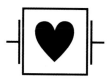

This can be Class I or II equipment powered by mains with an internal electrical power source, but considered safe for direct connection to the heart. Isolated circuits are used. There is no risk of electrocution by leakage currents (allows 0.05 mA per electrode for Class I and 0.01 mA per electrode for Class II). This provides a high degree of protection against electrical shock. This is used in ECG leads, pressure transducers and thermodilution computers.

The equipment may be provided with defibrillator protection.

Attention!

DANGER

The user must consult the accompanying documents. A black triangle on a yellow background with an exclamation mark means that there is no standardized symbol for the hazard.

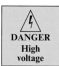
DANGER
High
voltage

DANGER
240 volts

DANGER
Electrocution
risk

DANGER
415 volts

High voltage and risk of electrocution.

Protective Earth

The equipment itself has its own earth connection via the green-and-yellow lead in the conventional three-pin plug. The earth lead is connected to the external case of the equipment so reducing it to zero potential. Although this provides some protection it does not guarantee it.

Functional Earth

This is part of the main circuit. The current is returned via the neutral wire back to the substation and so to earth. In effect, all conventional electrical circuits have functional earth. It is necessary for proper functioning of electrical equipment and is not a safety feature. On older equipment, the same symbol may have been used to denote protective earth.

Additional Protective Earth

This equipment carries an additional protective earth. This protects against electric shock in cases of a single fault condition.

Equipotentiality

This is used to ensure that all metalwork is normally at or near zero voltage. Therefore, under fault conditions, all the metalwork will increase to the same potential. Simultaneous contact between two such metal appliances would not cause a flow of current because they are both at the same potential, therefore no shock results. This provides some protection against electric shock by joining together all the metal appliances and connecting to earth.

Drip Proof, Splash Proof, Water Tight

Depending on the nature and use of the equipment, some are drip proof, splash proof or water proof.

Off, On

Anaesthetic-Proof Equipment

AP equipment standards are based on the ignition energy required to ignite the most flammable mixture of ether and air. Can be used within 5–25 cm of gas escaping from a breathing system. Its temperature should not exceed 200°C. It is a less stringent requirement.

Anaesthetic-Proof Equipment Category G

APG standards are based on the ignition energy required to ignite the most flammable mixture of ether and oxygen. Can be used within 5 cm of gas escaping from a breathing system. The temperature should not exceed 90°C. This is a more stringent requirement as the energy level should be less than 1 mJ.

CE

This is one of the most important symbols. It means conformity according to the Council of Europe Directive 93/42/EEC concerning medical devices.

Isolated or floating circuit

This is a safety feature whereby current is not allowed to flow between the electrical source and earth. These circuits are used to isolate individual equipment. An isolating transformer is used with two coils insulated from each other. The mains circuit is earthed whereas the patient's circuit is not earthed, so floating. As current flows through the mains coil (producing an electromagnetic field), a current is induced in the patient's coil. To complete the patient's circuit, the wires A and B should be connected. Contact with wire A or B alone will not complete a circuit, even if the subject is earthed.

Current-operated earth leakage circuit breakers (COELCB)

These safety features are also known as an **earth trip** or **residual circuit breakers**. They consist of a transformer with a core that has an equal number of windings of a live and neutral wire around it. These are connected via a third winding to the coil of a relay that operates the circuit breaker. Under normal conditions, the magnetic fluxes cancel themselves out, as the current in the live and neutral wires is the same. In the case of a fault (e.g. excessive leakage current), the current in the live and neutral wires will be different so resulting in a magnetic field. This induces a current in the third winding causing the relay to break circuit. The COELCB are designed to be very sensitive. A very small current is needed to trip the COELCB (e.g. 30 mA) for a very short period of time reducing the risk of electrocution.

Maintenance of equipment

Two factors should be checked during the maintenance of equipment (details of the tests are beyond the scope of this book).

1. Earth leakage – the maximum current allowed is less than 0.5 mA. Devices that are connected directly to the patient's heart should have a leakage current of less than 10 mA.

2. Earth continuity – the maximum resistance allowed is less than 0.1 Ω.

Hazards of electrical shock

An electric shock can occur whenever an individual becomes part of the electric circuit. The person has to be in contact with the circuit at two points with a potential difference between them for the electrons to flow. This can happen either with a faulty high leakage current or by a direct connection to the mains. Mains frequency is very dangerous as it can cause muscle spasm or tetany. As the frequency increases, the stimulation effect decreases but with an increase in heating effect. With a frequency of over 100 kHz, heating is the only effect. Electric shock can happen with both AC and DC. The DC required to cause ventricular fibrillation is very much higher than the AC.

If a connection is made between the live wire and earth, electricity will flow through that connection to earth. This connection can be a patient or member of staff. Mains supplies are maintained at a constant voltage (240 V in the UK). According to Ohm's law, current flow is ∝ 1/impedance. A high impedance will reduce the current flow and vice versa. The main impedance is the skin resistance which can vary from a few hundred thousand ohms to one million ohms. Skin impedance can be reduced in inflamed areas or when skin is covered with sweat.

Current density is the amount of current per unit area of tissues. In the body, the current diffusion tends to be in all directions. The larger the current or the smaller the area over which it is applied, the higher the current density.

Regarding the heart, a current of 100 mA (100 000 μA) is required to cause ventricular fibrillation when the current is applied to the surface of the body. However, only 0.05–0.1 mA (50–100 μA) is required to cause ventricular fibrillation when the current is applied directly to the myocardium. This is known as **microshock**.

Methods to reduce the risk of electrocution

- General measures: adequate maintenance and testing of electrical equipment at regular intervals, wearing antistatic shoes and having antistatic flooring in theatres.
- Ensuring that the patient is not in contact with earthed objects.
- Equipment design: all medical equipment used in theatres must comply with British Standard 5724 and *International Electro-technical Committee* (IEC) 60601-1 describing the various methods used for protection and the degree of protection (see above).
- Equipotentiality (see above).
- Isolated circuits (see above).
- Circuit breakers (COELCB) (see above).

Electricity can cause electrocution, burns or ignition of a flammable material so causing fire or explosion. Burns can be caused as heat is generated due to the flow of the current. This is typically seen in the skin. Fires and explosions can occur through sparks caused by switches or plugs being removed from wall sockets skin and igniting inflammable vapours.

Damage caused by electrical shock can occur in two ways.

1. Disruption of the normal electrical function of cells. This can cause contraction of muscles, alteration of the cerebral function, paralysis of respiration and disruption of normal cardiac function resulting in ventricular fibrillation.
2. Dissipation of electrical energy throughout all the tissues of the body. This leads to a rise in temperature due to the flow of electrons, and can result in burns.

The severity of the shock depends on:

1. The size of current (number of amperes) per unit of area.
2. Current pathway (where it flows). A current passing through the chest may cause ventricular fibrillation or tetany of the respiratory muscles leading to asphyxia. A current passing vertically through the body may cause loss of consciousness and spinal cord damage.
3. The duration of contact. The shorter the contact, the less damage caused.
4. The type of current (AC or DC) and its frequency. The higher the frequency, the less risk to the patient. A 50 Hz current is almost the most lethal frequency. The myocardium is most susceptible to the arrthymogenic effects of electric currents at this frequency and muscle spasm prevents the

victim letting go of the source. As the frequencies increase to >1 kHz, the risks decrease dramatically.

THE EFFECTS OF ELECTROCUTION

As a general guide to the effect of electrocution, the following might occur:

- 1 mA–tingling pain
- 5 mA–pain
- 15 mA–tonic muscle contraction and pain
- 50 mA–tonic contraction of respiratory muscles and respiratory arrest
- 75–100 mA–ventricular fibrillation.

The body can form part of an electrical circuit either by acting as the plate of a capacitor (capacitance coupling) without being in direct contact with a conductor or as an electrical resistance (resistive coupling).

Resistive coupling

This can be caused by:

- faulty equipment allowing a contact with a live wire if it touches the casing of the equipment
- leakage current. As there is no perfect insulation or infinite resistance, some small currents will flow to earth because the equipment is at a higher potential than earth.

Diathermy

Diathermy is frequently used to coagulate a bleeding vessel or to cut tissues. Unipolar diathermy is commonly used. As the current frequency increases above 100 kHz (i.e. radiofrequency), the entire effect is heat generating.

Components

1. Diathermy active or live electrode.
2. Patient's neutral or passive plate.
3. Diathermy case where the frequency and voltage of the current used can be adjusted. An isolating capacitor is situated between the patient's plate and earth.

Mechanism of action

1. Heat is generated when a current passes through a resistor depending on the current density (current per unit area). The amount of heat generated (H) is proportional to the square of current (I^2) divided by the area (A) ($H = I^2/A$). So the smaller the area, the greater the heat generated. The current density around the active electrode can be as much as 10 A/cm^2 generating a heating power of about 200 W.
2. A large amount of heat is produced at the tip of the diathermy forceps because of its small size (high current density). Whereas at the site of the patient's plate, because of its large surface area, no heat or burning is produced (low current density).
3. A high frequency current (in the radiofrequency range) of 500 000 to more than 1 000 000 Hz is used. This high frequency current behaves differently from the standard 50 Hz current. It passes directly across the precordium without causing ventricular fibrillation. This is because high frequency currents have a low tissue penetration without exciting the contractile cells.

4. The isolating capacitor has low impedance to a high frequency current, i.e. diathermy current. The capacitor has a high impedance to 50 Hz current thus protecting the patient against electrical shock.
5. Earth-free circuit diathermy can be used. The patient, the tip of the diathermy forceps and the patient plate are not connected to earth. This reduces the risk of burns to the patient. This type of circuit is known as a floating patient circuit.
6. Cutting diathermy uses a continuous sine waveform at a voltage of 250–3000 V. Coagulation diathermy uses a modulated waveform. Coagulation can be achieved by fulguration or desiccation. Blended modes (cutting and coagulation) can be used with a variable mixture of both cutting and coagulation.
7. Bipolar diathermy does not require a patient plate. The current flows through one side of the forceps, through the patient and then back through the other side of the forceps. The current density and heating effect is the same at both electrodes. Usually low power can be achieved from a bipolar diathermy with good coagulation effect but less cutting ability. Bipolar diathermy is frequently used during neurosurgery or ophthalmic surgery.

Problems in practice and safety features

1. If the area of contact between the plate and patient is reduced, the patient is at risk of being burned at the site of the plate. If the plate is completely detached, current might flow through any point of contact between patient and earth, for example earthed ECG

electrodes or temperature probes. Modern diathermy machines do not function with any of the above.
2. Electrical interference with other electrical monitoring devices. The use of electrical filters can solve this problem.
3. Interference with the function of cardiac pacemakers. Damage to the electrical circuits or changes in the programming can occur. This is more of a hazard with cutting diathermy than with coagulation diathermy. Modern pacemakers are protected against diathermy.
4. Fires and explosions may be caused by sparks igniting flammable material such as skin cleansing solutions or bowel gas.

> Diathermy
> - High frequency current is used.
> - An isolating capacitor is used to protect the patient against mains frequency current.
> - Floating patient circuit (earth-free circuit) is used.
> - There is a high current density at the tip of the diathermy forceps generating heat.

Static electricity

Measures to stop the build-up of static electricity in the operating theatre are necessary to prevent the risk of sparks, fire and explosions. The electrical impedance of equipment should allow the leakage of charge to earth, but should not be so low that there is a risk of electrocution and electrical burns.

Some of the measures used to prevent the build-up of static electricity are:

1. Tubings, reservoir bags and face masks are made of carbon-containing rubber; they are black in colour with yellow labels.
2. Staff wear anti-static footwear.
3. Trolleys have conducting wheels.
4. The relative humidity in the operating theatre is kept at more than 50% with a room temperature of more than 20°C.

With modern anaesthesia, the significance of these measures is questionable as the flammable inhalational agents (e.g. ether and cyclopropane) are not used any more.

Lasers

Lasers are being used more frequently, both in and outside the operating theatre. Lasers have the ability to cut tissue with precision with almost perfect haemostasis. They are used in thoracic surgery (excision of central airway tumours such as bronchial carcinoma), ENT (e.g. excision of vocal cord tumours), gynaecology (excision of endometriosis), urology (benign prostatic hyperplasia), skin lesion and myopia. Basic knowledge of laser principles is essential for both patient and staff safety.

Laser stands for light amplification by the stimulated emission of radiation. Laser produces a non-divergent light beam of a single colour or frequency (monochromatic) with a high-energy intensity and has a very small cross-sectional area. The energy of the beam depends on the frequency.

Types of laser

- *Solid-state laser* such as the Nd-YAG laser that emits light at 1064 nm (infrared).
- *Semiconductor laser* such as the gallium arsenide (GaAs) laser. The power output tends to be low.
- *Liquid laser*.
- *Gas laser* such as the helium-neon laser (emits red light), carbon dioxide laser (emits infrared light) and argon lasers (emits green light).

Problems in practice and safety features

Increasing the distance from the laser offers little increase in safety as the laser is a high-energy non-divergent beam.

1. Permanent damage to the eye retina or the head of the optic nerve can be caused by laser beams in the visible portion. Infrared light can cause damage to cornea, lens and aqueous and vitreous humours. All staff should wear eye protection appropriate for the type of laser and within the laser-controlled area. This should offer adequate protection against accidental exposure to the main beam. Spectacles do not give reliable peripheral visual field protection.
2. Burning can be caused if the laser hits the skin.
3. A non-water based fire extinguisher should be immediately.
4. All doors should be locked and all windows covered in order to protect those outside the operating theatre.

Table 14.1 shows the different classes of laser products.

AIRWAY LASER SURGERY

There is a high risk of fire due to the combination of an oxygen-enriched environment and the very high thermal energy generated by the laser. The risk can be reduced by avoiding the use of nitrous oxide, the use of lower oxygen concentrations (25% or less), the use of the

Table 14.1 Classification of laser products

Class 1	Power not to exceed maximum permissible exposure for the eye, or safe because of engineering design.
Class 2	Visible laser beam only (400–700 nm), powers up to 1 mW, eye protected by blink-reflex time of 0.25 sec.
Class 2m	As Class 2, but not safe when viewed with visual aids such as eye loupes.
Class 3a	Relaxation of Class 2 to 5 mW for radiation in the visible spectrum (400–700 nm) provided the beam is expanded so that the eye is still protected by the blink reflex. Maximum irradiance must not exceed 25 W/m for intrabeam viewing. For other wavelengths, hazard is no greater than Class 1.
Class 3b	Powers up to 0.5 W. Direct viewing hazardous. Can be of any wavelength from 180 nm to 1 mm.
Class 4	Powers over 0.5 W. Any wavelength from 180 nm to 1 mm. Capable of igniting inflammable materials. Extremely hazardous.

laser-resistant tracheal tubes, protecting other tissues with wet swabs and using non-reflective matt-black surgical instruments so reducing reflection of the main laser beam.

If fire occurs, the laser should be switched off and the site of surgery flooded with saline. The breathing system should be disconnected and the tracheal tube removed. The patient can then be ventilated with air using a bag-valve-mask system.

FURTHER READING

Boumphrey S, Langton JA. Electrical safety in the operating theatre. BJA CPED Reviews 2003;3:10–14.

Kitching AJ, Edge CE. Laser and surgery. BJA CPED Reviews 2003;8:143–146.

Safety testing of medical and electrical equipment. www.ebme.co.uk/arts/safety/index.htm.

MCQs

In the following list which of the statements (a) to (e) are true?

1. Concerning electric current
   a) Inductance is a measure of the ability to store a charge.
   b) Mains current in the UK is at a frequency of 50 Hz.
   c) The leakage current of a central venous pressure monitoring device should be less than 10 mA.
   d) Current density is the current flow per unit of area.
   e) In alternating current, the flow of electrons is in one direction.

2. Electrical impedance
   a) When current flow depends on the frequency, impedance is used in preference to resistance.
   b) The impedance of an inductor to low frequency current is high.
   c) Isolating capacitors in surgical diathermy are used because of their low impedance to high frequency current.
   d) With ECG, skin electrodes need a good contact to reduce impedance.
   e) Ohms are the units used to measure impedance.

3. Which of the following statements are correct?
   a) With equipotentiality, all metal work is normally at or near zero voltage.
   b) Functional earth found on medical devices acts as a safety feature.
   c) Ohm's law states that electric resistance = current × potential difference.
   d) Type CF equipment can be safely used with direct connection to the heart.
   e) Defibrillators can not be used with Type B equipment.

4. Electrical shock
   a) It does not happen with direct current.
   b) The main impedance is in the muscles.
   c) A current of 50 Hz is lethal.
   d) A current of 100 mA applied to the surface of the body can cause ventricular fibrillation.
   e) It can result in burns.

5. Diathermy
   a) The current density at the patient's plate should be high to protect the patient.
   b) An isolating capacitor is incorporated to protect the patient against low frequency electrical shock.
   c) A floating patient circuit can be used.
   d) Filters can reduce interference with ECG.
   e) A current of 50 Hz is used to cut tissues.

Answers

1. Concerning electric current
   a) *False. Inductance occurs when a magnetic field is induced as electrons flow in a wire. The ability to store a charge is known as capacitance. In an inductor, the impedance is proportional to the frequency of the current. In a capacitor, impedance is inversely proportional to the current frequency.*
   b) *True. The frequency of the mains supply in the UK is 50 Hz. At this relatively low frequency, the danger of electric shock is high.*
   c) *True. A central venous pressure monitoring device can be in direct contact with the heart. Ventricular fibrillation can occur with very small current, between 50 and 100 mA, as the current is applied directly to the myocardium (microshock). Such devices should have a leakage current of less than 10 mA to prevent microshock.*
   d) *True. The amount of current flow per unit of area is known as the current density. This is important in the function of diathermy. At the tip of the diathermy forceps the current density is high so heat is generated. At the patient plate, the current density is low and no heat is generated.*
   e) *False. In alternating current, the flow of electrons reverses direction at regular intervals. In the UK, the AC is 50 cycles per second (Hz). In direct current, the flow of electrons is in one direction only.*

2. Electrical impedance
   a) *True. Impedance is the sum of the forces that oppose the movement of electrons in an AC circuit. In capacitors, the impedance is low to high frequency current and vice versa. The opposite is correct in inductors.*
   b) *False. Inductors have low impedance to low frequency current and vice versa.*
   c) *True. Capacitors have low impedance to high frequency current and high impedance to low frequency current. The latter is of most importance in protecting the patient from low frequency current. High frequency currents have low tissue penetration without exciting the contractile cells, allowing the current to pass directly across the heart without causing ventricular fibrillation.*
   d) *True. The skin forms the main impedance against the conduction of the ECG signal. In order to reduce the skin impedance, there should be good contact between the skin and the electrodes.*
   e) *True. Ohms are used to measure both impedance and electrical resistance. Ohm = volt/ampere.*

3. Which of the following statements are correct?
   a) *True. Equipotentiality is a safety feature when, under fault conditions, all metalwork increases to the same potential. Current will not flow during simultaneous contact between two such metal appliances as they are both at the same potential and no shock results.*
   b) *False. Functional earth is not a safety feature. It is necessary for the proper functioning of the device. It is part of the main circuit where the current, via the neutral wire, is returned to the substation and so to earth.*
   c) *False. Ohm's law states that the potential difference (volts) = current (ampere) × resistance (ohms).*
   d) *True. Type CF equipment can be used safely in direct contact with the heart. The leakage current is less than 50 μA in Class I and less than 10 μA in Class II, providing a high degree of protection against electrical shock.*
   e) *False. Type B equipment can be provided with defibrillator protection. The same applies to Type BF and Type CF equipment.*

4. Electrical shock

a) *False. Electric shock can happen with direct current although the amount of current required to cause ventricular fibrillation is much higher than that of alternating current.*

b) *False. The main impedance is in the skin and not the muscles. Skin impedance is variable and can be from 100 000 to 1 000 000 Ω depending on the area of contact and whether or not the skin is wet.*

c) *True. The severity of the electric shock depends on the frequency of the current. The lower the frequency, the higher the risk. A current of 50 Hz is almost the most lethal frequency.*

d) *True. A current of 100 mA, when applied to the surface of the body, can cause ventricular fibrillation. Most of the current is lost as the current travels through the body and only 50–100 μA are required to cause ventricular fibrillation.*

e) *True. The electrical energy is dissipated throughout the tissues of the body leading to a rise in temperature and resulting in burns.*

5. Diathermy

a) *False. In order to protect the patient from burns, the current density at the plate should be low. The same current is passed through the tip of the diathermy forceps where the current density is high, thus producing heat. The current density at the plate is low because of its large surface area.*

b) *True. The isolating capacitor protects the patient from low frequency current (50 Hz) shock because of its high impedance to low frequency currents. It has low impedance to high frequency (diathermy) currents.*

c) *True. A floating patient circuit can be used to reduce the risk of burns. The diathermy circuit is earth free. The patient, the tip of the diathermy forceps and the patient's plate are not connected to earth.*

d) *True. Diathermy can cause electrical interference with ECG and other monitoring devices. The use of electrical filters can solve this.*

e) *False. Very high frequency current (in the radiofrequency range) of 500 000 to 1 000 000 Hz is used. This high frequency current behaves differently from the standard 50 Hz current; because of its low tissue penetration it passes directly through the heart without causing ventricular fibrillation.*

Appendices

APPENDIX A

Checking Anaesthetic Equipment, 3, 2004

(Reproduced with the permission of The Association of Anaesthetists of Great Britain and Ireland)

Membership of the working party

Dr John A Carter, Chairman
Dr Richard JS Birks, Honorary
  Treasurer
Ex officio
Dr Peter GM Wallace, President
Professor Michael Harmer, President
  Elect
Dr David J Wilkinson, Vice President
Dr David K Whitaker, Honorary
  Secretary
Dr Alastair Chambers, Assistant
  Honorary Secretary
Dr Stephanie K Greenwell,
  Honorary Membership Secretary
Dr David Bogod, Editor in Chief,
  Anaesthesia

In addition, advice and input
are acknowledged from members
of the Safety Committee and the
Standards Group of the Association,
Anaesthetic Equipment Officers,
members of the British Anaesthetic
and Respiratory Equipment
Manufacturers Association, and
members of the Department of
Health Expert Group on Blocked
Anaesthetic Tubing.
  This document has been endorsed
by Sir Liam Donaldson, the Chief
Medical Officer, and the Royal
College of Anaesthetists.

January 2004
To be revised by 2009

Contents

Section 1: Introduction

To check the correct functioning of
anaesthetic equipment before use
is a mandatory procedure. In 1997
the Association of Anaesthetists
of Great Britain and Ireland
published the second edition of
its 'Checklist for Anaesthetic
Machines' which gained widespread
acceptance in the profession. This
document recognized that changes
in anaesthetic equipment and the
introduction of microprocessor-
controlled technology would
necessitate continued revision of
the document in the future. This
new edition further updates the
procedures recommended in 1997.
  The principles set out in
previous booklets have governed
amendments to this new edition. It
must be emphasized that a major
contributory cause of anaesthetic
misadventures, resulting at worst in
hypoxic brain damage or death, has
been the use of anaesthetic machines
and/or breathing systems which
had not been adequately checked
beforehand by an anaesthetist. It is
the responsibility of all Trusts and

other Hospitals to ensure that all
personnel are trained in the use and
checking of relevant equipment.
This is usually devolved to the
Department of Anaesthesia, but
where such a department does not
exist other arrangements must be
made. The use of checklists and
associated procedures is an integral
part of training in Anaesthesia, and
as such is part of the Royal College
of Anaesthetists' Competency Based
Training.
  This checking procedure is
applicable to all anaesthetic
machines, should take only a few
minutes to perform, and represents
an important aspect of patient safety.
It is not intended to replace any
pre-anaesthetic checking procedures
issued by manufacturers, and
should be used in conjunction with
them. For example, some modern
anaesthetic 'workstations' will enter
an integral self-testing cycle when
the machine is switched on, in which
case those functions tested by the
machine need not be re-tested by
the user. The intention is to strike
the right level of checking so that
it is not so superficial that its value
is doubtful, nor so detailed that the
procedure is impracticable.
  The checking procedure covers
all aspects of the anaesthetic delivery
system from the gas supply pipelines,
the machine and breathing systems,
including filters, to connectors
and airway devices. It includes an
outline check for ventilators, suction,
monitoring and ancillary equipment.
  There must be a system of
implementing the routine checking
of anaesthetic machines by trained
staff according to the checklist,
together with the manufacturer's
instructions, in every environment
where an anaesthetic is given.
**A record should be kept, with the
anaesthetic machine, that this has
been done.**
  In addition, Trusts, Independent
Hospitals, Service Hospitals and
other organizations must ensure

that all machines are fully serviced at the regular intervals designated by the manufacturer and that a service record is maintained. Since it is possible for errors to occur in the reassembly of machines, it is essential to confirm that the machine is correctly configured for use after servicing. The 'first user' check after servicing is therefore especially important and must be recorded.

Faults may develop during anaesthesia which were either not present or not apparent on the preoperative equipment check. These may include pipeline failure, electrical failure, circuit disconnections etc. In the event of any mishap it should not be presumed that the equipment is in the same state as when checked before the start of the case.

The checking procedure described in this publication is reproduced in an abbreviated form as a laminated sheet entitled 'Checklist for Anaesthetic Equipment 2004'. This laminated sheet should be attached to each anaesthetic machine and used to assist in the routine checking of anaesthetic equipment.

Section 2: Procedures

The following checks should be carried out at the beginning of each operating theatre session. In addition, specific checks should be carried out for each new patient during a session on any alteration or addition to the breathing system, monitoring or ancillary equipment.

Implementation of these checks is the responsibility of the anaesthetist, who must be satisfied that they have been carried out correctly. In the event of a change of anaesthetist during an operating session the checked status of the anaesthetic equipment must be agreed.

Before using any anaesthetic equipment, ventilator, breathing system or monitor, it is essential to be fully familiar with it. Many of the new anaesthetic 'workstations' are complex pieces of machinery. It is essential that anaesthetists have a full and formal induction on any machines they may use. A short 'run-through' prior to an operating session is not acceptable.

The anaesthetic machine should be connected directly to the mains electrical supply (where appropriate), and only correctly rated equipment connected to its electrical outlets. Multi-socket extension leads must not be plugged into the anaesthetic machine outlets or used to connect the anaesthetic machine to the mains supply.

To check the correct function of the oxygen failure alarm involves disconnecting the oxygen pipeline on some machines, whilst on machines with a gas supply master switch, the alarm may be operated by turning the master switch off. Because repeated disconnection of gas hoses may lead to premature failure of the Schrader socket and probe, the following guidelines recommend that the regular pre-session check of equipment includes a 'tug' test to confirm correct insertion of each pipeline into the appropriate socket.

It is therefore recommended that, in addition to these checks, the oxygen failure alarm must be checked on a weekly basis by disconnecting the oxygen hose whilst the oxygen flowmeter is turned on, and a written record kept. In addition to sounding an alarm which must sound for at least 7 seconds, oxygen failure warning devices are also linked to a gas shut off device. Anaesthetists must be aware both of the tone of the alarm and also what gases will continue to flow with the make of anaesthetic machine in use.

A. ANAESTHETIC MACHINE

Check that the anaesthetic machine and relevant ancillary equipment are connected to the mains electrical supply (where appropriate) and switched on. Switch on the gas supply master switch (if one is fitted). Check that the system clock (if fitted) is set correctly. Careful note should be taken of any information or labelling on the anaesthetic machine which might refer to its current status.

B. MONITORING EQUIPMENT

Check that all monitoring devices, especially those referred to in the AAGBI Monitoring Standards document, are functioning and that appropriate parameters have been set before using the anaesthetic machine. This includes the cycling times, or frequency of recordings, of automatic non-invasive blood pressure monitors. Check that gas sampling lines are properly attached and free from obstruction or kinks. In particular check that the oxygen analyser, pulse oximeter and capnograph are functioning correctly and that appropriate alarm limits for all monitors are set.

C. MEDICAL GAS SUPPLIES

1. Identify and take note of the gases which are being supplied by pipeline, confirming with a 'tug test' that each pipeline is correctly inserted into the appropriate gas supply terminal.

2. Check that the anaesthetic apparatus is connected to a supply of oxygen and that an adequate reserve supply of oxygen is available from a spare cylinder.

3. Check that adequate supplies of any other gases intended for use are available and connected as appropriate. All cylinders should be securely seated and turned **off** after checking their contents.

4. Carbon dioxide cylinders should not normally be present on the anaesthetic machine. A blanking plug should be fitted to any empty cylinder yoke.

5. Check that all pressure gauges for pipelines connected to the anaesthetic machine indicate 400–500 kPa.

6. Check the operation of flowmeters, where these are present, ensuring that each control valve operates smoothly and that the bobbin moves freely throughout its range without sticking. If nitrous oxide is to be used the anti-hypoxia device should be tested by first turning on the nitrous oxide flow and ensuring that at least 25% oxygen also flows. Then turn the oxygen flow off and check that the nitrous oxide flow also stops. Turn on the oxygen flow and check that the oxygen analyser display approaches 100%. **Turn off all flow control valves.** (Machines fitted with a gas supply master switch will continue to deliver a basal flow of oxygen.)

7. Operate the emergency oxygen bypass control and ensure that flow occurs without significant decrease in the pipeline supply pressure. Ensure that the emergency oxygen bypass control ceases to operate when released.

D.　VAPORIZERS

1. Check that the vaporizer(s) for the required volatile agent(s) are fitted correctly to the anaesthetic machine, that any back bar locking mechanism is fully engaged and that the control knobs rotate fully through the full range(s). Ensure that the vaporizer is not tilted. **Turn off the vaporizers.**

2. Check that the vaporizer(s) are adequately but not over-filled and that the filling port is tightly closed.

3.
  (i) Set a flow of oxygen of 5 litres/min and, with the vaporizer turned off, temporarily occlude the common gas outlet. There should be no leak from any of the vaporizer fitments and the flowmeter bobbin (if present) should dip.

  (ii) Turn each vaporizer on in turn and repeat this test. There should be no leak of liquid from the filling port. **After this test, ensure that the vaporizers and flowmeters are turned off.**

  (iii) Should it be necessary to change a vaporizer at any stage, it is essential to repeat the leak test. Failure to do so is a common cause of critical incidents.

  (iv) Removal of a vaporizer from a machine in order to refill it is not considered necessary.

  (v) Vaporizers must always be kept upright since tilting can result in the subsequent delivery of dangerously high concentrations of vapour.

E.　BREATHING SYSTEM

1. Check all breathing systems which are to be employed. They should be visually and manually inspected for correct configuration and assembly. Check that all connections within the system and to the anaesthetic machine are secured by 'push and twist'. Ensure that there are no leaks or obstructions in the reservoir bags or breathing system and that they are not obstructed by foreign material. Perform a pressure leak test on the breathing system by occluding the patient-end and compressing the reservoir bag. Breathing systems should be protected at the patient-end when not in use to prevent the intrusion of foreign bodies.

2. Bain-type and circle co-axial systems - perform an occlusion test on the inner tube and check that the adjustable exhaust valve, where fitted, can be fully opened and closed.

3. Check the correct operation of the unidirectional valves in a circle system.

4. If it is intended to use very low fresh gas flows in a circle breathing system, there must be a means to analyse the oxygen and vapour concentration in the inspiratory limb. (Under other circumstances these may be monitored at the anaesthetic machine fresh gas outlet.)

5. A new, single-use bacterial/viral filter and angle piece/catheter mount must be used for each patient. It is important that these are checked for patency and flow, both visually and by ensuring gas flow through the whole assembly when connected to the breathing system.

F. VENTILATOR

1. Check that the ventilator is configured correctly for its intended use. Ensure that the ventilator tubing is securely attached. Set the controls for use and ensure that adequate pressure is generated during the inspiratory phase.
2. Check that disconnect alarms are present and function correctly.
3. Check that the pressure relief valve functions correctly at the set pressure.

G. SCAVENGING

Check that the anaesthetic gas scavenging system is switched on and functioning. Ensure that the tubing is attached to the appropriate exhaust port of the breathing system, ventilator or anaesthetic workstation.

H. ANCILLARY EQUIPMENT

1. Check that all ancillary equipment (such as laryngoscopes, intubation aids e.g. intubation forceps, bougies, etc.) which may be needed is present and in working order. Ensure that all appropriate sizes of face masks, laryngeal masks, airways, tracheal tubes and connectors are available, and checked for patency at the point of use.
2. Check that the appropriate laryngoscopes function reliably.
3. Check that the suction apparatus is functioning and all connections are secure; test for the rapid development of an adequate negative pressure.
4. Check that the patient trolley, bed or operating table can be rapidly tilted head-down.

I. SINGLE USE DEVICES

Any part of the breathing system, ancillary equipment or other apparatus that is designated 'single-use' must be used for one patient only, and not re-used. Packaging should not be removed until the point of use for infection control, identification and safety. (For details of decontamination of reusable equipment, see the AAGBI Infection Control document.)

J. MACHINE FAILURE

In the event of failure some modern anaesthetic workstations may default to little or no flow. It is essential that an alternative oxygen supply and means of ventilation (e.g. self-inflating bag, circuit and oxygen cylinder, which must be checked as functioning correctly with an adequate supply of oxygen) are always readily available. Consideration should be given to alternative methods of maintaining anaesthesia in this situation.

K. RECORDING AND AUDIT

A clear note must be made in the patient's anaesthetic record, that the anaesthetic machine check has been performed, that appropriate monitoring is in place and functional, and that the integrity, patency and safety of the whole breathing system has been assured. There must also be a logbook kept with each anaesthetic machine to record the daily pre-session check and weekly check of the oxygen failure alarm. Documentation of the routine checking and regular servicing of anaesthetic machines and patient breathing systems should be sufficient to permit audit on a regular basis.

The Association of Anaesthetists of Great Britain and Ireland cannot be held responsible for failure of any anaesthetic equipment as a result of a defect not revealed by these procedures.

BIBLIOGRAPHY

Hazard notices and safety warnings
HN(84)13 HAZARD Health Service Management. Selectatec Vaporizer Systems. London: Department of Health, 1984.
SAFETY ACTION BULLETIN Anaesthetic Vaporizers: servicing. SAB(88)72. London: Department of Health, 1988.
HN 1993(4) March 1993. Anaesthetic Machines – Service induced fault. Transposition of gas pipelines within anaesthetic machine.
SAFETY NOTICE MDA SN(96)36 1996 Demountable anaesthetic agent vaporizers. MDA DB 2000(04) August 2000.

Single-use medical devices
Implications and consequences of Re-use. HN 2001(05) November 2001. Anaesthetic Breathing System Components – risk of blockages from intravenous administration (giving) set caps.
MDA 2003(039) 6 November 2003. Anaesthetic Vaporizers – risk of overdose of anaesthetic agent due to overfilling of the vaporizer.

Books
Infection Control in Anaesthesia. 2002. Association of Anaesthetists of Great Britain and Ireland, 21 Portland Place, London W1B 1PY. www.aagbi.org/pdf/Infection.pdf
Recommendations for Standards of Monitoring during Anaesthesia and Recovery. 2000. Association of Anaesthetists of Great Britain and Ireland, 21 Portland Place, London W1B 1PY. www.aagbi.org/pdf/Absolute.pdf
Moyle JTB, Davey A. In: Ward C (ed). Ward's Anaesthetic Equipment, 4th edn. London: Saunders, 1988.

*Editorials, reviews, reports
and original work*

Bergman IJ, Kluger MT, Short TG. Awareness during general anaesthesia: a review of 81 cases from the Anaesthetic Incident Monitoring Study. Anaesthesia 2002;57:549–556.

Birks RJS. Editorial: Safety matters. Anaesthesia 2001;56:823–824.

Blunt MC, Burchett KR. Editorial: Variant CJD and disposable anaesthetic equipment – balancing the risks. British Journal of Anaesthesia 2003;90:1–3.

Brahams D. Anaesthesia and the law. Awareness and pain during anaesthesia. Anaesthesia 1989;44:352.

Bridgland IA, Menon DK. Editorial: Monitoring medical devices: the need for new evaluation methodology. British Journal of Anaesthesia 2001;87:678–681.

Caplan RA, Vistica MF, Posner KL, Cheney FW. Adverse anesthetic outcomes arising from gas delivery equipment: a closed claims analysis. Anesthesiology 1997;87:741–748.

Carter JA, McAteer P. A serious hazard associated with the Fluotec Mk 4 vaporizer. Anaesthesia 1984;39:1257–1258.

Clayton DG, Barker L, Runciman WB. Evaluation of safety procedures in Anaesthesia and Intensive Care. Anaes and Int Care 1993;21:670–672.

Cooper JB, Newbower RS, Kitz RJ. An analysis of major errors and equipment failures in anesthesia management: considerations for prevention and detection. Anesthesiology 1984;60:34–42.

Craig J, Wilson ME. A survey of anaesthetic misadventures. Anaesthesia 1981;36:933–936.

Cundy JF, Baldock G. Safety check procedures in anaesthetic machines. Anaesthesia 1982;37:161–169.

Fasting S, Gisvold SE. Equipment problems during anaesthesia – are they a quality problem? British Journal of Anaesthesia 2002;89:825–831.

Gilron I. Anaesthesia equipment safety in Canada: the role of government regulation. Canadian Journal of Anaesthesia 1993;40:987–992.

Holland R. 'Wrong gas' disaster in Hong Kong. Anesthesia Patient Safety Newsletter 1989;4:26.

Lawes EG. Hidden hazards and dangers associated with the use of HME/filters in breathing circuits. British Journal of Anaesthesia 2003;91:249–264.

Lunn JN, Mushin WW. Mortality associated with anaesthesia. London: The Nuffield Provincial Hospitals Trust, 1982.

Olympio MA, Goldstein MM, Matheys DD. Instructional review improves performance of anesthesia apparatus checkout procedures. Anesthesia and Analgesia 1996;83:618–622.

Page J. Testing for leaks. Anaesthesia 1977;32:673.

Schreiber PJ. Con: there is nothing wrong with old anesthesia machines and equipment. Journal of Clinical Monitoring 1996;12:39–41.

Spittal MJ, Findlay GP, Spencer I. A prospective analysis of critical incidents attributable to anaesthesia. International Journal of Quality Health Care 1995;7:363–371.

Sprague DH, Archer GW. Intra-operative hypoxia from an erroneously filled liquid oxygen reservoir. Anesthesiology 1975;42:360–364.

The Westminster Inquiry. Lancet 1977;ii:175–176.

Webb RK, Russell WJ, Klepper I, Runciman WB. The Australian Incident Monitoring Study. Equipment failure: an analysis of 2000 incident reports. Anaesthesia International Care 1993;21:673–677.

Wilkes AR. Breathing System Filters. British Journal of Anaesthesia CEPD Review 2002;2:151–154.

Wilkes AR, Benbough JE, Speight SE, Harmer M. The bacterial and viral filtration performance of breathing system filters. Anaesthesia 2000;55:458–465.

APPENDIX B

Recommendations for Standards of Monitoring During Anaesthesia and Recovery 3 December 2000

(Reproduced with the permission of the Association of Anaesthetists of Great Britain and Ireland.)

Summary

The Association of Anaesthetists of Great Britain and Ireland regards it as essential that certain core standards of monitoring must be used whenever a patient is anaesthetized. These standards should be uniform irrespective of duration or location of anaesthesia.

1. The anaesthetist must be present throughout the conduct of an anaesthetic.
2. Monitoring devices must be attached before induction of anaesthesia and their use continued until the patient has recovered from the effects of anaesthesia.
3. The same standards of monitoring apply when the anaesthetist is responsible for a local anaesthetic or sedative technique for an operative procedure.
4. All information provided by monitoring devices should be recorded in the patient's notes. Trend display and printing devices are recommended as they allow the anaesthetist to concentrate on managing the patient in emergency situations.
5. The anaesthetist must check all equipment before use. All alarm limits must be set appropriately. Infusion devices and their alarm settings must be checked before use. Audible alarms must be enabled when anaesthesia commences.
6. The recommendations state the monitoring devices which are essential and those which must be immediately available during anaesthesia. If a monitoring device deemed essential is not available and anaesthesia continues without it, the anaesthetist must clearly state in the notes the reasons for proceeding without the device.
7. Additional monitoring may be necessary as adjudged by the anaesthetist.
8. Only a brief interruption of monitoring is acceptable if the recovery area is immediately adjacent to the operating theatre. Otherwise monitoring should be continued during transfer to the same degree as any other intra or inter hospital transfer.

Introduction

The presence of an appropriately trained and experienced anaesthetist is the main determinant of patient safety during anaesthesia. However, human error is inevitable, and many studies of critical incidents and mortality associated with anaesthesia have shown that adverse incidents and accidents are frequently attributable, at least in part, to error by anaesthetists.[1,2]

Instrumental monitoring will not prevent all adverse incidents or accidents in the peri-operative period. However, there is substantial evidence that it reduces risks of incidents and accidents both by detecting the consequences of errors, and by giving early warning that the condition of a patient is deteriorating for some other reason. The introduction of modern instrumental monitors halved the number of intra-operative cardiac arrests in one study,[3] and the decrease was due almost entirely to a decrease in cardiac arrests from preventable respiratory causes. After the introduction of minimal monitoring standards in one American group of hospitals, the numbers of serious accidents and deaths were reduced substantially.[4] The Australian Incident Monitoring Study found that 52% of incidents were detected first by a monitor;[5] in more than half of these cases, the pulse oximeter or capnograph detected the first changes. It was calculated that a combination of pulse oximetry, capnography and blood pressure monitoring should detect 93% of serious incidents in the large majority of cases before organ damage occurs.

The use of pulse oximetry shortens the time to detection of critical events.[6] The introduction of pulse oximetry decreased the number of patients admitted unexpectedly from the operating theatre to the intensive care unit.[7] In a randomized, controlled study,[8,9] the use of pulse oximetry reduced the number of episodes of hypoxaemia and the number of patients suffering myocardial ischaemia during anaesthesia and resulted in increases in the flow of oxygen used in the recovery area, the number of patients discharged to the ward with supplemental oxygen and the number of patients treated with naloxone.

There has never been a randomised, prospective study of instrumental monitoring in anaesthesia, proving conclusively that outcome is influenced. The overwhelming view is that such a study would be unethical and the circumstantial evidence that is available indicates clearly that the use of such monitoring improves the safety of patients. Consequently, it is appropriate that the AAGBI should make clear recommendations about the standards of monitoring which anaesthetists in the United Kingdom must use.

The anaesthetist's presence during anaesthesia

An anaesthetist of appropriate experience must be present throughout general anaesthesia, including any period of cardiopulmonary bypass. The anaesthetist must undertake frequent clinical observations as well as reviewing the information provided by monitoring devices. The same standards must apply when an anaesthetist is responsible for a local anaesthetic or sedative technique for an operative procedure. When there is a known potential hazard to the anaesthetist, for example during imaging procedures, facilities for remotely observing and monitoring the patient must be available.

Accurate records of the measurements provided by monitors must be kept. It is recognized that contemporaneous records may be difficult to keep in emergency circumstances. Many modern monitoring displays provide trend or printing facilities which help in subsequent retrieval of information. Printed records must be attached securely to hand-written records and any artifacts noted.

Handing over responsibility for a patient under anaesthesia should be avoided if at all possible. However, during long procedures primary responsibility may have to be passed to another anaesthetist. If so, hand-over time must be sufficient to appraise the incoming anaesthetist of all information concerning the patient's anaesthesia and the time and details noted in the anaesthetic record.

Very occasionally, an anaesthetist working single handedly may be called upon to attend a life-threatening emergency nearby. Leaving an anaesthetised patient in these circumstances is a matter for individual judgement. If this should prove necessary, the surgeon must stop the operation; another medical practitioner (usually the surgeon) must formally assume responsibility for the patient and a trained anaesthetic assistant must be instructed to observe the patient's vital signs and report them to the responsible doctor.

Monitoring the anaesthetic equipment

It is the responsibility of the anaesthetist to check all equipment before use as recommended in Checklist for Anaesthetic Apparatus.[10] Anaesthetists must ensure that they are familiar with all equipment that they intend to use and that they have followed any specific checking procedure recommended by individual manufacturers. During anaesthesia, it is important to monitor continuously the continuity of the oxygen supply and the correct function of the breathing system.

Oxygen supply

The use of an oxygen analyser with an audible alarm is essential during anaesthesia. It must be placed in such a position that the composition of the gas mixture delivered to the patient is monitored continuously. The positioning of the sampling port will depend on the breathing system in use. Oxygen analysers must be available whenever anaesthesia is administered.

Breathing systems

During spontaneous ventilation, observation of the reservoir bag may reveal a leak, disconnection, high pressure or abnormalities of ventilation. Carbon dioxide concentration monitoring will detect most of these problems. Capnography is therefore an essential part of routine monitoring during anaesthesia.

Alarms

Anaesthetists must ensure that all alarms are set at appropriate values. The default alarm settings incorporated by the manufacturer are often inappropriate and during the checking procedure the anaesthetist must review and reset the upper and lower limits as necessary. Audible alarms must be enabled when anaesthesia commences.

When intermittent positive pressure ventilation is used during anaesthesia, airway pressure alarms must also be used to detect excessive pressure within the airway and also to give warning of disconnection or leaks. The upper and lower alarm limits must be reviewed and set appropriately before anaesthesia commences.

Vapour analyser

The use of a vapour analyser is essential during anaesthesia whenever a volatile anaesthetic agent is in use.

Infusion devices

When any component of anaesthesia (hypnotic, analgesic, muscle relaxant) is administered by infusion, the infusion device unit must be checked before use. Alarm settings and infusion limits must be verified and set to appropriate levels before commencing anaesthesia. It is essential to verify that these drugs are delivered to the patient. The infusion site should therefore be visible and must be checked regularly to ensure that extravasation does not occur. The anaesthetist must be fully familiar with the particular device being used before using it.

Monitoring the patient

During anaesthesia, the patient's physiological state, depth of anaesthesia and function of equipment need continual assessment. Monitoring devices supplement clinical observation in order to achieve this. The anaesthetist should make observations of the patient's mucosal colour, pupil size, response to surgical stimuli and movements of the chest wall and of the reservoir bag and should undertake palpation of the pulse, auscultation of breath sounds and where appropriate, measurement of urine output and blood loss. A stethoscope must always be available.

MONITORING DEVICES

The following monitoring devices are essential to the safe conduct of anaesthesia. If it is necessary to continue anaesthesia without a particular device, the anaesthetist must clearly record the reasons for this in the anaesthetic record.

Induction of anaesthesia

1. Pulse oximeter
2. Non-invasive blood pressure monitor
3. Electrocardiograph
4. Capnograph

The following must also be available:

- A nerve stimulator whenever a muscle relaxant is used
- A means of measuring the patient's temperature.

During induction of anaesthesia in children and in uncooperative adults, it may not be possible to attach all monitoring before induction. In these circumstances monitoring must be attached as soon as possible and the reasons for delay recorded in the patient's notes.

For very short procedures e.g. electro-convulsive therapy (ECT) and orthopaedic manipulations under general anaesthesia the above monitoring standards for induction of anaesthesia will suffice under normal circumstances.

If the patient remains in the anaesthetic room for a prolonged period after induction of anaesthesia, for example siting of lines, then monitoring standards must equate to those for maintenance of anaesthesia as described below.

Maintenance of anaesthesia

1. Pulse oximeter
2. Non-invasive blood pressure monitor
3. Electrocardiograph
4. Capnograph
5. Vapour analyser

The following must also be immediately available:

- A nerve stimulator whenever a muscle relaxant is being used
- A means of measuring the patient's temperature.

Recovery from anaesthesia

A high standard of monitoring should be maintained until the patient is fully recovered from anaesthesia. Clinical observations must be supplemented by the following monitoring devices:

1. Pulse oximeter
2. Non-invasive blood pressure monitor.

The following must also be immediately available:

- Electrocardiograph
- Nerve stimulator
- Means of measuring temperature
- Capnograph.

If the recovery area is not immediately adjacent to the operating theatre, or if the patient's general condition is poor, adequate mobile monitoring of the above parameters will be needed during transfer. The anaesthetist is responsible for ensuring that this transfer is accomplished safely.

Facilities and staff needed for the recovery area are detailed in the Association booklets, *The Anaesthesia Team* and *Immediate Post Anaesthetic Recovery*.[11,12]

Regional techniques and sedation for operative procedures

Patients must have appropriate monitoring, including the following devices:

1. Pulse oximeter
2. Non-invasive blood pressure monitor
3. Electrocardiograph.

Additional monitoring

Some patients will require additional, mainly invasive, monitoring; for example, of vascular or intracranial pressures, cardiac output or biochemical variables.

Monitoring during transfer

It is essential that the standard of care and monitoring during transfer is as high as that applied in the controlled operating theatre environment and that personnel with adequate knowledge and experience accompany the patient.[13]

The patient should be physiologically stable on departure. Prior to transfer, appropriate monitoring must be commenced. Oxygen saturation, electrocardiogram and arterial pressure should be monitored in all patients. It may be necessary in selected patients to monitor central venous pressure, pulmonary artery wedge pressure and/or intracranial pressure. A monitored oxygen supply of known content sufficient to last the maximum duration of the transfer is essential for all patients. If the patient's lungs are ventilated, airway pressure, tidal volume and expired carbon dioxide concentration should be continuously monitored.

There are monitoring problems which are specific to transfer particularly if this involves an ambulance journey. The diagnosis of arrhythmias may be impossible in the presence of movement artifacts. Few devices can be relied upon to give accurate non-invasive arterial pressure measurements during transfers and invasive arterial pressure monitoring should be considered for all patients.[14,15]

All monitors must be easily accessible and have clearly visible, illuminated displays. It is preferable that all monitoring functions are combined in one robust, battery operated monitor of reasonable weight and size.

Anaesthesia outside hospital

The Association's view is that the standards of monitoring used during general and regional analgesia and sedation should be exactly the same in all locations.[16]

References

1. Buck N, Devlin HB, Lunn JN. Report on the confidential enquiry into perioperative deaths. London: Nuffield Provincial Hospitals Trust, The King's Fund Publishing House, 1987.
2. Webb RK, Currie M, Morgan CA et al. The Australian Incident Monitoring Study: an analysis of 2000 incident reports. Anaesthesia and Intensive Care 1993;21:520–528.
3. Keenan RL, Boyan CP. Decreasing frequency of anesthetic cardiac arrests. Journal of Clinical Anesthesia 1991;3:354–357.
4. Eichhorn JH, Cooper JB, Cullen DJ, Maier WR, Philip JH, Seeman RG. Standards of patient monitoring during anesthesia at Harvard Medical School. Journal of the American Medical Association 1986;256:1017–1020.
5. Webb RK, Van der Walt JH, Runciman WB et al. Which monitor? An analysis of 2000 incident reports. Anaesthesia and Intensive Care 1993;21:529–542.
6. McKay WP, Noble WH. Critical incidents detected by pulse oximetry during anaesthesia. Canadian Journal of Anaesthesia 1988;35:265–269.
7. Cullen DJ, Nemaskal JR, Cooper JB, Zaslavsky A, Dwyer MJ. Effect of pulse oximetry, age, and ASA physical status on the frequency of patients admitted unexpectedly to a post-operative intensive care unit. Anesthesia and Analgesia 1992;74:181–188.
8. Moller JT, Pedersen T, Rasmussen LS et al. Randomized evaluation of pulse oximetry in 20,802 patients. I. Design, demography, pulse oximetry failure rate, and overall complication rate. Anesthesiology 1993;78:436–444.
9. Moller JT, Johannessen NW, Espersen K et al. Randomized evaluation of pulse oximetry in 20,802 patients. II. Perioperative events and postoperative complications. Anesthesiology 1993;78:444–453.
10. Checklist for Anaesthetic Apparatus. Association of

Anaesthetists of Great Britain and Ireland, London, 1997.

11. The Anaesthesia Team. Association of Anaesthetists of Great Britain and Ireland, London, 1998.

12. Immediate Post Anaesthetic Recovery. Association of Anaesthetists of Great Britain and Ireland, London, 1993.

13. Recommendations for the Transfer of Patients with Acute Head Injuries to Neurosurgical Units. Neuroanaesthesia Society of Great Britain and Ireland and Association of Anaesthetists of Great Britain and Ireland, London, 1996.

14. Guidelines for Transfer of the Critically Ill Adult in the UK. Intensive Care Society, London, 1987.

15. Wallace PGM. Transfer of the critically ill patient. In: Bion J (ed.) Intensive Care Medicine. London: BMJ Books, 1999; 404–413.

16. Surgery and General Anaesthesia in General Practice Premises. Association of Anaesthetists of Great Britain and Ireland, London, 1995.

APPENDIX C

Graphical symbols for use in labelling medical devices

Batch code

Can be autoclaved

Cannot be autoclaved

REF

Catalogue number

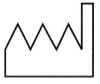

Certified to British Standards

Date of manufacture

Expiry date

SN

Serial number

Do not reuse (single use only)

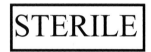

Sterile

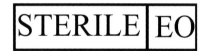

Method of sterilization using ethylene oxide

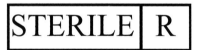

Method of sterilization using irradiation

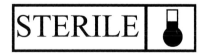

Method of sterilization using dry heat or steam

APPENDIX D

Sterilization and cleaning of medical equipment

There are two steps to processing equipment that are used during clinical and surgical procedures. Cleaning is the first and the most important step followed by either sterilization or disinfection.

1. **Cleaning:** is the removal of foreign material (e.g. dirt or micro-organisms) from an object and usually involves a detergent or enzymatic pre-soak. Cleaning can be either manual or mechanical. The latter includes ultrasonic cleaners or washer/disinfectors that may facilitate cleaning and decontamination.
2. **Decontamination:** is using physical or chemical means to remove, in-activate, or destroy pathogens on a surface. Decontamination can comprise cleaning, disinfection or sterilization as appropriate.
3. **Disinfection:** is a chemical or physical (thermal) process that destroys pathogens. Thermal disinfection is more reliable and can be achieved by boiling or by moist heat at 70–100°C. Chemical disinfectants are used for heat-sensitive equipment (e.g. endoscopes). Disinfectants are chemical agents that destroy most pathogens but may not kill bacterial spores. There is a broad spectrum of chemical disinfectants that have different antimicrobial activities. Most of them do not necessarily kill all micro-organisms present but instead reduce their numbers to a level that is not harmful. Chemical disinfection should only be used if heat treatment is impractical. Examples are glutaraldehyde 2% for 20 minutes, hydrogen peroxide 6–7.5% for 20–30 minutes, peracetic acid 0.2–0.35% for 5 minutes and orthophthalaldehyde (OPA) for 5–12 minutes.
4. **Pasteurization** (heat disinfection): heating to 60–100°C for approximately 30 minutes to reduce the number of pathogens by killing a significant number of them. The higher the temperature, the shorter the time needed.
5. **Sterilization** is a process that achieves the complete destruction or killing of all microorganisms, including bacterial spores. It can be accomplished by steam under pressure (autoclaving), dry heat (hot air oven), and the use of chemicals such as ethylene oxide gas (which is mainly used in industry).

Steam sterilization is the most common and popular method. It is reliable, non-toxic, inexpensive, sporicidal, and has rapid heating and good penetration of fabrics. The steam must be applied for a specified time so that the items reach the required temperature. For unwrapped items:

121°C for 20 minutes at 1.036 bar above atmospheric pressure.
134°C for 3–4 minutes at 2.026 bar above atmospheric pressure.

Steam sterilization

Advantages	Disadvantages
Highly effective	Items must be heat and moisture resistant
Rapid heating and penetration of instruments	Does not sterilize powders, ointments or oils
Non-toxic	
Inexpensive	Needs good maintenance
Can be used to sterilize liquids	

Dry heat sterilization (hot air oven): a constant supply of electricity is needed. Used for reusable glass, metal instruments, oil, ointments and powders.

Ethylene oxide can be used to sterilize most equipment that can withstand temperatures of 50–60°C. However, it should be used under carefully controlled conditions because it is extremely toxic and explosive. Although it is very versatile and can be used for heat-sensitive equipment, fluids and rubber etc., a long period of aeration (to remove all traces of the gas) is required before the equipment can be distributed. The operating cycle ranges from 2 to 24 hours and it is a relatively expensive process. Bacterial spore tests are used to monitor sterilization with ethylene oxide.

Monitoring the effectiveness of sterilization

To ensure that sterilization has been successful, the process of sterilization (not the end product) is tested. Indicators have been developed to monitor the effectiveness of sterilization by measuring various aspects of the process.

Mechanical indicators

These indicators, which are part of the autoclave or dry-heat oven itself, record and allow the observation of time, temperature, and/or pressure readings during the sterilization cycle.

Chemical indicators

There are various chemical indicators such as:

- Tape with lines that change colour when the intended temperature has been reached.
- Pellets in glass tubes that melt, indicating that the intended temperature and time have been reached.

- Indicator strips that show that the intended combination of temperature, time and pressure has been achieved.
- Indicator strips that show that the chemicals and/or gas are still effective.
- Chemical indicators are available for testing ethylene oxide, dry heat and steam processes. These indicators are used internally, placed where steam or temperature take longest to reach, or put on the outside of the wrapped packs to distinguish processed from non-processed packages.

Biological indicators

These indicators use heat-resistant bacterial endospores to demonstrate whether or not sterilization has been achieved. If the bacterial endospores have been killed after sterilization, you can assume that all micro-organisms have been killed as well. After the sterilization process the strips are placed in a broth that supports aerobic growth and are incubated for 7 days. The advantage of this method is that it directly measures the effectiveness of sterilization. The disadvantage is that this indicator is not immediate, as are mechanical and chemical indicators. Bacterial culture results are needed before sterilization effectiveness can be determined.

FURTHER READING

Manual of Sterilization, Disinfection and Cleaning of Medical Equipment: Guidance on Decontamination from the Microbiology Advisory Committee (UK) to Department of Health, Medical Devices Agency. www.mhra.gov.uk

www.ems.org.eg/esic_home/data/giued_part1/Cleaning.pdf

APPENDIX E

Latex allergy

Allergy to natural rubber latex has become a major source of concern for patient safety in clinical practice and a potentially serious occupational hazard to operating theatre staff. It is estimated that 8% of the general population in the United States are allergic to products containing latex and thus subject to severe intra-operative allergic reactions. In France, it is estimated that 16.6% of anaphylactoid reactions during anaesthesia are due to latex allergy, second only to reactions due to muscle relaxants.

Latex is a milky liquid derived from the *Hevea brasiliensis* rubber tree. It contains a mixture of lipids, sugars and proteins. In addition, several chemicals are added to this liquid during its transportation, processing and manufacturing. Allergic reactions seem to be against proteins naturally present, which constitute about 1% of liquid latex sap. A protein of a molecular weight of 14 000 Daltons seems to be the major allergen.

The use of latex in medical equipment has increased dramatically since the 1980s following health legislation introduced recommending the use of latex gloves to prevent transmission of blood-borne pathogens, such as HIV and hepatitis B, during medical procedures. This resulted in a global demand for latex medical gloves resulting in changes in quality during manufacture.

Clinical manifestations

1. *Irritant contact dermatitis* is the most common reaction. It is a non-allergic condition following chronic exposure to latex gloves. Dry, crusty and itchy skin predominantly affects the hands. The symptoms resolve when contact with latex ceases.
2. *Delayed type IV hypersensitivity (allergic contact dermatitis)* is a chemical reaction resulting from exposure to substances incorporated in the harvesting, processing and manufacturing of latex. It is a cell mediated allergic reaction. Rash, dryness and itching occur within 24–48 hours after exposure to latex. This may progress to skin blistering and spread to surround areas of contact.
3. *Immediate type I hypersensitivity* is the most serious reaction but the least common. It is an IgE-mediated response triggering the release of inflammatory mediators with a massive release of histamine at a local or whole body level. This results from binding of the latex allergen to sensitized receptors on mast cells. The symptoms may begin within minutes or a few hours following exposure to latex equipment. They can vary from skin redness and itching (local or generalized), rhinitis, conjunctivitis, bronchospasm and laryngeal oedema, to life-threatening anaphylactic shock.

Exposure to latex can be via cutaneous (gloves), inhalation of airborne particles, intravascular (cannulae, giving sets, syringes), internal tissue (surgical equipment), mucous membrane (mouth, rectum, vagina, urethra, eyes and ears) and intrauterine routes.

High risk individuals are:

1. Health care workers such as theatre staff.
2. Children and young adults with cerebral palsy and spina bifida. This is due to the increased early exposure to latex with repeated bladder catheterization and multiple surgical procedures. About 40% of spina bifida patients have IgE antibodies specific for latex.
3. Atopic individuals.
4. Those with allergy to certain foods such as avocado, banana, chestnut, kiwi, potato, tomato and nectarines.

Diagnosis can be made clinically, by skin prick testing, skin patch testing and radio-immunoassay test (RAST).

Management

The American Academy of Allergy and Immunology and the American Society of Anesthesiologists recommend:

1. Patients in high risk groups should be identified with careful history.
2. All patients, regardless of risk status, should be questioned about history of latex allergy. High risk patients should offered testing for latex allergy.
3. Patients who have suggestive history and/or confirmatory laboratory findings must be managed with complete latex avoidance
4. Procedures on all patients with spina bifida, regardless of history, should be performed in a latex-free environment.
5. When possible, patients should be scheduled for elective surgery as the first case of the day with induction done in theatre with minimal staff present. 'Latex Allergy' signs should be posted on all operating theatre doors.
6. Preview all equipment to be used. A cart containing latex-free equipment should accompany the patient throughout their hospital stay.
7. Patients identified as latex allergic (by history or testing) should be advised to obtain a Medic Alert bracelet and

self-injectable epinephrine with medical records appropriately labelled.

Contact dermatitis and Type IV reactions are treated by avoiding irritating skin cleansers and the use of topical corticosteroids application.

Type I latex reactions are managed according to their severity. This can include antihistamines, topical nasal and systemic steroids, H_2 blockers, oxygen, bronchodilators, tracheal intubation and epinephrine.

Filters used in anaesthesia have been shown to prevent the spread of airborne latex particles thus protecting patients against inhalation exposure.

A special 'latex allergy trolley' should be made with suggested items:

- Glass syringes unless latex-free plastic syringes are available
- Drugs in latex-free vials; stoppers can be removed and drugs drawn up
- IV giving sets without latex injection ports. Use three-way stopcocks or tape all injection ports and do not use them
- Cotton wool or similar as a barrier between skin and latex-containing items
- Silicone resuscitation bags
- Neoprene/latex-free sterile gloves
- Plastic face masks
- Teflon cannulae

APPENDIX F

Directory of Manufacturers

Abbott Laboratories Ltd
Abbott House, Norden Road,
Maidenhead, Berkshire SL6 4XE UK
01628 773355
www.abbott.com

SLE Ltd (for Acutronic products)
Twin Bridges Business Park,
232 Selsdon Road, South Croydon,
Surrey CR2 6PL, UK
0208 681 1414
www.sle.co.uk & www.acutronic-
medical.ch

Medtronic Physio Control (for
Ambu products)
Leamington Court, Andover Road,
Newfound, Basingstoke RG23 7HE
UK
01256 782727
www.physiocontrol.com

Anaequip UK
Back Lane, Worthen, Shrewsbury,
Shropshire SY5 9HN UK
01743 891342
www.anaequip.com

Roche Diagnostics Ltd (for AVL
products)
Bell Lane, Lewes, East Sussex
BN7 1LG UK
01273 480444
www.roche.com

Blease Medical Equipment Ltd
Unit 3, Beech House, Chiltern Court,
Asheridge Road, Chesham, Bucks
HP5 2PX
01494 784422
www.spacelabshealthcare.com

B. Braun Medical Ltd
Thorncliffe Park, Sheffield S35 2PW
UK
0114 225 9000
www.bbraun.co.uk

Cook Medical
O'Halloran Road
National Technology Park
Limerick, Ireland
www.cookmedical.com

Datex-Ohmeda Medical Equipment
Supplies Ltd
71 Great North Road, Hatfield,
Herts AL9 5EN UK
01707 263570
www.gehealthcare.com

Gambro Ltd
Unit 1, 47 Leeson's Hill,
St Marys Cray, Kent BR5 2LF UK
01689 836121
www.gambro.com

Intavent Orthofix Ltd
5 Burney Court, Cordwallis Park,
Maidenhead, Berkshire SL6 7BZ UK
01628 594500
www.intaventorthofix.com

Keymed (Medical & Industrial
Equipment) Ltd (for Olympus
products)
Keymed House, Stock Road,
Southend-on-Sea, SS2 5QH UK
01702 616333
www.keymed.co.uk

Penlon & East Healthcare Ltd
Abingdon Science Park, Barton Lane,
Abingdon, Oxon
OX14 3PH UK
01235 547000
www.penlon.com

Siemens Medical Solutions
Siemens House, Oldbury, Bracknell
Berkshire RG12 8FZ UK
01344 396000
www.medical.siemens.com

Tyco Healthcare UK Ltd (for
Mallinckrodt & Kendall products)
154 Fareham Road, Gosport,
Hampshire PO13 0AS UK
01329 224000
www.tycohealthcare.com

Intersurgical
Crane House, Molly Millars Lane,
Wokingham, Berkshire RG41 2RZ
UK
0118 965 6300
www.intersurgical.com

Smiths Graseby Ltd
Colonial Way, Watford, Herts
WD2 4LG UK
01923 246434
www.smiths-medical.com

Smiths pneuPAC Ltd
Crescent Road, Luton, Beds
LU2 0AH UK
01582 453303
www.smiths-medical.com

Smiths Portex
Hythe, Kent
CT21 6JL UK
01303 260551
www.smiths-medical.com

Glossary

Absolute pressure This is the total pressure exerted on a system; i.e. the gauge pressure plus atmospheric pressure.

Absolute pressure = gauge pressure + atmospheric pressure

Absolute temperature This is the temperature measured in relation to the absolute zero using the Kelvin temperature scale with the absolute zero, or 0K, that corresponds to −273.15°C.

Absolute zero is the temperature at which molecular energy is minimum and below which temperatures do not exist.

Cardiac index is the cardiac output divided by the body surface area. Normally, it is about 3.2 L/min/m^2.

Dead space That volume of inspired air that does not take part in gas exchange. It is divided into:

1. *Anatomical dead space* That part of the patient's respiratory tract into which fresh gases enter without undergoing gas exchange. Gases are warmed and humidified in the anatomical dead space.
2. *Alveolar dead space* That part of the lungs where perfusion is impaired resulting in ventilation/perfusion mismatch.

End-tidal gas concentration This is an estimation of the alveolar gas composition. In cases of severe ventilation/perfusion mismatch, it is an inaccurate estimation of the alveolar gas composition.

FGF Fresh gas flow from the anaesthetic machine or other source supplied to the patient.

Flow The amount of fluid (gas or liquid) moving per unit of time.

1. *Laminar flow* Flow (through a smooth tube with no sharp edges or bends) is even with no eddies. Laminar flow can be described by the Hagen–Poiseuille equation.

$$Q = \frac{\pi P r4}{8\eta l}$$

where
Q = flow
P = pressure across tube
r = radius of tube
η = viscosity
l = length of tube

2. *Turbulent flow* Flow through a tube with a constriction (an orifice) is uneven and eddies occur.
   In this situation, flow (Q) is:
   proportional to the square of the radius of the tube $\propto r^2$
   proportional to the square root of the pressure gradient (P) $\propto \sqrt{P}$
   inversely proportional to the length of the tube (l) $\propto \frac{1}{1}$

   inversely proportional to the density of the fluid (ρ) $\propto \frac{1}{\rho}$

FRC The functional residual capacity. It is the sum of the expiratory reserve volume and the residual volume. In an adult male, it is normally about 2.5–3 litres.

Gas laws

Dalton's law of partial pressures In a mixture of gases, each gas exerts the same pressure which it would if it alone occupied the container.

Boyle's law At a constant temperature, the volume of a given mass of gas varies inversely with the absolute pressure.

$$\text{Volume} = \text{constant} \times \frac{1}{\text{pressure}}$$

Charles' law At a constant pressure, the volume of a given mass of gas varies directly with the absolute temperature.

$$\text{Volume} = \text{constant} \times \text{temperature}$$

Gay-Lussac's law At a constant volume, the absolute pressure of a given mass of gas varies directly with the absolute temperature.

$$\text{Pressure} = \text{constant} \times \text{temperature}$$

Humidity
1. *Absolute humidity* The mass of water vapour present in a given volume of air. The unit is mg/L.
2. *Relative humidity* The ratio of the mass of water vapour in a given volume of air to that required to saturate the same volume at the same temperature. The unit is %.

I/E ratio The ratio of the length of inspiration to the length of expiration, including the expiratory pause. The commonly used ratio is 1:2.

Implantation testing (IT) In order to ensure that tracheal tubes are safe for use in the human body, tube material is cut into strips and inserted usually into rabbit muscle. After a period of time the effect of the implant on the tissue is compared to controls.

IPPV Intermittent positive pressure ventilation includes both controlled and assisted ventilation. The pressure within the lung increases during inspiration (e.g. 15–20 cmH₂O) and decreases during expiration to atmospheric pressure. This reverses the pressures found during spontaneous ventilation.

Latent heat of vaporization The energy needed to change a substance from liquid to gas, without changing its temperature.

Minute volume The sum of the tidal volumes in one minute. It is the tidal volume × respiratory rate.

Oscilloscope A device capable of displaying recorded electrical signals. It is particularly useful in displaying high frequency signals and allowing analysis of their shapes.

Partial pressure The pressure exerted by each gas in a gas mixture.

PCWP Pulmonary capillary wedge pressure is a reflection of the pressure in the left atrium. It is obtained by using a balloon-tipped flow-guided pulmonary artery catheter.

PEEP Positive end-expiratory pressure where the pressure during expiration is prevented from reaching atmospheric pressure (zero). It prevents the closure of airways during expiration thus improving oxygenation.

Plenum A chamber where the pressure inside is greater than the pressure outside. Most modern vaporizers are plenum vaporizers where compressed gases are driven under pressure over or through a liquid anaesthetic.

Pulmonary vascular resistance (PVR)[1] The resistance against which the right heart pumps. The unit is dyne/s/cm⁻⁵.

Pulse pressure The difference between the arterial systolic and diastolic pressures.

SI units

Length	Metre, m
Mass	Kilogram, kg
Time	Second, s
Electric current	Ampere, A
Thermodynamic temperature	Kelvin, K
Luminous intensity	Candela, cd
Amount of substance	Mole, mol

Other units are derived, e.g.

pressure (force + area)	Pascal, P
Force	Newton, N
Volume	cubic metre, m³

SIMV Synchronized intermittent mandatory ventilation where the patient is allowed to breathe spontaneously between the preset mechanical breaths delivered by the ventilator. The ventilator synchronizes the patient's spontaneous breaths if they coincide.

Stroke volume The amount of blood expelled from a ventricle at each beat. In an adult it is about 70–125 mL.

$$\text{Stroke volume} = \frac{\text{cardiac output}}{\text{heart rate}}$$

Systemic vascular resistance (SVR)[2] The resistance against which the left heart pumps. The unit is dyne/s/cm⁻⁵.

Tidal volume This is the volume of a single breath. It is about 10 mL/kg body weight.

Transducer A device which changes one form of energy to another. An example is the pressure transducer used to measure pressures in the body. Mechanical energy is converted to electrical energy.

Venturi principle A constriction in a tube causing an area of low pressure leading to the entrainment of a fluid (gas or liquid) via a side arm.

1. PVR =

$$\frac{\text{mean pulmonary artery pressure} - \text{left atrial pressure}}{\text{cardiac output}} \times 80 \ (\text{correction factor})$$

   Normally, PVR = 80–120 dyne/s/cm⁻⁵.

2. SVR =

$$\frac{\text{mean arterial pressure} - \text{right atrial pressure}}{\text{cardiac output}} \times 80 \ (\text{correction factor})$$

   Normally, SVR = 1000–1500 dyne/s/cm⁻⁵.

Index